Cardiorenal Syndrome

"About 35.5 million U.S. adults are estimated to have kidney disease – that's more than 1 in 7 (14%).

Kidney disease, also known as 'chronic kidney disease' (CKD), causes more deaths each year than breast cancer or prostate cancer. It is the under-recognized public health crisis.

About 9 in 10 adults with kidney disease do not know they have it.

People with kidney disease may not feel ill, or notice symptoms, until the disease is advanced.

Kidney disease is the 8th leading cause of death in the U.S."
— National Kidney Foundation; 2025

"Chronic kidney disease is a worldwide public health problem associated with a poor prognosis and high mortality. Dietary management plays an important role in the prevention and treatment of chronic kidney disease."
— Healthy adult vegetarians have better renal function than matched omnivores: a cross-sectional study in China; *BMC Nephrology* journal; July 2020

Heart disease is the number one killer of Americans. About 7% of adult Americans have some form of coronary heart disease. According to the U.S. Centers for Disease Control and Prevention, in 2023, 919,032 people died from cardiovascular disease. That's the equivalent of 1 of every 3 deaths.

According to the American Heart Association, about 82.6 million people in the U.S. have one or more forms of cardiovascular disease. These include coronary heart disease, stroke, hypertension, and congestive heart failure. There are also congenital defects and hypertension, and illnesses and environmental pollutants that can damage the cardiovascular system.

About 90% of heart disease is preventable, including through diet, exercise, a regular sleep pattern, and avoiding addictive substances. Kidney disease can be prevented or slowed by the same measures.

Over 60% of those with chronic kidney disease also have cardiovascular disease, with cardiovascular disease being the leading cause of death among them. The combination is called cardiorenal syndrome, with disease in one organ stressing and increasing the risk of disease in the other.

KIDNEY HEART HEALTH NUTRITION

PREVENTION & MANAGEMENT OF CHRONIC & DEGENERATIVE CONDITIONS

Daniel John Carey

AUTHOR OF PLANT-BASED REGENERATIVE NUTRITION

Kidney Heart Health Nutrition
By Daniel John Carey

Disclaimer:

This book is sold for information purposes only. How you interpret and utilize the information in this book is your decision. Neither the author nor the publisher and/or distributor will be held accountable for the use or misuse of the information contained in this book. This book is not intended as medical advice because the author and publisher of this work are not recommending the use of chemical drugs or surgery to alleviate health challenges, but encourage readers to research and seek their own health solutions. This book also does not stand as legal advice, or suggest the breaking of any laws. Because of the way people interpret what they read, and take actions based on their own intellect and life situations – which are not in the author's, publisher's, and/or distributor's control – there is always some risk involved; therefore, the author, publisher, and/or distributor of this book are not responsible for any adverse effects or consequences from the use of any suggestions, foods, substances, products, procedures, practices, or lifestyles described hereafter. It is up to each person to do research, and to consult with professionals, specialists, and caretakers of their choice to experience the life they hope for.

ISBN: 978-1-884702-05-1

First Edition: 2025
Published by: Oakonic, POB 1272, Santa Monica, CA 90406-1272, USA

Table of Contents

The global costs of kidney disease are skyrocketing

In the U.S., about 555,000 people are on dialysis. Over 200,000 are living with a kidney transplant.

According to the Centers for Disease Control and Prevention, in 2019, treatment for Medicare beneficiaries with chronic kidney disease (CKD) cost $87.2 billion, and treatment for people with end-stage kidney disease (ESKD) cost an additional $37.3 billion.

The U.S. spends several times more on kidney disease than it does on the budget of NASA ($25.4 billion).

The kidney disease issues isn't limited to America. It is global. Largely due to dietary and lifestyle choices, lack of exercise, and addictions.

One in seven Americans has kidney dysfunction, and heart disease is the number one killer

Most commonly, those with heart disease or kidney disease have some stage of the other.

Nearly 50% of American have some stage of cardiovascular disease.

Why are heart disease and kidney disease so common? The rest of this book will help to explain. Read and learn. And take actions to protect your health.

"Heart disease, along with stroke, which is the fifth leading cause of death, claimed more lives in 2021 in the U.S. than all forms of cancer and chronic lower respiratory disease combined.

More than half of people in the U.S. (51%) do not know that heart disease is the leading cause of death in the country, according to a recent Harris Poll survey conducted on behalf of the American Heart Association in November 2023. Yet, heart disease has now been the #1 killer or more than a century, according to the 2024 Heart Disease and Stroke Statistics: A Report of U.S. and Global Data from American Heart Association.

On average, someone dies of cardiovascular disease every 34 seconds in the U.S."

– More than half of U.S. adults don't know heart disease is leading cause of death, despite 100-year reign; American Heart Association Newsroom; Jan. 2024

As I'm writing this in 2025, statistics from the National Kidney Foundation claim that one in seven Americans has some form of chronic kidney disease.

Globally, the number of adults with some level of kidney disease is estimated to be about 10% of the population.

In the past several months, at least a dozen people have told me they have been diagnosed with kidney disease, or someone close to them has.

"Eating more plant-based foods such as vegetables and grains in place of animal-based foods such as red meat may help prevent and slow the progression of chronic kidney disease, type 2 diabetes, high blood pressure, and kidney disease.

Studies show that eating whole grains, nuts, fruits, and vegetables is one of the most important ways to keep kidneys healthy."
– Plant-based Diet and Kidney Health; National Kidney Foundation; 2025

Diabetes and cardiovascular disease are listed as the chief causes of kidney disease. What brings on those conditions, and/or makes them worse: an unhealthful diet.

In 2025, it is estimated that, globally, 830,000 million people have diabetes. There are different kinds of diabetes brought on by some combination of causes, from genetic to environmental to food and lifestyle choices. They respond well to dietary, exercise, sleep, and other patterns.

According to the U.S. Centers for Disease Control and Prevention, about 1 in 20 adults age 20 and older have some level of coronary artery disease.

"Plant-based diets can help improve blood pressure, control high blood sugar (if you have diabetes), and maintain a healthy weight. Plant-based diets can help prevent other medical problems, such as heart disease, and help to manage or slow the progression of kidney disease."
– Plant-based Diet and Chronic Kidney Disease; UC Davis Health; 2025

It can be said an unhealthful diet is the chief cause of both kidney and heart disease, with genetics being secondary. There are also certain chemical and industrial toxins, types of viruses, bacteria, mold, or other contagions, and also drug and alcohol addictions, and prescription drugs that can damage the heart, kidneys, and other organs.

"In addition to their role in regulating the body's fluid composition, the kidneys produce hormones that influence a host of physiological processes, including blood pressure regulation, red blood cell production, and calcium metabolism. Besides producing hormones, the kidneys respond to the actions of regulatory hormones produced in the brain, the parathyroid glands in the neck, and adrenal glands located atop the kidneys."
– Alcohol's Impact on Kidney Function; Alcohol Health and Research World journal; 1997

Many people have a combination of factors going on, relating to why they have kidney and/or heart disease. These play roles in what can make their conditions worse, or what will improve them.

In addition to an unhealthful diet, both lack of exercise and a bad sleep schedule can trigger and magnify kidney and heart problems. So can hypertension, diabetes, and many other chronic and degenerative conditions, as well as everything from tobacco, alcohol, and drug use, and environmental factors.

"In recent years, a growing body of evidence has emerged on the benefits of plant-based diets for the prevention and treatment of lifestyle diseases. In parallel, data now exist regarding the treatment of chronic kidney disease, and its most common complications with this dietary pattern. Improving the nutrient quality of foods consumed by patients by including a higher proportion of plant-based foods while reducing total and animal protein intake may reduce the need for or complement nephroprotective medications, improve kidney disease

complications, and perhaps favorably affect disease progression and patient survival."
— Plant-based Diets for Kidney Disease: A Guide for Clinicians; *American Journal of Kidney Diseases*; Oct. 2020

Anyone diagnosed with kidney and/or heart disease, and who is interested in improving their condition would be wise to improve their diet, learn what food really is, and what is not food. This in an era when everywhere we turn there are unhealthful foods being promoted, sold, and consumed. It is easy to fall into eating foods that damage health.

I am someone who found out 40 years ago that I have genetic kidney issues. At the same time, part of my kidney problems were diet-related. I learned kidney disease could play a role in cardiovascular disease, and other health problems, including everything from chronic and degenerative conditions of the brain and nerves, to the stomach and intestines, to the parathyroid and eyes, to the bones and skin. All of the body systems and tissues rely on each other.

Kidney disease and heart disease and prevention are something I have been learning about for decades.

What I've observed is: The kidney disease industry is growing, as are the heart disease, and cancer industries. It doesn't have to be this way.

The kidney disease industry is intertwined with the cardiovascular disease, bone disease, liver disease, autoimmune disorder, neurodegeneration, and cancer industries.

People with one health problem often have others, or soon will – unless they take preventive measures. Nutrition, exercise, quality of sleep, and reducing toxins are keys to those measures.

With kidney and cardiovascular functions so reliant on each other, a person diagnosed with problems with either will need to address their health in relation to both.

"Chronic kidney disease represents a major public health burden that affects 10% of the general population worldwide, amounting to 800 million individuals, and has emerged as one of the leading causes of mortality; predictions suggest that chronic kidney disease will become the fifth highest cause of years of life lost globally by 2040. Hypertension, diabetes, metabolic syndrome, and obesity represent the most important risk factors for chronic kidney disease, and the adoption of a healthy diet may reduce the incidence of these pathologies and prevent damage to the kidneys.

It is known that chronic kidney disease (defined as a reduction in the estimated filtrate rate and/or the presence of albuminuria-proteinuria) increases the risk of death, cardiovascular disease, and hypertension, and predisposes individuals to the progression of kidney disease to end-stage renal disease.

Chronic kidney disease also correlates with the onset of anemia; metabolic acidosis, which predisposes individuals to hyperkalemia; the retention of uremic toxins, including phosphorus; and hyperphosphatemia, which contributes to high blood levels of Fibroblast growth factor 23, low levels of 1.25-dihydroxy vitamin D3, and secondary hyperparathyroidism, which leads to mineral bone disease (osteoporosis and a high risk of bone fractures), vascular calcifications, and cardiovascular events that cause a dramatic increase in healthcare costs. Pharmacological therapies (erythropoietin, phosphate, and potassium binders, calcium mimetics, etc.) and renal replacement therapies (hemodialysis, peritoneal dialysis, and renal transplant) that are used for the advanced stages of CKD are expensive. Individuals with advanced CKD are also at high risk of developing a spectrum of nutritional disturbances. Dietary changes represent a low-cost and powerful means of mitigating metabolic abnormalities in CKD and may also help to reduce the pill burden on and healthcare costs incurred by nephropathy patients.

Recently, plant-based diets have received increasing interest because they have been associated with favorable effects on health. Moreover, growing evidence suggests that plant-based diets may have favorable effects on kidney health through primary and secondary prevention."

– The Role of Plant-Based Diets in Preventing and Mitigating Chronic Kidney Disease; *Journal of Clinical Medicine*; Sept. 2023

Your condition

If you suspect you have kidney issues, see a doctor. Undergo a physical, and have the blood and urine tests, and an ultrasound – and possibly other images – done to determine what might be causing the problems.

A doctor may refer you to a dietician or nutritionist, who will help you get your diet on track to help your condition.

That is on you do to.

This book is not a replacement for a physical, blood and urine tests, or ultrasound, or other medical imaging, diagnostic, and monitoring techniques.

"A proper renal diet is extremely important for patients with chronic kidney failure. Many health care professionals have shown that a carefully planned vegetarian diet is adequate in managing chronic kidney failure.

It is vital that a renal patient's food and fluid intake be overseen by a nephrologist and a registered dietitian familiar with vegan diets. These professionals can help manage kidney disease with appropriate vegan food and fluid choices."

– Menu Selection for Vegan Renal Patients, by Nancy Berkoff, RD, EdR; Vegetarian Resource Group; 2009

To find a plant-based dietician, including to schedule a video consultation, see: PlantBasedRDs.com.

Also check out the site of Michele Crosmer, RD, CSR at PlantBasedKidneys.com. Michele also has the YouTube channel: Eat For Your Kidneys.

"In the wake of the huge increase in diabetes and obesity in recent years, more people than ever are being diagnosed with chronic kidney disease, a progressive, incurable disease that causes kidney failure. Chronic kidney disease is especially dangerous because patients rarely notice any symptoms, until the disease reaches its later stages. When the damage is no longer reversible."

– Dr. Dira Sooparth, Nephrologist; Bumrungrad International Hospital; Jan. 2019

The undone

A book like this could never be finished. This is because there is so much to learn about health and nutrition, and more is to be discovered, that, for this book to be more complete, it would be volumes of work containing thousands of pages – with regular updates. And then, new additions in expanded volumes to include updates.

I worked for this book to provide what I thought is helpful information to learn about kidney and heart health, while also encouraging readers to do their own research to find what is best for their situation.

Part of the book tells some of my story, and how I ended up writing this book.

People with kidney and/or cardiovascular disease often also have other health conditions. What is good for kidney and heart health is also good for health in general.

I hope you find this book to be helpful in avoiding kidney, cardiovascular, autoimmune, neurological, and other health problems.

The kidney disease industry

If you are ever in a large town or city, count the hospitals, medical centers, dialysis clinics, and pharmacies you see during one day.

There are reasons people so often see doctors, take prescriptions, undergo medical procedures, and have surgeries, and are caught in a loop of health concerns.

The main reason chronic and degenerative diseases are so common relates more to a combination of food choices and physical fitness, rather than to anything else. Genetics are part of it, but many genetic conditions can be set off by a bad diet and unfortunate lifestyle choices – including lack of exercise, and using addictive substances ruinous to health.

Always listed in the top ten diseases are kidney disease, and cardiovascular disease, and what is often experienced by people with those diseases: diabetes.

In May 2025, The World Health Organization listed the top causes of death in 2021 as:
1) Ischemic heart disease
2) COVID-19
3) Stroke
4) Chronic pulmonary disease
5) Lower respiratory disease
6) Trachea, bronchus, lung cancers
7) Alzheimer's disease or other dementias
8) Diabetes mellitus
9) Kidney disease
10) Tuberculosis

Treating people with kidney and cardiovascular problems is big business. Over-the-counter medications, natural treatments, pharmaceutical drugs, dialysis, and kidney or heart transplants bring billions of dollars into the global medical marketplace. It financially pays off for the "healthcare" executives, institutional investors, and stockholders.

It repeatedly is reported that people with kidney disease often have a variety of health conditions, especially cardiovascular disease and some level of diabetes. All three diseases have been on the rise, for decades, and in tune with the increased popularity of truly toxic, mass marketed, junk and otherwise ultra-processed foods.

"A 2022 study found that those who eat a lot of processed foods had a 24% risk of kidney disease. These foods are heavily processed and packed with artificial additives, added sugar, refined carbs, unhealthy fats, and sodium, but are low in fiber, protein, and essential nutrients."
    – 10 Common Habits That May Harm Your Kidneys; National Kidney Foundation; June 2016

"Diabetes prevalence has increased in recent decades in the context of significant diet changes, including reduced consumption of vegetables, fruits, and legumes, coupled with increased consumption of animal-derived and processed food products. A plant-based eating pattern is associated with a significantly lower prevalence of type 2 diabetes, compared with nonvegetarian diets, and there is strong evidence supporting the use of a plant-based eating pattern in clinical practice for individuals with type 2 diabetes. The American Association of Clinical Endocrinologists and the American College of Endocrinology, as well as the American College of Lifestyle Medicine, recommend a plant-based eating pattern as a key component of lifestyle therapy for patients with type 2 diabetes. Both the American and Canadian Diabetes Associations include vegetarian and vegan eating patterns among those shown to improve glycemic control, body weight, and cardiovascular risk factors. In addition to these organizations that support a plant-based diet for diabetes, the USDA lists a Healthy Vegetarian Dietary Pattern as an example of a healthy meal plan in the 2020-2025 Dietary Guidelines for Americans."
    – Perspective: Plant-Based Eating Pattern for Type 2 Diabetes Prevention and Treatment: Efficacy, Mechanisms, and Practical Considerations; *Advances in Nutrition* journal; June, 2021

As the book details, a clean, plant-based diet rich in whole plant matter, and free of processed and sugary, salty, and chemically saturated foods, and damaged oils is beneficial for reducing the incidence, progression, and intensity of kidney and cardiovascular disease, immune disorders, and other chronic and degenerative health conditions.

"Chronic kidney disease (CKD) and its effect on cardiovascular disease resulted in 2.6 million deaths and 35.8 million disability-adjusted life years. It has become a global public health problem with a high disease burden. Diabetes, hypertension, obesity, hyperlipidemia, advanced age, and smoking have been identified as traditional risk factors for CKD. Trace elements such as zinc, manganese, iron, and selenium, have also been reported to be involved in the progression of CKD."
    – Association between Selenium Status and Chronic Kidney Disease in Middle-Aged and Older Chinese Based on China Health and Nutrition Survey Data; *Nutrients Journal*; June 2022

If you have kidney or cardiovascular disease, there are many issues to consider. These are serious health issue, and the causes, symptoms, and intensity of the diseases likely are highly related to your diet.

While this book goes into a wide variety of issues related to kidney and heart disease, I'm aiming to provide you with a well-rounded view of what the diseases are, and how you can take steps to improve your health so you are less likely to experience a variety of conditions, including autoimmune disorders, including diabetes, lupus, arthritis, asthma, and others.

Businesses are investing in the kidney and heart disease industries because they see them growing. They want part of that money. They are "growth industries" for investors.

In a nation with a medical industry ruled by corporations, profiting off ailing people is the American way. At least this is so for certain companies, and their executives.

Dialysis

If you are on dialysis, or have undergone a kidney transplant, this doesn't mean you made the wrong choice. Don't feel as if you failed, or were fooled, or simply made a bad decision. There were many layers of things that played into your situation, and many of those were not in your control – including your genetics, and what you started out eating as a child. Unfortunately, childhood nutrition can play a role in a person's health for the rest of their life.

For some people dialysis is the right choice. As is a kidney transplant for other people.

No matter what medical procedure a person undergoes, there are always risks – including the risk of doing something they might not have needed.

For me, decades ago, doctors were pressuring me to go onto dialysis and to chase after getting a kidney transplant. They also wanted to remove my parathyroid. I didn't undergo any of those procedures.

Looking into the history of dialysis has been interesting.

Dialysis can save a person's life. And allow them to manage their health as they pursue a kidney transplant.

Under some health conditions, people are temporarily placed on dialysis. One of those conditions for undergoing temporary dialysis could be drug addiction. Another could be severe bodily injuries, which could require giving the kidneys some assistance in clearing waste products.

Father of dialysis

When I hear of an invention strictly credited to a man, I wonder what it could mean, and if there were others involved in the invention process, including women, assistants, or even servants who may have played a key role.

Some people consider the "father of dialysis" to be Thomas Graham, an 1800s Scottish professor of chemistry at Anderson's College (now the Royal College of Science and Technology), and then at the University College, London. He developed ways of separating dissolved substances through permeable membranes, including filtering salt from water. Some of his numerous discoveries relating to liquification, diffusion, osmosis, colloidal phenomena, thermodynamics, the law of expansion, and the constitution of matter all played roles in what was eventually to become kidney dialysis.

Early experiments with dialysis

In the late 1800s, anesthetized animals were used in the development of the early dialysis devices, which used a cellulosic membrane to filter the blood. To prevent the blood from clogging, they used an anticoagulant extracted from the saliva of leeches, but later switched to heparin – which is still in use.

The first humans to receive dialysis were in Germany. The procedures were performed in 1924 by Georg Haas at the University of Giessen, and more patients in 1928. The treatments ultimately failed.

The other "father of dialysis"

Some consider the "father of dialysis" to be Dutch physician Willem Johan Kolff. He developed the first artificial kidney (dialyzer) in 1943, with the first human patients treated in 1945. He had spent years working at the University of Groningen Hospital in the Netherlands, and later at a Dutch hospital. His original, crude invention to clean waste products from the blood used a washing machine, sausage skins, juice cans, and other materials. By 1945, Kolff had developed the machine to the point it was helping to save lives. They were in limited use, and few patients benefited.

Kolff continued his work at Mt. Sinai Hospital in New York, where he worked after hours to avoid the administrators who had doubts about his dialyzer machine.

Kolff-Brigham artificial kidney

By 1954, working with staff of Peter Brent Brigham Hospital in Boston, Kolff had developed a stainless steel dialyzer that was used by the first kidney transplant patient. The machine was called the "Kolff-Brigham artificial kidney," which removed excess water and uremic toxins from the blood. At least 22 hospitals in the U.S. and other countries began using the machine.

Kolff also played a key role in developing the heart-lung machine, and the artificial heart.

The artificial kidney machines remained in limited use through the 1950s and into the 1960s.

Into the 1970s, dialysis was limited because of cost, and it required patients to sit for about twelve hours.

Scribner shunt

In 1960, Belding Hibbard Scribner, David Dillard, and Wayne Quinton improved the artificial kidney, inventing the "Scribner shunt" using Teflon tubing to allow for repeated access to the same blood vessel for dialysis treatment.

The first patient to receive the Scribner shunt was Clyde Shields of Seattle. As the first "chronic dialysis patient," Shields lived 11 years with the shunt, until he passed away from vascular disease.

The Scribner shunt eventually faded from use as newer ways of access were developed in 1966 by James Camino and Michael Brescia, surgically altering a vein in the arm to allow for repeated use.

First dialysis clinic

By 1962, Scribner and company had opened the Seattle Artificial Kidney Center, which was the first dialysis clinic. As more clinics were opened, they changed the name to Northwest Kidney Centers.

Deciding which patients lived: the American Society for Artificial Internal Organs

With limited machines available, there was the dilemma of which patients would be treated using them, a concern Scribner expressed when addressing the 1964 American Society for Artificial Internal Organs. He then established a bioethics committee who would decide which patients were best for dialysis treatment. The committee literally decided who lived, and who died.

Dialysis machines evolved, clinics opened

As dialysis machines, medical technology, and kidney therapies continued to evolve, the time it took to undergo dialysis was reduced, as were costs.

By the year 2000, dialysis machines were commonly available in hospitals, and in highly profitable dialysis clinics. This was just in time for chemically-saturated, mass marketed junk and processed foods and canned and bottled, health-depleting garbage drinks to become broadly available.

The popular consumption of horribly toxic foods and drinks continues, and has increased the number of people seeking treatment for largely avoidable, noncommunicable, chronic, and degenerative kidney, cardiovascular, autoimmune, and other conditions, including nerve and brain issues, and cancer.

"Ultra-processed foods are becoming dominant in the global food supply. Prospective cohort studies have consistently found an association between high consumption of ultra-processed food and increased risk of several noncommunicable diseases and all-cause mortality.

Ultra-processed foods [UPFs] are heavily marketed and dominate the global food supply. The increase in their consumption globally over the last decades is mostly represented in by the low- and middle-income countries gradually replacing their traditional diets predominantly made of fresh foods and culinary preparations. UPFs represent over half of the energy content of the diets in many high-income countries, and consumption is high in almost all population subgroups. UPF intake starts early in life, and frequently, children and adolescents proportionally consume more UPF than adults in many countries, likely representing a higher risk of noncommunicable diseases in adulthood."
– Premature Mortality Attributed to Ultra-processed Food Consumption in 8 Countries; *American Journal of Preventive Medicine*; April 2025.

Popularity of dialysis

Considering the popularity of dialysis, isn't it interesting how common it now is? It has grown rapidly in the past few decades, and now dialysis clinics are common around U.S. cities, and many towns.

In 2022, the U.S. dialysis industry was worth more than $36 billion.

For hospitals, it is financially smart to provide dialysis. One patient can bring in nearly $100,000 per year.

What dialysis doesn't do

A dialysis machine doesn't do all a kidney can do. It doesn't produce the hormones a healthy kidney produces. Those are hormones that help balance the rest of the system, and trigger the bone marrow to produce blood cells.

A dialysis machine doesn't eliminate excess fat and cholesterol from the blood, or remove environmental toxins. It doesn't cure you of diseases.

Being on dialysis doesn't mean you can eat high protein, or junk foods, or toxic drinks.

A dialysis machine filters the blood of urea and potassium, and helps to balance the proteins and electrolytes. You get hooked to the machine a few times every week, and you are reliant on it to stay alive.

Eventually, you might get a kidney transplant – if a match is found through an organ donor (someone who has died), or through a live donation (person willing to give you one of their kidneys – who then will have some level of health concerns.).

"The most dangerous condition for the development or worsening of cardiovascular disease is dialysis, therefore, an early transplantation is recommended to avoid long-term consequences of dialysis. However, transplantation does not represent a definitive solution because cardiovascular risk persists after kidney transplantation. In case of necessity of a long-term dialysis, a careful follow-up and management of hypertension, dyslipidemia, abnormal mineral metabolism, inflammation, and other dialysis complications is a must."
– Cardiovascular risk in children: a burden for future generations; *Italian Journal of Pediatrics*; April 2022

Wall Street is depending on you to get kidney disease

In 1979, Medical Ambulatory Care, Inc. was founded as a subsidiary of National Medical Enterprises, which, in 2025, is Tenet Healthcare.

In 1994, 70% of Medical Ambulatory Care was purchased by DLJ Merchant Banking, and DLJ became Total Renal Care Holdings, Inc. The company began selling its stock in October 1995. In 1998 it purchased another dialysis chain called Renal Treatment Centers. After selling the treatment centers outside of the U.S., the company name was changed to DaVita Inc, and it purchased another company called Gambro Healthcare.

Kickbacks to doctors

People who think they are pressured by certain doctors to undergo unnecessary medical treatments, take note: DaVita paid $350 million in 2014 to settle claims it had paid kickbacks to doctors.

Did the kickbacks to doctors stop? That is, in relation to dialysis or services or medical products related to dialysis.

There is this press release from July 2024 by the U.S. Department of Justice. In part, it says:

"DaVita Inc., headquartered in Denver, Colorado, has agreed to pay $34,487,390 to resolve allegations that it violated the False Claims Act by paying kickbacks to induce referrals to DaVita Rx, a former subsidiary that provided pharmacy services for dialysis patients, and paying kickbacks to nephrologists and vascular access physicians to induce the referral of patients to DaVita's dialysis centers.

The Anti-Kickback Statute prohibits anyone from offering or paying, directly or indirectly, ay remuneration – which includes money or other thigs of value – to induce referrals of patients or of items or services covered by Medicare, Medicaid, and other federally funded programs.

The United States alleges that DaVita paid kickbacks to a competitor to induce referrals to DaVita Rx to serve as a "central fill pharmacy," or prescription fulfillment provider, for that competitor's Medicare patients' prescriptions. In exchange, DaVita paid to acquire certain European dialysis clinics and agreed to extend a prior commitment to purchase dialysis products from the competitor. DaVita would not have paid the price that it did for these deals without the competitor's commitment to refer its Medicare patients' prescriptions to DaVita Rx in return.

The United States further alleges that DaVita provided management services to vascular access centers owned by physicians in a position to refer patients to DaVita's dialysis clinics. DaVita paid improper remuneration to these physician-owners I the form of uncollected management fees to induce referrals to DaVita's dialysis centers.

Finally, the United States alleges that DaVita paid improper remuneration to a large nephrology practice to induce referrals to DaVita's dialysis clinics. DaVita gave the practice a right to refusal to staff the medical director position at any new dialysis center that opened near the nephrology practice and paid the practice $50,000 despite the practice's decision not to staff the medical director for those clinics.

'Improper financial arrangements between Medicare providers can distort the healthcare marketplace,' said Principal Deputy Assistant Attorney General Brian M. Boynton, head of the Justice Department's Civil Division. 'We will hold accountable healthcare providers that seek to generate business by paying unlawful remuneration.'

'Medicare patients should be able to trust their healthcare providers not to pay illegal kickbacks to induce referrals,' said Acting U.S. Attorney Matthew Kirsch for the District of Colorado. 'This resolution reflects the seriousness of the government's determination to restore integrity to the healthcare marketplace.'

'Illegal kickback payments corrupt the market for health care services and cause harm and financial loss to Medicare and other federally funded health care programs.' Said Special Agent in Charge Linda Hanley of the Department of Health and Human Services Office of Inspector General. Our ongoing enforcement efforts aim to safeguard the integrity of taxpayer-funded health care programs, like Medicare and Medicaid, while curbing schemes that unduly influence patients' and doctors' health care options."

– DaVita to Pay Over $34 Million to Resolve Allegations of Illegal Kickbacks; U.S. Department of Justice press release; July 2024, updated Feb. 2025

That's not all of the corruption in the kidney disease industry. It also goes into the pharmaceutical industry and its kidney-related drugs. The following is some of what has gone on. I doubt this type of activity has been stopped. It often takes years of corruption to take place, before it gets reported. Then an investigation has to take place, before charges can be made. Then corporate attorneys fight the charges. And many people make money along each step of the way.

"The U.S. government has sued Novartis Pharmaceuticals Corp., claiming it gave kickbacks to pharmacies to switch kidney transplant patients from competitors' drugs to its own. The civil healthcare fraud lawsuit in U.S. District Court in Manhattan has sought unspecified damages and civil penalties for a scheme that the government said has been carried out since 2005.

U.S. Attorney Preet Bharara said on Tuesday that the company used the 'lure of kickbacks disguised as rebates' to turn 20 or more pharmacies into a sales force for its drug, Myfortic. He said the company's actions caused the public to pay tens of millions of dollars for kickback-tainted drugs dispensed by pharmacists who had buddied up to Novartis. Bharara said Novartis is a repeat offender, having settled fraud charges based on kickbacks less than three years ago.

The government said Novartis offered one pharmacist a 'bonus' rebate amounting to several hundred thousand dollars to 'shoulder the burden' of switching 700 to 1,000 transplant patients to Myfortic."
– U.S. government sues Novartis for kickbacks in kidney drug; *The Times of India*; April 2013

How do you know if you were a patient pressured to undergo a procedure, or to otherwise receive any sort of medical "care" – or medicine – so a medical facility, and/or a doctor, or a pharmacy – or company of any sort – could get a kickback from a company? I don't know.

Considering how much has been paid in penalties by various companies, it is blatantly obvious that many people have undergone invasive medical procedures and/or have been prescribed certain medicines so those working in some area of the disease industry could financially benefit.

DaVita's path to dominance in the dialysis industry

DaVita paid $450 million in 2015 to settle allegations it has disposed of drugs and then billed U.S. federal government programs for the loss.

DaVita spent billions to purchase other companies, including Healthcare Partners in 2012, Colorado Springs Health Partners in 2014, The Everett Company Clinic Medical Group in 2016, and WellHealth Quality Care in 2017.

By early 2025, DaVita apparently held 37% of the U.S. dialysis market. As I'm writing this paragraph in 2025, the company has about 2,700 outpatient centers in the United States, with an estimated 200,800 patients. They had an additional 367 centers in 11 other countries, with about 50,000 patients.

In the United States, DaVita is largely dependent on government insurance programs. By 2025, about 65% of its revenues were from Medicare and other government programs. Private insurance companies pay a higher rate, making the company more money per patient when a patient is with a commercial insurance plan.

DaVita is a publicly traded company, and is on the Fortune 500, which is a list of the most prosperous publicly traded companies.

At the end of 1995, DaVita stock was trading on the New York Stock Exchange for $2. For five years, the stock barely rose, even dropping to .96¢ in May 2000. Then, it began to rise. By the end of 2000, it was worth over $5 per share. By the end of 2003, it had more than doubled to over $12. By the end of 2007, it was $28. By the end of 2011, $38.24. In 2015 it went to over $83. In 2021 it was $133. In early 2025 the stock had reached $173. After the company's earnings missed expectations, billionaire Warren Buffet's company Berkshire Hathaway sold DaVita stock in February 2025, and the stock dropped to $147.

The global dialysis industry

Other top dialysis management, product, and supply business in the U.S., and other countries, include U.S. Renal Care, Dialysis Clinic Inc., Sotera Health, AMN Healthcare Services, Satellite Healthcare, Baxter International, B. Braun Melsungen, Quest Diagnostics, Chemed CorVel, Amedisys, and Becton, and the current largest dialysis company: Fresenius Medical Care, and its affiliate NxStage Medical. Each of these companies, and others, are financially reliant on at least a steady number of kidney patients. And, for the financial gains of investors, preferably a growing number of kidney patients. They are depending on more people getting kidney disease.

"How much is the global dialysis market worth? Fortune Business Insights says the global market stood at $95.22 billion (U.S. currency) in 2023, and is projected to reach $181.16 billion by 2032. What was the value of the dialysis market in North America in 2023? In 2023, the market value stood at $48.73 billion.

The prevalence of chronic kidney disease is rising at a significant rate, which in turn, has increased patient visits to renal therapy clinics over the last decade. Rise in the number of patients opting for this treatment have increased the demand for products, such as dialysate and hemodialysis machines. As a result of this, key companies are launching new products in the market, and expanding their services, thereby accelerating the market growth.

In May 2022, Diaverum announced the acquisition of booknowmed.com, the world's leading renal care booking website that allows patients to browse through over 400 dialysis clinics across 54 countries.

As per the data published by the United States Renal Data Systems, in its 2023 annual report, in 2021, the number of prevalent USRD patients in the U.S. was 808,536.

In April 2022 Fresenius Medical Care North America received the U.S. FDA 510(k) clearance for its VersiPD Cylcer System, which is a portable automated peritoneal dialysis system.

In July 2020, Baxter announced a partnership with Aryogo Health, Inc. to provide digital health solutions for home dialysis. The aim of this strategic

13

partnership was to deliver advanced digital health solutions that train and empower patients with kidney failure."
– Dialysis Market Size, Share & Growth; *Fortune Business Insights*; Nov. 2024

The above article goes on and on about how many companies have been investing to make money from the kidney disease industry.

Isn't it interesting that financial publications are publishing articles about the money to be made in the growing kidney disease industry?

Home dialysis

With technological advancements, home dialysis has gained popularity among people on dialysis. Belding Scribner helped develop a portable dialysis machine.

In the U.S. about 20% of dialysis patients undergo dialysis at home. The rest go to dialysis clinics, or to hospitals to undergo dialysis.

It doesn't have to be this way

Kidney disease, dialysis, kidney transplants, and early deaths from kidney failure don't have to be this common. Nor do the profits of the medical industry in relation to kidney disorders.

For you, the person you see in the mirror, you can reduce your chances of ending up on dialysis. IF you take the necessary steps to reduce your risks of experiencing kidney disease, and/or to manage – and perhaps improve – the level of kidney function you now have. I'm someone who has done it.

If you are on dialysis, or perhaps have already had a transplant, there are also ways to better manage your health so you are in fact healthier. Including through dietary and exercise choices.

Money pouring in

The money coming into the medical industry to "treat" patients experiencing various forms of kidney disorders trickles not only into hospitals, dialysis clinics, and the various doctors and staff involved in the kidney industry, it also flows into the various companies making the dialysis machines, and all the technology, medical supplies, products, and pharmaceuticals used in relation to kidney patients, and also the real estate of the clinics.

Instead of becoming more common, kidney disease could be decreasing – IF people would be more proactive in maintaining their kidney health through diet, exercise, and lifestyle choices.

Problem number one in relation to the growing number of people experiencing kidney disease seems to be: dietary choices, as junk and otherwise ultra-processed foods have become so common across the globe.

Trillion-dollar medical industry

For those wanting to learn ways of avoiding the nutritional ignorance feeding much of the trillion-dollar hospital, pharmaceutical, and disease industries, in addition to this book, I wrote the book *Plant-based Regenerative Nutrition*. You might also find it helpful to watch videos and read articles on the two sites NutritionFacts.org, and ForksOverKnives.com.

Do what is right for you

To be clear: None of this is to say you should, or should not go onto dialysis, or should, or should not, undergo a transplant. Nor is it saying you should, or should not, take certain medications.

This also is not saying dialysis and/or a kidney transplant are never needed to keep someone alive.

Do what is right for you.

I'm telling my experience with my situation.

They pressured me

I had spent years being pressured by doctors to go onto dialysis. This included two doctors one day telling me I needed to come in the next morning to undergo arm and leg surgeries to prepare a port in my arm so I could start getting dialysis. I refused. I didn't feel it was right for me.

It's now been more than 35 years since the last time I refused to be put onto dialysis.

For many years now tests show my kidney function as what doctors describe as "normal."

Those doctors telling me "or, you will die" if I didn't go onto dialysis were not doing what was right for me. Being told by the nephrologist "you're going to die," when I said I would not be back the next day for the arm and leg surgery was not helpful. I told him "I don't think I'm going to die." He seemed beyond displeased, and appeared to be angry as he got on the phone in front of me to speak with the urologist to tell him I was refusing their advice. But why such a response? Was he angry because I was doing what wasn't right for me? Maybe, from what he knew with his training and experience, he was doing what was right for me. Or, was he angry because his sales tactics didn't work on me?

Perhaps the doctors telling me those things were doing what they felt was best for my health. Or, maybe they were being given kickbacks for putting people onto dialysis. I will never know. Those doctors are all dead.

No body shaming

Often, you can glance at someone and know they have not been following a nutritious diet, or getting adequate exercise, but have been doing the opposite. This isn't meant to body shame, which is cruel. You never know what someone has gone through in their life – including what sort of health problems and life trials they have experienced – or are experiencing.

Cruel comments about a person's physical appearance are not necessary, or helpful. By saying cruel things to people, you only reveal who you are, and the type of work you need to do on yourself.

When I see people struggling to exercise, including someone unlikely to have been taking care of themselves, it is inspiring. The person straining to ride a bike, struggling to jog, or to do any sort of exercise outdoors is living their life. Silently cheer them on.

You might be a person struggling to get into an exercise routine – and away from an excuse routine. Get outdoors – or to a gym – and exercise. Do not concern yourself with others judging you. If they don't like to see it, they can look the other way. You also might be the encouragement needed for others who see you exercising. Be strong, and improve your nutrition, fitness, and life.

"To eat is a necessity, but to eat intelligently is an art."
– François de la Rochefoucauld

Kidney health and global health

Health is a broad spectrum issue composed of our own nutrition, which is reliant on the environment, clean water, healthy soil, stable climate, robust and diverse wildlife populations, and a vast number of plants able to thrive. It all ties in with our kidneys, liver, digestive tract, heart, brain, muscles, bones, and other organs and tissues, and how sustainably we live, and our ability to survive.

As someone who has genetic kidney issues, I have had to learn to keep my kidneys functioning at a healthful level. That is, through a clean diet rich in nutrients, free of garbage, and with daily exercise. Over the past decades I've learned about the food system, and how it is connected to how humans impact everything from the bottoms of the seas to the grassland meadows, to the mountain forests, and all life forms on Earth. What ends up in the environment also ends up in us, and in wildlife, and impacts our health, as well as the health of everything from the fish of the seas to the creatures on the land, and those that fly.

The way I see it, my health, the health of humanity, and the health of wildlife and the climate are all linked. So this book touches on all of these issues.

CKD: chronic kidney disease: inherited, or developed

Chronic kidney disease can be a contributor to and/or related to high blood pressure, low blood count, bad nutrient absorption, dysbiosis of the gut flora, blood sugar issues, nerve damage, weakened bones, anemia, and blood vessel disease, including of the heart.

Chronic kidney disease can be inherited as a genetic disorder, or developed during life from an unhealthy diet, drug and/or alcohol addictions, as well as from kidney stones, infections, inflammation, high blood pressure, diabetes, chemical injury, and/or a combination of lack of exercise, bad sleeping patterns, obesity, and general health neglect.

High blood pressure and diabetes are of the most common conditions causing kidney damage, including to the hundreds of thousands of nephrons in the kidneys, which are the microscopic filters that both eliminate toxins and reabsorb electrolytes.

The most unhealthful community in the U.S. has been identified as those living in Kentucky. Consider what they eat as being in alignment with what to consume to experience debilitating diseases: fried food, meat, sugar, and few fresh fruits and vegetables. They also commonly lack in adequate exercise, and have a propensity for being overweight. According to the 2020 census, there were 41.2 new cases of colorectal cancer per 100,000 people in Kentucky.

"Two-thirds of adults in Kentucky are overweight, less than a tenth eat a sufficient amount of fruits and vegetables, and more than a third are not getting enough exercise.

Kentucky is known for having some of the poorest diets, which includes a regular consumption of fried foods, meats, and bread. Fried foods and over-processed meats, in particular, can expose one's body to carcinogens that have been linked to colorectal cancer, as well as various other cancers."
– Fried Chicken, Colon Cancer, Kentucky, and Everything In Between, by Parker Lynch; ColonCancerFoundation.org; Feb. 2024

A clean, plant-based diet avoids all animal protein, processed foods, clarified sugars, garbage breads (see information about potassium bromate and cancer), and unhealthful baked items, and fried and sautéed (or otherwise damaged or rancid) oils. A clean, plant-based diet nurtures healthy gut microbiota, improves digestion, builds a healthy stomach and intestinal lining, and greatly reduces the risks of experiencing inflammation, high blood pressure, cardiovascular and kidney disease, kidney stones, colon and other cancers, and autoimmune disorders.

"Western diets are characterized by the consumption of large amounts of animal protein, which leads to an increase in the excretion of calcium, oxalate, and uric acid in the urine, consequently predisposing individuals to kidney stones."
– Probiotics in the Prevention of the Calcium Oxalate Urolithiasis; *Cells* journal; Jan. 2022

"Vegetarian and vegan diets are associated with anti-inflammatory effects partly because they exclude meat products, which contain pro-oxidant substances. Meat, especially processed meat, can lead to oxidative stress due to the presence of heme iron [blood iron] and other compounds, which promote lipid peroxidation, enhancing the proinflammatory environment.

Vegetarian and vegan diets have gained popularity not only for ethical and environmental reasons, but also for their potential health benefits. Among these benefits, their anti-inflammatory and antioxidant properties are particularly remarkable. Hence, vegetarian and vegan diets have been pointed out by the previous literature as rich in various bioactive compounds that contribute to their health benefits."
– Impact of Vegan and Vegetarian Diets on Neurological Health: A Critical Review; *MDPI* journal of the Multidisciplinary Digital Publishing Institute; Feb. 2025

Iron and nutrients

Those with concerns about getting enough iron may want to consult with their doctor and/or nutritionist. Look at blood test results to see if they actually do have inadequate iron – or other nutrients.

The nutrition blood test is called a CMP (comprehensive metabolic panel). It measures substances including electrolytes, enzymes, proteins, and other nutrients. It is done as part of a physical, and helping to manage cardiovascular, kidney, autoimmune, and other health issues.

It is easy to get iron on a vegan diet. Research "vegan sources of iron." Also consider taking a vegan iron supplement, which is iron sourced from plants.

Vegan iron supplements are free of problematic heme iron (blood iron) from animals, an oxidative stressor that builds and plays into cardiovascular events.

I've followed a vegan for decades, regularly have a CMP done, and have not tested low in nutrients.

I do occasionally take B12, zinc, a vegan iron supplement, a vegan D3 supplement, and CoQ10. More on this later in the book.

Diabetes, a link in the disease chain

A clean, plant-based diet lowers the risk of experiencing type 2 diabetes, reduces adverse impacts of type 1 diabetes, and helps to bring the weight to a healthful level.

According to the International Diabetes Federation, as of 2019, diabetes had been diagnosed in about 9.3% of the global population. It is a disease so linked to kidney and cardiovascular health that studies done on one disease often mention the other. Diabetes contributes to about 12% of global healthcare costs, causes disabilities including blindness and loss of limbs, and annually plays a leading role in about 15 million deaths.

If you have diabetes, it doesn't mean you will have a shorter than normal lifespan, or that related diseases have to rule your life. By taking advantage of advances in medical technology, along with following a healthy diet, getting exercise, and avoiding harmful substances, you can lead a life less troubled by your condition – and be more healthful than people who do not have diabetes.

Studies conducted in a variety of countries are revealing what dietary choices are better for those with diabetes.

The members of the Seventh-day Adventist religion are known for avoiding meat and animal products. They have been studied because they often also have much lower rates of diabetes.

"In 1985, Snowdon and Phillips first reported a strongly positive association between meat consumption and diabetes prevalence in 25,698 men and women from California who were followed for 21 years in the Adventist Mortality Study. Fifty per cent of this cohort reported following a vegetarian diet. Age-adjusted diabetes prevalence ratios in participants who consumed meat 6 or more times per week were 1.9 for men and 1.6 for women, compared with vegetarians. Fraser reported similar findings from the Adventist Health Study, in which men and women meat consumers reported a 97% and 93% greater diabetes risk, respectfully, compared with vegetarian participants. Vang et al. followed 8,401 Adventists, all of whom were free of diabetes at study onset, for 17 years. After controlling for differences in body weight, those who consumed any type of meat (including poultry) at least once a week had a 38% increased risk of developing diabetes during the follow-up period, compared with those who consumed no meat."

– Perspective: Plant-Based Eating Pattern for Type 2 Diabetes Prevention and Treatment: Efficacy, Mechanisms, and Practical Considerations; *Advances in Nutrition* journal; June, 2021

Your microorganisms: the gut microbiota

Later in the book, a little about what your gut biome does is explained. This includes about the vitally important short-chain fatty acids (SCFAs) produced by the fermentation of plant fiber in your digestive tract. Among the benefits of SCFAs are a healthy colon, and prevention of colon cancer, and other cancers. SCFAs can help eliminate tumor cells.

If you want to strengthen your immune system, a key above all else is to improve your gut biome. You do this by following a high-fiber diet, including soluble and insoluble fiber. And eliminating foods that do not have fiber, which are meat, dairy, and eggs.

"The human gut is the largest organ with immune function in our body, responsible for regulating homeostasis of the intestinal barrier. A diverse, complex, and dynamic population of microorganisms, called microbiota, which exert a significant impact on the host during homeostasis and disease, supports this role. In fact, intestinal bacteria maintain immune and metabolic homeostasis, protecting our organism against pathogens. The development of numerous inflammatory disorders and infections has been linked to altered gut bacteria composition or dysbiosis. Multiple factors contribute to the establishment of the human gut microbiota. For instance, diet is considered as one of the many drivers in shaping the gut microbiota across the lifetime."
  – The Immune System through the Lens of Alcohol Intake and Gut Microbiota; *International Journal of Molecular Science*; July 2021

The microorganisms in your gut feast on what you eat. A key is feeding them a variety of plants, from green leafy and other vegetables, as well as fruits, sprouts, nuts, beans, legumes, grains, and seeds, and fermented foods. There is also fiber in mushrooms, although they are a fungus, and contain a variety of nutrients.

There are ways of preparing foods that make them more nutritious, including soaking some, sprouting some, and fermenting others. These ways of preparing foods also help the varieties of microorganisms in the gut, and their function. The book goes into this.

There are also microorganisms in your tract that help to prevent kidney stones.

The more animal protein you consume increases the likelihood you will form kidney stones, and to have other kidney issues, and cardiovascular disease, and to experience numerous other chronic and degenerative diseases.

Most people in modern society are eating exactly what degrades the gut microbiome, and harms all areas of their health. This includes eating substances increasing the likelihood of experiencing leaky gut syndrome, which plays into a wide variety of health issues, including mood disorders, autoimmune issues, insulin issues, skin issues, muscle strength issues, bone density and function, and cardiovascular, liver, spleen, pancreas, and kidney disease, and neurodegeneration.

"Red meat was a strong driver of omnivore microbiomes, with corresponding signatures of microbes negatively correlated with host cardiometabolic health. Conversely, vegan signature microbes were correlated with favorable cardiometabolic markers.

The gut microbiome plays an integral role in human health that can be modified by diet. For example, fermentation of otherwise indigestible plant polysaccharides by gut microbes contributes to a healthy, non-inflamed gut barrier and maintenance of gut homeostasis through the production of short-chain fatty acids (SCFAs) and immune system crosstalk, Moreover, plants contain polyphenols, the products of plant secondary metabolism, that are known to promote beneficial bacteria that prevent inflammation, enhance the gut barrier, and hinder potential pathogens.

By contrast, a diet rich in animal foods leads to increased protein fermentation, which may result in a leaky mucosa, local systemic inflammation, and reduced production of SCFAs. For example, the breakdown of certain animal proteins is linked to the synthesis of gut microbial trimethylamine (TMA), which is oxidized in the liver to trimethylamine N-oxide (TMAO). TMAO has been implicated in various (cardio)vascular diseases and is a potential contributing factor in colorectal cancer."

   – Gut microbiome signatures of vegan, vegetarian, and omnivore diets and associated health outcomes across 21,561 individuals; *Nature Microbiology* journal; Jan. 2025

The gastrointestinal tract is where your health, or the degradation of it, is staged.

There are so many digestive, nutrient metabolism and absorption, toxin breakdown, immune system, emotion molecule, and other processes the microorganisms of the gut biome do that it is beyond the scope of this book to explain.

Your gut biome consists of tens of trillions of microorganisms in your intestinal tract. As someone with kidney disease, or cardiovascular disease, or diabetes – or any health concern – it would be wise to have some understanding of the gut biome.

You can nurture a healthful, diverse gut biome through wise food, exercise, sleep, and lifestyle choices.

"The diet is a crucial factor determining the functionality of gut microbiota and its qualitative and quantitative composition. An individual microbial pattern can promote health, or be detrimental. For example, an imbalance of the gut microbiota, called dysbiosis or dysbacteriosis, is associated with the development of metabolic syndrome, cardiovascular disease, inflammatory bowel disease, and neurological disorders. So, we are what we eat."

   – Glucoraphanin conversion into sulforaphane and related compounds by gut microbiota; *Frontiers of Physiology* journal; Feb. 2025

As explained later in the book, the metabolites of intestinal bacteria help to reduce the risk of experiencing everything from neurological disorders, cardiovascular disease, kidney disease, liver disease, autoimmune disorders, inflammation, and various types of cancer.

"Microorganisms within the human intestine ferment carbohydrate sources, which reach the colon into the short-chain fatty acids (SCFA) acetate, propionate, and butyrate. These small organic acids have been shown in animal studies to regulate incretin or gut hormone production, thereby controlling satiety and food intake. They also stimulate the gut hormone glucagon-like peptide-2, which is involved in maintaining gut barrier function, a defense mechanism, which can impede the uptake of inflammatory compounds such as lipopolysaccharide (LPS) from the gut lumen that trigger the low-grade chronic inflammation and subsequent insulin resistance associated with obesity and cardiovascular disease. Similarly SCFA have been shown to regulate adipocyte hormone production, not least of leptin, the obesity hormone, and to control inflammatory processes in adipose tissue, processes intimately involved in cardiovascular disease risk, and possibly also impact the way energy is stores or burned in the body controlling adiposity and thermogenesis."

– The way to a man's heart is through his gut microbiota – dietary pro- and prebiotics for the management of cardiovascular risk, by Karen M. Tuohy, Francesca Fava, and Roberto Viola; *Proceedings of the Nutrition Society* journal; Feb. 2014

"Short-chain fatty acids are important metabolites produced by gut microbes. As the second-largest genome and ninth-largest system in the human body, the intestinal microbiota is critical for maintaining health. Bacterial imbalances and their metabolites lead to various diseases, including obesity, type 2 diabetes, non-alcoholic fatty liver disease, chronic kidney disease, pneumonia, and schizophrenia. SCFAs affect the occurrence and development of various diseases in several ways. Among the diseases, SCFAs mainly exert their effects by enhancing intestinal barrier function, inhibiting the inflammatory response, promoting apoptosis, increasing the expression of GPCRs (G protein-coupled receptors), affecting histone acetylation, and regulating immunity."

– Short-chain fatty acids in diseases; *Cell Communication and Signaling* journal; Aug. 2023

You need the fiber from plants in your diet for the microorganisms in your intestinal tract to digest certain nutrients, and to produce (metabolize) other nutrients.

The microorganisms in the gut include bacteria, archaea (similar to – but distinctly different from – bacteria, but both archaea and bacteria are prokaryotes), fungi, and viruses. Those organisms are the components of what is the *gastrointestinal metagenome*. Yes, we depend on those organisms for our health.

What you eat either nurtures a healthful gut biome, or damages it, and your health – including of your kidneys, cardiovascular system, immune system, muscles, bones, nerves, and brain, and all parts of you, including your hormonal balance.

"Over the past few years, it has become general knowledge that the gut microbiome plays an important role in a person's overall health.

Past studies show that an imbalanced gut microbiome may lead to health issues such as inflammatory bowel disease (IBD), type 2 diabetes, cardiovascular disease, and depression.

'We know that the gut microbiome, with its roles in breaking down certain compounds and synthesizing other molecules mediates part of the effect that diet has on our body and our health,' Nicola Segata, PhD, professor and principal investigator at the Department of Cellular Computational and Integrative Biology (CIBIO) at Universita di Trento in Italy explained.

In fact, when examining the gut microbiomes of vegans, the researchers observed that they included several species of helpful bacteria, such as Bacteroides and Firmicutes phyla. These bacteria aid in producing short-chain fatty acids, such as butyrate, which is associated with beneficial effects on gut health, including inflammation reduction."

– Vegan vs. vegetarian vs. omnivore: Does diet type have a big impact on gut health? by Corrie Pelck; *Medical News Today*; Jan. 2025

Chronic kidney disease is increasingly common

It is estimated that about 15% of Americans have CKD, and most people who have it do not know they do. They have not been diagnosed, don't know the symptoms, or otherwise are unaware of their condition.

Statistics indicate that, because of the popularity of unhealthful foods, unfortunate lifestyle choices, lack of exercise, and bad sleeping patterns, the number of people with CKD is growing.

Ingesting animal protein increases kidney disease risk

A diet rich in animal protein is high in saturated fat and cholesterol. Both of those increase the risk of cardiovascular disease, and cancers, especially of the organs, blood, and brain.

"Plant-based diets confer various health benefits, including lowering the risk of cardiovascular disease and certain cancers.

We found that participants with a higher plant protein intake had a lower risk of developing chronic kidney disease. Our finding suggests that a higher dietary intake of plant-based protein may be beneficial for kidney health, and provides insight into dietary interventions to prevent chronic kidney disease in primary care settings."
– Association of Plant Protein Intake With Risk of Incident Chronic Kidney Disease: A UK Biobank Study; *American Journal of Kidney Diseases*; Dec. 2023

"There has been accumulating evidence that animal protein consumption may have detrimental effects on vascular health, potentially contributing to the development of kidney disease."
– Seung Hyeok Han, MD, PhD, University Hospital, Seoul, Korea

Age plays a role

The older you get, the chances of having CKD increases. Especially with what people are eating today.

It is estimated that nearly 40% of people over age 65 have CKD. Many do not know it, until they understand the symptoms, undergo the tests to be diagnosed, or they end up hospitalized with one or more complication related to kidney disease.

Untreated or unmanaged kidney disease, diabetes, and high blood pressure can lead to kidney failure. This can result in a person going onto dialysis, or undergoing a kidney transplant. Or experiencing whatever is the mystery of death.

As I was growing up, I did not know why my sides hurt. I did not know why I sometimes peed what looked like pure blood, nor did I tell anyone about that, or know that I should. Peeing what looked like blood was so common for me that I thought everyone experienced it. I was wrong. I didn't know about my kidney disease until I was in my early 20s.

Diet-induced disease

If you are eating a junk diet, the result is an unhealthy digestive tract, liver, kidneys, pancreas, and spleen, and lymph and cardiovascular systems. You likely have a variety of some level of health problems relating to what you are eating and drinking, including everything from your skin, eyes, and digestive and reproductive organs, to your muscles, nerves, brain, blood, and lymph system, and your bone marrow function.

All of your systems work in unison. Your diet is key to helping everything from your organs, gut biome, digestion, bones, muscles, and nerves, all the way to the function of every one of your cells.

Medication review after diet change

If you are taking numerous medications, it could be time to review the necessity for them, with your healthcare provider. This is especially so if you are cleaning up your diet, getting into daily exercise, and working to become more healthful.

Taking numerous pharmaceutical drugs can tax both the kidneys and liver, sometimes doing more harm than good. Especially if you are taking drugs you don't need.

The liver and kidneys are both involved with eliminating toxins, including unnatural substances, and they treat pharmaceutical drugs as foreign materials.

This is not saying to avoid all pharmaceutical drugs. Do what is best for you.

The sickness loop

People in North America who consume the most fast food meat are also more likely to consume the most pasteurized dairy, synthetic food chemicals, fried foods, extracted oils, and ultra-processed foods, and the most corn syrup, white sugar, rice syrup, and other clarified sugars. These are the same people who are most likely to experience common maladies – which then funds the highly polluting medical and pharmaceutical industries. It is the sickness loop.

Your health problems aren't only about you

The medical industry produces an abundance of trash.

Medical trash and pharmaceutical residues are a global pollution issue. The production and use of the pharmaceutical drugs, medical devices, and single-use plastic medical supplies impact the water, land, air, wildlife, climate, and you, and future generations of humans and wildlife.

Profound, transformational improvements

When choosing a low-fat, clean diet rich in raw fruits and vegetables, you are likely to experience health in relation to the nourishing diet.

If you previously followed a horrible diet, and switched to a clean, plant-based diet free of processed, clarified, and chemical ingredients, your health, energy, and brain function can undergo profound improvements.

As you change your life and become different from what you used to be, you may find yourself getting attention you had not been accustomed to receiving. When people are familiar with seeing you maintain a certain lifestyle and appear one way, and they then see you have physically transformed, they also might feel uncomfortable. You will be breaking from the role you had been playing. People will have to re-cast you in their mind as no longer being the person they thought you were – and perhaps the person they thought you could never be.

Completely changing your diet to the being the most healthful way available to you will make a huge difference in many areas of your life. When provided with high-quality nutrition, the body will change to a state in tune with those nutrients.

The power to heal

Within the body is an amazing power to heal, to detoxify the cells, to reform the tissues, and to reconfigure the shape of the organs, and to produce a healthful and balanced level of hormones and other substances. Providing the body with a clean diet is a key to what can fuel the power.

"You can't turn back the clock. But you can wind it up again."
– Bonnie Prudden

When you become more healthful, people notice. Your skin, shape, and movement change. Your confidence and energy improve. It is then when people may be interested in what you had been doing to improve.

Those who are used to experiencing health problems, and who then switch to a clean diet can undergo such a change in health they will need to reconsider the medications they had been taking, and "medical" treatments they had been undergoing. Their blood pressure, cholesterol, and sugar levels will improve, as will their gut biome, digestion, and nutrient absorption. Their weight likely will change. If they had been taking prescription drugs, their medical provider will have to be informed. Medications likely will need to be adjusted, or halted.

As you follow a clean diet your life will change. This is especially true if you had been eating devitalized, unhealthful, deadening, fried, and processed foods saturated with what dulls health.

Things leading to – or associated with – CKD include one or more of these:
- Long-term or overuse of NSAIDs (non-steroidal anti-inflammatory drugs = over the counter painkillers)
- Bad diet
- Lack of exercise
- High blood pressure
- Substance abuse
- Kidney, bladder or otherwise urinary tract infections
- Autoimmune disorders, including diabetes, arthritis, and lupus
- Inflammation
- Leaky gut and an unhealthful gut biome
- Genetic predispositions
- Stress
- Pollution
- Contagions
- Continued exposure to toxic food additives, and farming, landscaping, and industrial chemicals (including those in some paints, soaps, cleansers, makeup, perfumes and colognes, and in other household and "personal care" items).

What keeps coming up in relation to kidney and cardiovascular health is: diet. And exercise.

How this book came to be

After over 30 years of following a clean diet to maintain my health, and to improve my kidney function, I thought maybe it would be a good idea to put together something about what I've learned so it could help others.

This book goes into more than the kidney issues, but covers a wider variety of things. This is so because what is good for the kidneys is also good for the digestive tract, and the heart, liver, pancreas, adrenal glands, brain and nerves, lungs, skin, and other organs, and the lymph, blood, and other systems – including the bones as they are part of the blood system because the bone marrow makes blood. Coincidentally, this way of eating is also healthier for the environment, for farmers, for people living in farm communities, and for wildlife, and the climate.

After following a plant-based diet for decades, it isn't something I think much about doing. It simply is what I do. I avoid eating anything born, hatched, or spawned, and anything containing eggs, or dairy (milk, cheese, cream, butter, whey, casein, yogurt, and kefir). I avoid highly processed foods, those containing artificial ingredients, and those that have been grilled, broiled, seared, fried, and those sautéed in oil.

When is my protein deficiency going to kick in?

People often ask if I'm getting enough protein. As if they suddenly become nutritionists once they find I don't eat animal protein. So many people don't know what proteins consist of, or how they are formed within the system, that I assume anyone asking me that question is also unaware of what proteins consist of.

When is my protein deficiency going to kick in? Never. By eating a wide variety of plants, I get all the amino acids I need for making proteins.

As I explain throughout the book, a diet high in animal protein taxes the kidneys, increases the risks of experiencing kidney disease, and enables the disease process to progress into end stage kidney disease (ESKD).

Metabolic acidosis

One thing a clean, plant-based diet does for the kidneys is it reduces stress on them, including by reducing blood urea nitrogen, the acidity of the body, inflammation, and the amount of work the kidneys have to do.

Types of acidosis include diabetic ketoacidosis, hyperkalemia, lactic acidosis, metabolic acidosis, and renal tubular acidosis. Metabolic acidosis is experienced by as many as 15% of people who have chronic kidney disease as their kidneys are not filtering are not balancing the pH of the body. This can play into other conditions experienced with CKD, including anemia, cardiovascular disease, bone loss, dysbiosis, malnutrition, muscle atrophy, parathyroid disorders, and others.

"In people with CKD who develop metabolic acidosis, the kidneys can't remove enough acid from the body. A buildup of acid disrupts the typical acid-base (pH) balance in the body. Along with abnormally high acid levels, people with metabolic acidosis have abnormally low levels of bicarbonate in their blood."
– How is Sodium Bicarbonate Used to Treat Kidney Disease?, by Steve Barry, ELS; Healthline.com; April 2024

"Including a higher proportion of foods with natural alkali, such as fruits and vegetables, a vegan diet is nearly acid neutral. Plant-based foods can be used to reduce both the dietary acid load and the severity of metabolic acidosis. Similarly, a low protein intake in patients with advanced nondialysis chronic kidney disease has also been shown to attenuate the severity of metabolic acidosis. NHANES III data have shown that, among 1,486 adult participants with chronic kidney disease, higher dietary acid load ascertained by 24-hour dietary recall was strongly associated with development of end stage kidney disease [ESKD] over a median follow-up of 14.2 years. Compared with participants whose dietary acid consumption was in the lowest tertile, those with dietary acid consumption in the highest tertile had triple the risk of incidence of ends stage kidney disease, even after accounting for differences in sociodemographics, nutritional factors, clinical factors, baseline estimated glomerular filtration rate (eGFR), proteinuria, and serum bicarbonate levels."

    – The Effects of High-Protein Diets on Kidney Health and Longevity; *Journal of American Nephrology*; July 2020

Many people experience a variety of health issues indicating kidney disease, but they don't know they have kidney disease. Once they understand what the signs are of kidney disease, and that their health issues can be linked, they then can learn what can be done to address their health issues. As most people with some stage of kidney disease don't know they have it, the sooner they know, the better – before the damage becomes irreversible.

Born this way, and didn't know it

I was born with bad kidneys. It's genetic. I traced my ancestry, and found people on my mother's, mother's side who also had kidney issues.

I didn't know it then, but the foods I ate growing up worked to magnify my kidney problems. Although not rich in today's version of fast food or junk food, I did eat an abundance of animal protein. My diet was also lacking in fresh vegetables and fruit.

Although I was in kidney pain in my childhood – and had other symptoms I didn't know were symptoms – I didn't know my kidneys were the problem, until I was in my early 20s. I didn't even know the pain I was feeling was kidney pain. I went through childhood never having seen a doctor about the pain, or having anyone concerned with – or who spoke with me about – the pain. Mentioning the pain seemed only to be irritating, and nobody seemed interested in hearing about it.

No contact sports

As a child, I wanted to play baseball. But any kind of contact sport resulting in my torso being bumped was too painful – and I didn't know why.

Growing up while not being involved in any kind of contact sport meant missing out on a whole bunch of activities with other children, in school, and out. Part of that meant what I now see as being socially stunted.

Sports can be important for building friendships, social skills, rational, fitness, dexterity, a team spirit, and "sportsmanship" manners.

At times, if I was bumped there was a moment when the pain halted my breathing. I'd try to not show that I was in pain, but sometimes that was impossible. Maybe it appeared as if I was about to cry, for some reason that wasn't obvious. At times, I was mocked for that situation, likely because kids didn't know what was happening to me. Maybe it appeared bizarre, and therefore odd, unusual, dramatic, strange, and awkward. The kind of things kids who didn't know what was happening within me, or what it was about, would joke about. Not that I knew what was happening within me, because I didn't. All I knew was that there was too much pain.

I thought I was simply wimpy, and other boys were brave to put up with the pain I thought they were also experiencing when they were bumped. They made sports look like it was fun. I didn't know they weren't like me. I didn't know they weren't in pain when they were bumped into.

In 6th grade the middle-aged physical education teacher called me a sissy because I wouldn't play basketball. That wasn't helpful. He looked at me as if I was the pathetic one. I avoided him. As an adult, I now know he was wrong for treating a child that way. Maybe he thought it would motivate me to prove him wrong. He was wrong.

You'd think that maybe if a kid says it's too painful to play sports, the physical education teacher might want to figure out why.

I could have been diagnosed far earlier in my life. But what are the chances the doctors would have done what is right for me? Maybe it was better that I was not diagnosed into my adult life, so I could then do what I did, and figure out what is best for me, and decide which medical advice to refuse.

I grew up in one of those families where, for various reasons, a child rarely – or never – sees a doctor.

Discovery

In my early 20s, I went to a doctor because I had small lumps beneath the skin of my legs. Just as the little lumps had suddenly appeared, they went away. Doctors never identified the cause. Perhaps the problem was inflamed lymph nodes.

The doctors gave me tests that revealed other things, including blood in my urine.

They put me through tests, and took images.

The first doctor who saw the ultrasound images said he hadn't seen kidneys like mine, other than in text books. I wasn't sure how to respond to this. Congratulations, Mr. Doctor?

Other doctors wanted to see the images of my kidneys, and to talk with me. The hospital was part of Yale medical school. Maybe I had turned into some sort of specimen for them to examine for the students.

To be in, or not to be... plugged in

They wanted to put me on dialysis, with the aim of giving me a kidney transplant.

Being plugged to a machine at a dialysis clinic was the future they saw for me.

If I didn't do what they advised, they said I was unlikely to live long.

I didn't share their vision.

The dialysis procedure and the transplant didn't sound fun, or how I wanted to exist. I thought there must be another way, for me. I was stubborn, untrusting, and questioning. I'm glad I was. For me. Your condition might be completely different.

Genetically flawed

I was told my condition was genetic, because kidneys would only form this way. It wasn't a result of infection, illness, or chemical toxins, or other substances, or after-market experiences.

I also was told I have one working adrenal gland.

I barely mentioned any details about my situation to anyone. I mean, about what the doctors were telling me. I didn't want anyone freaking out on me about how terrible they thought it was. I didn't want to hear it, or to be pitied. Nor did I want anyone telling me what I should do, or telling me I was being irrational for not following doctor advice, and for being so questioning, and doubting.

For various reasons, the unreliable family I was born to was out of the picture. There was no family to discuss health things with. Only my brain to factor things. At times, it could be extremely frustrating, stressful, baffling, and saddening.

I had asked the doctors if I risked passing along my genetically screwed up kidneys and adrenal glands to any children I might have. Yes, they said.

I didn't want to put someone else through it.

Friends were getting married, and having babies, or simply having babies.

I told a girlfriend about my kidney situation, and that the doctors essentially had told me I was likely to die young. She told her mother. The mother became set against her daughter being involved with me. The mother wanted grandbabies, and ones without some genetic flaw. And she didn't want her daughter marrying some guy likely to die, leaving her as a single mother – with children stuck with problem kidneys. It was a harsh experience. The relationship ended.

I spent years mostly keeping quiet about my "genetic disorder," all while my kidney problems became worse, and medical expenses, and time spent in doctors' offices increased. Other people my age were starting to invest in stocks and real estate. My money was going to medical stuff. Days here and there off work added up to weeks, and, at times, months. Collectively, it ended up being years.

What the doctors were telling me about potentially dying if I didn't go onto dialysis – and then doing what I could to get a kidney transplant – shaded my existence. One solution they suggested was having a living relative donate a kidney.

I didn't know my relatives – other than I knew their history of substance abuse likely meant they were not kidney donation candidates.

I didn't know what to do, so I basically lived in denial.

The gentle – and sometimes strong – pain in my kidneys was increasingly bothersome.

I continued to sometimes have bloody urine. I kept quiet about this, too.

I never felt satisfied with the information I was getting from doctors. It was all perplexing. There was no Internet in those years to research stuff. I was stuck in a guessing game, denial, and an inner dialogue I didn't want to speak.

Pressure, and getting away from animal protein

Out of seven doctors involved in my kidney situation in the early years, one of the doctors asked me if the others were "pressuring" me to go onto dialysis, and to get a transplant. Yes, they were. With their added commentary that I would die, if I didn't go onto dialysis – and then, somehow, get a transplant.

Or, I would die... I kept thinking.

This one doctor said the only thing he sees that works for my sort of situation is a diet free of all animal protein.

I didn't know what that meant.

Didn't we need to eat at least some sort of animal protein in the form of meat, or eggs, or milk?

No, he said. We don't.

Carnivores: claws, razor teeth, and a more acidic digestive tract

Some people read the studies revealing the increased chronic and degenerative disease risk from eating beef, chicken, turkey, pork, and other meats, and reason that humans have always eaten meat. Not all humans have eaten meat. And they surely haven't eaten the amount of meat humans have gotten used to eating since the invention of household refrigerators.

Humans have the digestive juices and tract in alignment with plant-eaters like antelope, cows, deer, gorillas, goats, horses, rabbits, and other herbivores. True meat eating animals have a far more acidic digestive tract, and that is short, as in bears, cheetahs, cougars, coyotes, dingoes, foxes, hyenas, jaguars, leopards, lions, lynxes, margays, ocelots, oncillas, panthers, servals, tigers, and other carnivores, which all have claws, large, and pointed teeth, and jaws that open wide and can tear open flesh – which human teeth and jaws can't do.

Plant-based gladiators of ancient Rome

Even among who some consider to be the idealized athletes, the gladiators of Rome were vegetarians.

"The figure of gladiators recalls the ideas of strength, hard training, endurance, and deadly efficiency: a perfect fighting machine. Historically, a gladiator was a sort of sport hero, and gladiator's medicine probably one of the first forms of organized sports medicines. Statutes and painting of the ancient roman period tell us of this astonishing world of fighters.

Considering the modern diets of strength athletes, we should expect that gladiators had a high protein diet. However, analysis of their bones has put forward the hypothesis that gladiators were vegetarian athletes: in his accounts of Rome, the ancient historian Plinius refers to gladiators as 'hordearli' (barley-eaters).

Plants contain higher levels of strontium than animal tissues. People who consume more plants and less meat will build up measurably higher levels of strontium in their bones. Levels of strontium in the gladiators' bones were two times as high than the bones of contemporary Ephesians."

– The Best Athletes in Ancient Rome were Vegetarians; *Journal of Sports Science & Medicine*; Dec. 2008

Meat isn't a nutritional requirement for humans, including for growth, endurance, strength, or stamina. There is no "meat deficiency."

You are not a carnivore

I was relieved to hear we didn't have to eat meat. It wasn't something I liked cooking or eating, although I did – because I thought it was part of human nutritional needs. I began to understand I absolutely was nutritionally ignorant.

I had friends who liked eating steak, burgers, and other types of meat. I wasn't like them.

When I was 19 and 20, I had a friend five years older than me who was from New York. He ate steak and eggs every day. He claimed that is what New Yorkers eat. Eventually, at a relatively young age, he had a heart attack, nearly died, and then began following a plant-based diet. Then, another friend who ate meat and dairy for every meal experienced the same at age 29, spending three weeks in the hospital.

Little-by-little, I became more and more curious about the whole meat thing, why we eat it, and what it does to our health. This included wondering about what role animal protein plays in the rates of cardiovascular disease, heart attacks, strokes, cancers, and diabetes, arthritis, and other autoimmune diseases, and in kidney disease.

As I learned about nutrition, I also learned about the animal farming industry. What was it that we were doing to the animals? I studied up on how humans breed animals by the billions, raise them in confinement like prisoners, feed them most of the food grown on the planet, then slaughter billions of them every month (fish, birds, and mammals), cut them into pieces, and sell that "meat" as human food. All for amino acids (protein components) humans would be better off getting from plants.

For decades, studies have revealed benefits of a plant-based diet

There are many, many studies that have identified the benefits of a clean, plant-based diet. A botanical diet helps with everything from heart, liver, eye, brain, nerve, bone, eye, adrenal, spleen, pancreas, thyroid, and kidney health, to strengthening the microbiome and the autoimmune system, and helping with hormonal balance. Why that knowledge hasn't been more speedily making its way into the treatment of various diseases is a wonder. Some people view the slow adaptation as perhaps linked to what money could be made, or lost by the medical and pharmaceutical industries.

The benefits of the plant-based diet have been known for many decades. Later in the book, I give details of studies done many decades ago showing the benefits of a plant-based diet on kidney health.

A plant-based diet also benefits those with diseases by reducing their symptoms, as in this study revealed about arthritis:

"The notion that dietary factors may influence rheumatoid arthritis has been part of the folklore of the disease, but scientific support for this has been sparce. In a controlled, single-blind trial we tested the effect of fasting for 7 to 10 days, then consuming an individually adjusted, gluten-free, vegan diet for 3.5 months, and then consuming an individually adjusted lactovegetarian diet for 9 months on patients with rheumatoid arthritis. For all clinical variables and most laboratory variables measured, the 27 patients in the fasting and vegetarian diet groups improved significantly compared with the 26 patients in the control group who followed their usual omnivorous diet throughout the study period. One year after the patients completed the trial, they were reexamined. Compared with baseline, the improvements measured were significantly greater in the vegetarians who previously benefited from the diet."

— Rheumatoid arthritis treated with vegetarian diets; *American Journal of Clinical Nutrition*; Sept. 1999

Flavoring and eating meat

The day I wrote this page, I walked past a restaurant and stopped to watch a cook inside a window using a mallet to pound on chicken breast. He then rubbed herbs and salt onto the meat before tossing it into a pot.

I find it interesting that meat goes through so many flavoring and cooking processes to make it palatable.

We essentially flavor meat with herbs and spices, and sometimes fruits, and/or vegetables, which are all plants. What the aim seems to be is some sort of substance providing a taste sensation created by the right mixture of plants. Then, it is cooked to make it soft enough to eat.

Why are we breeding billions of animals to kill them to flavor their tissues to taste like a mixture of plants? Especially when we nutritionally don't need to be eating them? The more animal protein we eat, the more likely we are to host chronic, degenerative, and otherwise debilitating health problems. The more animal protein we eat, the more likely we are to experience events like heart attacks, strokes, blindness, and kidney failure.

Some people say humans are carnivores, but our teeth couldn't last long if we regularly tried to munch on untendered, uncooked meat, much less try to tear through the skin of an animal. Our fingernails can't tear through flesh, as the claws of carnivores easily can. We have teeth, jaws, hands, and a digestive tract unlike carnivores, and more along the lines of animals that eat leaves, fruits, and other plant matter. Even the acids and size of the human digestive tract are unlike a true carnivore.

Humans are peculiar creatures, often pretending to be something they are not. One thing humans are not is carnivores.

Among some people, not eating animal protein is viewed as odd, and the plant-based diet thought of as being for weak people. But there now are more and more professional athletes, from weight lifters and boxers, to basketball and football players, hockey and rugby players, wrestlers, marathon runners, bikers, tennis players, and Olympic gold medalists following plant-based diets, and succeeding in their sports.

It is time for people to learn about what nurtures a healthy body, and what degrades it. Especially if they want to avoid chronic, degenerative, and debilitating health problems so common in Western society.

Animal protein is problematic for health

More and more studies have been concluding humans do not need to be eating animal protein for excellent nutrition. More and more studies have also been concluding that eating animal protein can lead to a variety of degenerative and chronic conditions, including kidney and cardiovascular disease, and play a role in maladies as broad as diabetes, osteoporosis, cancer, brain and nerve issues, and other health problems.

"The pathophysiology of the association of animal protein with CKD remains unclear. One proposed mechanism is the link between animal protein consumption and hypertension, which observational studies and controlled trials have repeatedly demonstrated. Conversely, plant-based foods have been shown to have the opposite effect, so much so that emphasizing plant-based foods over animal-based foods is one of the principles of the Dietary Attempt to Stop Hypertension (DASH) diet. Animal protein consumption also may lead to weight gain, which might be another predisposing factor for kidney disease. Additionally, studies have demonstrated that, compared with intake of plant protein, intake of animal protein causes an imbalance in the composition of the gut microbiome by producing more ammonia and sulfur-based materials, and having a proinflammatory profile, which may result in reduced kidney function, and an increased risk of cardiovascular disease. Finally, high red meat intake has been associated with an increase in inflammation and oxidative stress, including upregulated inflammatory mediators such as NF-kB [a variety of proteins that help to control transcription of DNA, cell growth and function, cytokine production, and immunity and inflammatory responses] and inflammatory cytokines.

These differences between the effects of animal-based protein versus plant-based protein may favor the use of the latter in both CKD and ESKD [end-stage kidney disease]. Plant-based proteins have been previously described as being more than adequate for nutrition in these populations."
– The Effects of High-Protein Diets on Kidney Health and Longevity; *Journal of American Nephrology*; July 2020

Medical guessing game

With the other doctors leaving me feeling as if I only had the choices of drugs and surgeries, and experiencing degrading health as a dialysis patient who might or might not be sliced open to undergo a kidney transplant (which might fail), or experience death, the option the one doctor gave me of using what is now called a "plant-based diet" to help my situation sounded tremendously better than dialysis and a transplant.

The other doctors told me more discouraging stuff, including one doctor saying to me that "being a vegetarian would be really hard – especially on your social life. You'll never be able to eat in restaurants." He also said it would also make it more difficult on my social life at "the club." The club? He said "country club."

I've never been a member of a country club, and I didn't care about restaurants. I'm also not a restaurant type of person. I have worked in them. The food is grandly overpriced, and largely relies on salt, oil, and sugar. The goal of restaurant food is to provide luxury flavor and texture, which is not based on nutritional needs.

They gave me death timelines

There was also the pressure of likely death timelines the doctors were tossing around. The timelines ranged everywhere from – at one point – them telling me they didn't know if they would be able to keep me alive for more than a couple of days. Decades later, it seems they might have been wrong with that guess.

Mostly they were saying it could be weeks, or a couple months, maybe a couple years. One said, at the very most, I would live into my 50s. But, he said, I'd be really unhealthy and statistics are that I would not be making it to that age. I'm now in my 60s, and I bike, run, do yoga, hike, swim, and am quite active.

What kind of high-pressured marketing game were they involved in?

Was it about me being an income source for them, or was it about what was best for my health?

How much money were they aiming to make from me as their patient?

What if they were not as educated as they could be about solutions to my problem?

What if what they were advising me to do would shorten my life, rather than lengthen it?

What were the risks of doing what they advised, compared with the risks of not doing what they advised?

I wasn't getting answers from them, and I didn't want to participate in what they advised based on what seemed to be wild guesses.

Doctors of discouragement

The words of those doctors were discouragement paved with discouragement, coated with more discouragement.

It was grim and depressing, and made me sad and stressed and frustrated and perplexed. I was left to feel I was not going to experience the good life, but would be stuck going downhill into illness, frustration, sadness, and poverty.

The way my former girlfriend's mother responded to knowing about my genetic kidney issue made me feel as if I should never marry, as it would be unfair to leave someone as a young widow. I also felt as if I absolutely should not have children, as I would only be leaving them with genetic kidney disease. My life prognosis seems unpleasant, and people my age were making other decisions I could not make.

I wasn't having fun. I was in a situation, and didn't know what the solution could be.

Because of the experience with the girlfriend and her mother, I continued to barely discuss much of any details about my kidney situation with anyone. I didn't want pity, or pressure – or dismissal, or rejection.

I wanted to ignore it all. That wasn't possible. The constant subtle – and sometimes strong – pain in my kidneys, and the occasional bloody urine were reminders that all was not well in my torso.

What would my life be like if I did go onto dialysis, and if I had the kidney transplant? Couldn't those also fail me?

The answers the doctors gave me sounded more like guesses. Dreadful ones.

If you end up in the situation of having doctors saying the things they said to me, maybe your choice would be to follow their advice. Maybe, depending on your situation, it will be the right decision for you.

Do your research, get second opinions, and third, and fourth opinions, and do what you feel is best for you.

I took a guess, and chose to follow the advice of the doctor who said I should cut all animal protein from my diet. Because, why not? He said he saw it "work" with other people with kidney problems. Whoever they were.

Cheesy

By my early 20s, I was as close to a cheese addict as possible.

I had a girlfriend when I was 19 who loved cheese, and got me into all varieties of cheese.

Except brie. I hated brie. That stuff is wrong.

Later in the book, I tell about how dairy negatively impacts health. Dairy contributes to everything from osteoporosis to asthma, eczema, cardiovascular disease, heart attacks, strokes, organ and blood cancers, macular degeneration, colds, allergies, leaky gut, arthritis, and E.D. And mood swings. And diabetes. And kidney disease.

While cutting out milk and yogurt, I did continue to eat cheese. Less and less of it. Then, eventually, I stopped eating it. And my kidney function improved.

Egg McNever

Starting when I was little, my stomach said "no" to eggs. Eggs made me puke.

No matter how they were prepared: scrambled eggs, hardboiled eggs, egg salad, fried eggs, raw eggs in a smoothie, poached eggs, and egg sandwiches, eggs slathered with catsup, I hated the smell, flavor, texture, and everything about eggs.

When you grow up in a poverty-stricken household with troubled parents who have too many children to feed, you aren't to complain or refuse the food there. Do not make a scene. Don't express an opinion. Stay quiet, and eat. Don't be any sort of a spectacle, or problem.

I'd eat the scrambled eggs – or however they were prepared – and eventually end up in the bathroom with my head over the toilet. I'd never mention it. The puking also had to be done quietly.

When I saw the *Rocky* movie with the scene of Sylvester Stallone drinking raw eggs, I nearly hurled.

Luckily, as an adult, I could make my own food choices. Part of this meant banishing eggs. Forever, and ever.

Considering various studies concerning eggs consumption and human health, it's a good thing I gave up eggs.

"In the multivariable model with adjustment for age, sex, residence, education, income, interviewer, smoking, alcohol intake, intake of fruits and vegetables, grains, dairy, products, fatty foods, meat, energy intake, and BMI, there was a significant increase in the odds of cancers of the oral cavity and pharynx, upper

aerodigestive tract, colorectum, lung, breast, prostate, bladder, and all cancer sites combined with a high vs. low egg intake."
– Egg consumption and the risk of cancer: a multisite case-control study in Uruguay; *Asian Pacific Journal of Cancer Prevention*; 2009

Eggs have been linked to an increased risk of cancers of the bladder, breasts, colon, lungs, oral cavity, ovaries, pharynx, prostate, and upper digestive tract, and increasing the progression and lethality of cancer.

"Eggs are high in choline. Choline is converted in the gut into trimethylamine (TMA), which, after being oxidized by our liver into TMAO, may promote inflammation, and result in cancer progression."
– Do Eggs Cause Cancer & What Explains This Connection?, by Michael Greger, MD; NutritionFacts.org; Aug. 2023

There is enough evidence of problems with eggs that I don't want them in my foods. If even a little for people without cardiovascular and/or kidney disease, that little can mean a big difference in people who already are at risk of experience – or who have – cardiovascular or kidney disease, or other chronic and degenerative conditions.

Besides cancer, eggs increase the risk of heart disease, heart attacks and strokes, and kidney disease, nerve disorders, and diabetes and other autoimmune disorders.

"Egg yolk is a concentrated source of both phosphorus and the trimethylamine N-oxide precursor, choline, both of which may have potentially harmful effects in chronic kidney disease. The yolk is also an abundant source of cholesterol which has been extensively studied for its effects on lipoprotein cholesterol and the risk of cardiovascular disease."
– Egg Intake in Chronic Kidney Disease; Nutrients journal; Dec. 2018

"High levels of egg consumption are associated with an increased risk of type 2 diabetes in men and women."
– Egg Consumption and Risk of Type 2 Diabetes in Men and Women; *Diabetes Care*; Feb. 2009

Of course, research sponsored by the egg industry will tell you eggs are great for health.

The deer

I never much liked meat. By the time I was a teenager, I was eating less and less meat. It started after I was walking alone home from school while stomping on the thin ice shelf along the curb as the ice was being undermined by the water from melting snow. The water started to turn pink.

There was a thin stream of red liquid going down the center of a driveway. I stopped.

The stream led to the backyard where a dead deer was hanging by its hind legs in a tree. It's neck had been slit wide open, and the dripping blood had formed a puddle on the lawn.

The neighbors had gone hunting.

I had never hunted. I had never seen anything like the deer hanging upside down there, nearly decapitated.

The first animal death that impacted me was when my dog was killed when I was 8. That deer also made a big impact.

From nutritionally ignorant to my food revolution

I grew up in Ohio. It wasn't exactly a hot-spot to go through a dietary revolution. It especially was not a place for someone to consider not eating meat. Advertisements for meat were everywhere. Meat was always in the kitchen, and in the school cafeteria, and at picnics, and events. Everyone around me ate meat.

I was not familiar with the word *vegetarian*, and the word *vegan* wasn't something I had ever heard.

Nutrition wasn't a topic of conversation. "Eat your vegetables" was about as deep as nutritional advice went.

The "food pyramid" nonsense

For generations, nutrition information has been gained from information presented in TV and radio advertising, and print ads. What is advertised, and what stores and restaurants sell, has been what people eat.

If it can be sold, it's okay to eat, right? There are laws relating to protecting us from toxic food, right? Not quite, and often, not really.

Foods that are advertised, and many that are otherwise sold are often the foods to stay away from.

The way certain industries have promoted their food products has also been quite sneaky.

In American schools there was the "food pyramid" chart with teachers telling us to eat from the four food groups, including meat, eggs, and dairy.

I didn't know until I was an adult that the food pyramid was created by the animal farming industry. The promotional materials for the food pyramid were sent to schools, so teachers could hand out the animal farming propaganda to students. Teachers gave it to us, and it says to eat meat, dairy, and eggs. Therefore, that is what we should do. Right?

The food pyramid promoting meat, dairy, and eggs wasn't based on human nutritional needs. It was based on selling the products of the meat, dairy, and egg industries. In America, those industries receive what amounts to corporate welfare from the federal government. Part of that money goes into marketing and publicity for the products produced by the animal farming industry.

Today, people still believe the food pyramid is the nutritional standard to follow – or else you will be lacking in nutrition.

What you do by following the food pyramid is increase your risks of chronic and degenerative diseases – especially the more your diet relies on meat, dairy, and eggs.

There is no human meat deficiency, egg deficiency, or dairy deficiency. There is no animal protein deficiency.

Fast food

As a child, I didn't eat as much fast food or processed food as what people today consume. I also ate vastly less fast food than other kids I knew. But what I was eating was far from health-infusing. Because it was animal-protein heavy, as well as oily and sugary and salty, what I ate as a child was in tune with what brings about chronic and degenerative diseases, and, in the long-term, encourages heart attacks, strokes, cancers, diabetes, asthma, other maladies, and kidney problems.

It was the 70s, the rise of fast food was well underway. It seemed like there was a new junk food being broadly marketed every week. I did notice other families in the neighborhood eating more and more fast food, junk food, and packaged food. Maybe it was easier that way for the parents.

It became common to see famous people, and sports and music stars featured in fast food advertising. If they ate it, wasn't it also good for the rest of us? Would it make us glamorous, too? If sports stars ate the junk food, it was good, and healthy, right?

I was the generation that saw the rise of the ultra-processed food industry. Not only fast foods, colas, bottled drinks, and junk snacks, but "heat and serve" foods. It seemed every household in the neighborhood was buying this new thing called "a microwave." We didn't have a microwave.

We didn't eat the healthiest food, as much of it was based around meat. But it was healthier than what I saw some other families eating.

Slinging junk food

In high school, I worked at fast food joint. I didn't like the food, but working there was fun for a high school kid.

That food didn't smell like or seem like food. The meat was gross. As was everything else they sold.

Dealing with the gallons upon gallons of lard that dripped from the burgers and into a storage container made meat even less desirable to me – if that was possible.

I'd sometimes bring home large bags filled with burgers that didn't sell.

Butler

I knew how to make the foods my mother made, as I had often participated in making it. That came in handy when I moved to California, and worked various jobs.

By some fluke of L.A. weirdness, soon after I turned 20, I ended up living in a wealthy woman's mansion up on a hill in Bel Air. I had been hired to be her butler.

Being the butler involved making all of her food and maintaining the kitchen. I dressed in black and white, and had my hair cut short, the way she wanted it. Everything had to be done her way in what was essentially a luxury resort where she was the permanent – and only – guest.

It was surreal and bizarre. I grew up poor, but there I was living in a mansion in one of the most wealthy neighborhoods on the planet.

One thing it taught me was that mansions are a pain to maintain as it takes a staff of several people to keep things running smoothly.

I also learned wealthy people aren't necessarily the happiest people – and can be far less happy than some of the poorest people I've known.

I had to make breakfast, lunch, and dinner for the wealthy woman. There were certain recipes she had approved. It was the same breakfast every morning. I could get slightly creative with other meals.

37

She had some form of kidney disease, and blood sugar issues. I was too young and uneducated to understand the details. Her food was all part of a plan to remain healthy, and... sober.

From what I now know, the diet she was on was very much NOT what she should have been eating to keep her kidneys healthy.

Her former butler had quit. But he regularly phoned me to explain how to do the job, and to give me advice on how to deal with the woman.

I was purely a servant. I learned from the other staff to simply be agreeable and cooperative, and to put up with the mood swings. Pamper her. Don't interfere with the process of self-importance, or her focus on her global financial gains.

Eventually, after several months of being around her chemically-assisted roller coaster of mood swings, I quit.

L.A. can be a strange trip, as can wealthy people who like pills, and who start treating you as if you are a toy to manipulate.

Factoring a life path

I eventually started attending college as I worked various jobs.

I interned at a public radio station, where I wrote the morning news updates. It was interesting knowing millions of people were listening to my words being read on the radio.

I then got into working for newspapers, newsweeklies, and magazines.

I once started a monthly free parenting magazine delivered all over L.A., which I then sold out of. Probably odd for a young guy with no children. Being a young, single guy starting and running a parenting magazine was like being stuck in a TV sitcom.

When I was in my 30s, because of what I was learning about my own health, and as I was a member of a publishing association, I got into helping doctors and nutritionists to write books about nutrition and health.

My kidneys in my 20s

Besides other stuff going on, and trying to be a functional adult, having kidney problems throughout my 20s was my experience. At times it was the only thing I could experience, as sometimes I would be stuck in bed.

I was having fainting spells. Other times I would break out into drenching sweats. There were frustrating times where I had no energy. And, just as during my childhood, there were times of peeing what looked like pure blood, and not urine.

There was an increasing number of doctor visits, and being told I was on my way to becoming a diabetic.

There was kidney failure. And surgeries.

Age 29, death warmed over

When I was 29, days after one of the kidney surgeries, doctors and nurses said I had died. The nurse who was to get my corpse ready for transfer to the hospital morgue saw my eyes move. I guess I didn't die. Or, did I? Who knows. They say I did.

My girlfriend was out of town for weeks having to do with her job, and I didn't tell her the details of what happened to me in the hospital. I told her I had some kidney stones, which was only a small part of the problem. One thing they did during the surgery was remove some tissue blocking one kidney from draining, a birth defect. But there were complications. What was supposed to be one day in the hospital ended up being days, and more days, and then – according to the medical staff – death. Oops. No need for my girlfriend to know about that stuff. Nor did I tell other people.

My early version of "plant-based"

After that hospital experience, I thought I should more strongly follow the "no animal protein" diet thing the one doctor had advised me to follow.

I simply eliminated all animal protein from my diet. I only ate plants, and drank water.

As far as I knew, I didn't know other people who only ate plants. I also didn't know it was called "vegan." Nor did I know that term, or the term "plant-based."

I had next to no understanding of idea what excellent nutrition was. I had no idea what I was doing, other than I was only eating plants, and I was starting to feel better.

The Internet was in its beginning stages, and fairly useless. There was no easy way to research stuff. There were always "diet books" being sold, including by celebrities, but they seemed to be more puff than reality.

Mostly, what I was eating was chopped veggies, steamed rice, boiled beans, all mixed with salsa. I sometimes added avocado.

Other than cereal and water, and peanut butter sandwiches, and pasta with tomato sauce usually made from scratch, I mostly was eating the chopped veggies, rice, beans, and salsa for nearly every meal.

With that simple diet free of all animal protein, my health improved.

I had energy I didn't know what to do with.

I went from feeling like death warmed over, to jogging several miles per day. And often biking more than that.

I had other health problems, unrelated to my kidneys or nutrition. There was an accident, and a back injury, and facial surgeries to make me look like I had not been in an accident. There were years of horrible back pain. But my kidneys were being less and less of a problem, and less painful. There were fewer and fewer kidney stones, and fewer experiences of peeing blood. But there were lots of medical bills.

Medical poverty

Some of the people who read this book likely are or have gone through extreme financial situations. Especially in the U.S., where not everyone has access to medical care, and everything can quickly get complicated, including because treatments can get delayed, and health issues can worsen because of it.

At one point of my life, doctors were telling me I needed to have four vertebra fused, and have iron rods put in my back. I didn't do it.

They said I'd never run, bike, or walk without a cane. I didn't believe it.

I had already been through three kidney surgeries, and years of doctors saying I needed to go onto dialysis, and saying I needed a kidney transplant. I kept refusing their advice, including not going onto dialysis and not getting a transplant.

So, going through a back injury, with the doctors then saying I needed back surgery, was another load of medical drama.

Going through years of ongoing combinations of health drama, and medical poverty, while trying to have a life, and not wanting to share certain medical information with people who I thought would dismiss me, is no fun.

It's absolutely awful, frustrating, and dreary to have health problems, and to be in pain, and in severe financial stress. And to have doctors saying you are going to die, if you don't do as they advise. And other doctors saying you need to have back surgery. That was my life from my mid- to late-20s, and into my 30s.

Vegan

I continued to follow what I eventually learned was called a "vegan" diet. Through it, I met a variety of people also on the path for their own reasons, including some who had cancer, heart attacks, and other health issues.

I became occupied with learning about what I thought could help my kidney situation – in ways I was not being helped by doctors.

I began reading health and nutrition and medical books. Many, many books. Dozens of books. Into the hundreds of books. Sometimes I was reading more than one book per day. The city library and local university library were my hangouts, including as I began helping people to write books.

Publishing and book writing

I had already been in publishing – including working at newsweeklies, editing a local yoga magazine, and the experience of starting and selling the free monthly parenting magazine. I had also worked in the publicity department of a movie studio.

While working as what was essentially a ghost co-writer of books, I was sitting so much that, to get more movement, I got a job working nights at a vegan restaurant. Even though it was vegan, I wouldn't consider it to be "health food." There was LOTS of gluten, canola oil, salt, and stuff cooked to death, fried or sauteed in oil, and pretty much processed. It helped teach me the difference between healthy vegan food, and unhealthy vegan food.

Ghost co-writer

Helping people to write books started as a fluke when a doctor in the publisher association I had joined asked me to help him write his book. He told others, and some of them hired me to work on their books.

Some of the books I helped to write were novels. Some were recipe books. Most had to do with nutrition, or some aspect of medicine, or about the medical industry, or the life insurance or health insurance industries.

Things for me turned into a blur of helping one author after the other.

I was someone who could barely read until I was 13. Then, I started reading books, and often read the encyclopedias kept on a bookshelf in the family living room. Then there I was, in my 30s, writing books.

Because each book I worked on with various authors had its own set of issues needing to be explained, I had to learn enough to write about the topics. This meant I was spending many hours researching topics, and sometimes finding out so much about certain health issues I would end up informing a doctor I was working with about something they didn't know about their specialty.

Doctor, nope

I spent massive amounts of time in the local university medical library reading all sorts of medical and health reference books and journals. The library staff apparently thought I was a medical student, and they called me "doctor." I never corrected them.

Between a million other things happening, I continued improving my nutrition. I had a vegetable garden. I got a juicer, a good blender, and a bamboo cutting board, a dehydrator, a crock pot, and other equipment, and an excellent set of chef knives. I was eating a wider variety of fruits and vegetables, nuts, seeds, beans, sprouts, and seaweeds. Most of my diet was of unheated foods. I wrote down the recipes I made so I could repeat them.

For a long time, I was having monthly dinner parties, making too much food, and inviting anywhere from a few to dozens of people. Sometimes making the food all by myself. Sometimes I had a girlfriend who helped make the food. Other friends would also show up to help.

That is some of the background of how I ended up knowing this stuff, and how I could write this book.

Time to help others to avoid health problems like mine

With all I have learned about nutrition, I think the best I could do is share what I've learned. Especially if it helps people to avoid the medical problems I had experienced.

Now, 40 years after the first time doctors began telling me I needed to go onto dialysis and get a kidney transplant, my kidney function tests have been normal.

I recently sat with a doctor as he went through my latest tests, with him telling me he sees nothing of concern – other than… one of my ureter tubes has such a narrow area that it is interfering with drainage. It's something I've known about for years. It's a genetic defect. I'm currently planning on having a procedure to remove that part of the ureter tube.

Doctors ask me what I do to stay healthy. They tell me to keep doing it. It has helped me. Detailing it in this book hopefully will help you.

Encouraging vibrant health

As the book points out, there are awful choices a person can make while following a plant-based diet, and there are informed, wise, healthful food choices to be made.

This book isn't only about eating plant-based to help maintain kidney, heart, and other areas of health, but also about choosing less processed foods, choosing food less likely to contain problematic substances, and choosing foods containing what nurtures a higher level of health.

Changing your familiar diet: eating for nutrition

The message here is: Eat for nutrition, not for luxury.

You got used to a diet containing the substances that cause health problems. Now, get used to a diet that encourages vibrant health.

If you have had issues with acne, alcoholism, anxiety, asthma, eczema, celiac, colitis, dermatitis, fatigue, fibromyalgia, food allergies, food sensitivities, gluten sensitivity, heartburn, hepatitis, HIV infection, hives, indigestion, inflammatory arthritis, joint pain, juvenile idiopathic arthritis, kidney disorders, bowel inflammation, leaky gut syndrome, lupus, MS, pancreatitis, psoriasis, rashes, reflux, schizophrenia, Sjogren's syndrome, spondylarthritis, spondyloarthropathies, ulcers, urinary tract infections, or other health issues, you likely will find a favorable response to following a clean, plant-based diet free of damaged oils, and synthetic chemicals.

I did not say the diet can cure those conditions; however, many people have found following a clean diet cleared their body of – or greatly reduced – the symptoms of many ailments. To the point they consider themselves to be cured.

By cleaning up your diet, you might realize how certain foods had been causing or contributing to inflammation, irritation, digestive upset, insomnia, skin conditions, headaches, backaches, and other issues.

Diet is vastly important to kidney and heart health

Diet is vastly important to kidney and heart health, including to avoid experiencing kidney and cardiovascular disease, blood sugar issues, and to reduce the risks of autoimmune disorders like diabetes, lupus, certain types of arthritis, and skin conditions, and other maladies, including certain types of cancer. This is why most of this book is about the clean, plant-based nutrition necessary to maintain kidney health, heart health, bone health, blood sugar, stomach and intestinal functions, and the rest of your structures and systems. All areas of health are linked.

"Plant-based diets are associated with reduced risk of lifestyle-induced chronic diseases. The thousands of phytochemicals they contain are implicated in cellular-based mechanisms to promote antioxidant defense and reduce inflammation. While recommendations encourage the intake of fruits and vegetables, most people fall short of their target daily intake. Despite the need to increase plant-food consumption, there have been some concerns raised about whether they are beneficial because of the various 'anti-nutrient' compounds they contain. Some of these anti-nutrients that have been called into question include lectins, oxalates, goitrogens, phytoestrogens, phytates, and tannins. As a result, there may be select individuals with specific health conditions who elect to decrease their plant intake despite potential benefits. The purpose of this narrative review is to examine the science of these 'anti-nutrients' and weigh the evidence whether these compounds pose an actual health threat."
– Is There Such a Thing as "Anti-Nutrients"? A Narrative Review of Perceived Problematic Plant Compounds; *Nutrients Journal*; Sept. 2020

I use many quotations from various medical and science studies to back the claims. I did this so the book isn't simply my opinion. It relies on scientific findings.

No shame, no guilt

Nobody should feel shame or guilt about having kidney or heart disease, as shame and guilt in that way are not helpful. Nor should anyone project shame or guilt toward – or belittle – someone who has kidney or heart disease – or any chronic or degenerative condition.

One goal with this book is to help people find what is best for them, which concerns to discuss with their healthcare providers, and which changes to make to improve their health.

One thing this book encourages is avoiding foods that dull and diminish health, and that bring on health problems.

Highly marketed, processed, plasticized foods

Many have compared the products sold in supermarkets and restaurants as being equivalent to garbage. The products are so processed, preserved, and with synthetic chemicals that some call them *plasticized*.

When nutrient requirements of the human are taken into consideration, what is being sold as food is not what can be considered food. It is filler that might fill the stomach, but the nutrients humans need are lacking in many commercialized "foods."

Food advertising

Beginning in the 1950s, televisions became common in every household. With the TVs came a way to reach millions of people every day with commercials for unhealthful foods. TV shows were sponsored by food companies. Money from the food companies paid for the production of the most common TV shows. In this way, the TV stars were employees of the advertisers, as the studios were reliant on advertising. Companies realized that if you could get their products on screen, and in the hands of TV and movie stars, the product sales improved. A famous person being seen using a product spurred sales, which brought in money, which impressed stockholders.

Marketed foods and false claims in advertising

Refuse to buy into the false information various food companies use as they are trying to sell products filled with synthetic chemicals, chemically grown ingredients, and foods containing clarified sugars, bleached grains, overly processed ingredients, and unhealthful animal proteins and fats.

Simply choose what is presented by nature: A combination of edible plants, and especially if they are grown without using toxic chemicals.

Eating what is in tune with nature chemically and magnetically tunes us into nature, which truly is our natural state of being.

"When I buy cookies I eat just four and throw the rest away. But first I spray them with Raid so I won't dig them out of the garbage later. Be careful, though, because Raid really doesn't taste that bad."
– Janette Barber, writer and stand-up comic

Deadened, processed, and highly marketed foods

It is simple. If you eat a healthful diet, you will experience better health than if you eat junk. This concept isn't part of the commercial food marketing based on deception, greed, and nutritional ignorance. This is because people can't make money by simply telling you to eat organic fruits, vegetables, sprouts, nuts, beans, and seeds – other than organic farmers who deserve to be paid for their work.

Advertised foods are often what has been deadened through all the processing the ingredients are put through, and the synthetic chemicals in them. The more a person relies on mass-marketed corporate foods, the more likely their diet leads to diseases of affluence, including obesity, cardiovascular and kidney and liver and other organ diseases, and certain other types of dysfunction, and autoimmune disorders.

Tune out of the commercialized deception and confusion

If you are confused by the diet and health information you have heard and read of in the media, there is a reason you are confused. Commercials and monetized food systems are processes of manipulation, to get money from consumers so the corporations satisfy investors, and the corporate leaders can collect outlandishly larger yearly bonuses. It is a system using underpaid farmers who are put under suppressive contracts limiting what foods they can grow, where they can get their seed supplies, and to what companies they can sell their harvests to.

In today's world of nutrition, there are also predatory people on social media presenting themselves as nutrition experts, and with products to sell you. They have monetized their social media, and aim to get the most followers possible to click on their videos so the viewers see commercials. The viewership and the products they sell – including sponsor companies – are what they are about, more than providing accurate nutrition information. It's not about what is best for you, it's about fattening their bank account.

Forget about what advertising has told you about nutrition. When choosing food, simply stick with nature, and foods grown from the ground, that have roots, not eyes, or mothers.

This includes food for you, and anyone you are responsible for.

Ignore food advertising, and skip the processed foods

Skip over all of the processed foods you face at the supermarket, snack shops, and restaurants.

Know that even "salad bars" can contain a load of unhealthful ingredients, including canola oil, fried foods or otherwise damaged oils, as well as clarified sugars, overly salted foods, and synthetic chemical preservatives, dyes, flavors, scents, emulsifiers, and other substances that dull health.

Go straight to the produce section of your grocery store to find real food, as in fruits and vegetables.

Ask your local market to sell more organic produce – especially from regional produce farmers.

Where possible, shop at farmers' markets where regional farmers sell their harvest.

Join or start a CSA, or an organic food co-op.

Where possible, grow food.

Read up about the benefits of eating sprouts, and learn how to grow them. They are inexpensive, easy to grow, and filled with nutrients.

It's up to you to learn what benefits your health

When I first learned I have kidney problems, I was highly naïve about kidney health. I also was not being told a variety of important things. I quickly realized it was up to me to research and learn. Doctors and medical staff don't have hundreds of hours to teach each patient all they might want to take into consideration about health issues.

It is up to you to learn what benefits your health. And to act accordingly.

Financial profit in medicine

My situation left me wondering if the doctors received incentives for getting people to undergo the more intensive "treatments" – including dialysis and a kidney transplant.

Were the doctors being pressured to be financially high-performing for the hospital? I don't know.

Maybe it is wrong to have any shade of this assumption.

Or, is it?

Money-seeking institutional investors like Blackrock and Vanguard own a large chunk of the various "healthcare" and medical corporations, including hospital chains and medical insurance companies. And dialysis companies.

Institutional investors look for companies likely to have some sort of guarantee of a profit margin. How much of those profit expectations are then making it into what is expected of the doctors working at hospital chains owned by institutional investors?

Consider the annual pay, bonuses, benefits, and perks given to executives of hospital and other medical-related corporations.

The U.S. medical industry is a for profit system. As in, they make money from the patients and/or their "health" insurance. Medical facilities need patients, including those who undergo invasive and otherwise expensive procedures. Patients paying money – or their insurance coverage – are how the medical facility bills are paid, and how the doctors, nurses, other staff, and executives get paid.

Assassinating executives isn't the solution

As people have learned from the 2024 murder of United Healthcare CEO Brian Thompson by Luigi Mangione, some medical industry executives get paid tens of millions of dollars per year. This is so while many patients are denied medical care, and they die because of the denial. These deaths from denial of care go on as the companies appear to be focused on making money – not "losing" it by spending it on patient care.

Insurance companies very much do make money by denying and/or delaying – or approving the minimum of – "care."

As a result of insurance industry practices, many people experience ruinous health, financial, and other life problems. They, their families, and others suffer because of it. It is why some people consider Mangione to be a type of folk hero.

In reality, Mangione was a disturbed young man who murdered a man he had never met, leaving children without their father. Mangione ruined his own life. As a murderer, he will be stuck living out life within the sickly system that is the prison industry.

Getting financial profit out of medicine

Rather than murder someone, Mangione could have been active in helping to improve the system. That is, to get profit out of U.S. medical care, and establish a single-care national health plan. Two solutions are to get involved with Physicians for a National Health Program, and also the group Students for a National Health Program. See the sites for those groups, and consider getting involved.

Profit in the dialysis industry

Hospitals and dialysis companies make money by having numerous patients regularly undergoing procedures, including whatever utilizes the high-tech medical machinery the facilities have invested in. It's a business, after all. Businesses are set up to make money – from customers. Dialysis patients are the customers – usually with private or government insurance paying the for the treatment.

People caught up in health problems might find themselves wondering what sort of pressure – if any – the doctors on staff at hospitals are put under to get patients to undergo treatments. Maybe none. Or, maybe some. The patients also might wonder if some types of therapy or procedures are being denied simply because of cost, and not because of patient need.

I sure was being encouraged to go onto dialysis, and to get a transplant. It got to the point of feeling as if I was dealing with salespeople interested in a bonus – rather than doctors interested in what was best for my health.

Intuition

I'm glad I listened to my intuition, and refused the advice of doctors pushing me to go onto dialysis and a transplant. This is, for me. Your case might be very different. Perhaps you could benefit from choices unlike the ones I made.

Only one doctor was advising me against undergoing the procedures, as he encouraged dietary, exercise, and lifestyle solutions. I am glad I chose to listen to him.

I encourage you to do what is best for you.

More of what they didn't tell me

Some things doctors didn't tell me when they were pushing me to go onto dialysis as I was then to qualify for – and essentially chase after – undergoing a kidney transplant include:

• Many people put onto dialysis die within the first year. However, this statistic includes people in terrible health, including some who don't get proactive in taking charge of their health, and those who are eating a junk diet. And also people with substance addictions that have degraded their health, and damaged their cardiovascular system, intestinal function, and kidneys. It also includes people who didn't know they had kidney disease, until they were in the later stages. And it includes people with other serious health conditions.

- The five-year survival rate of someone on dialysis is only about 35%. Again, a whole variety of people are included in that percentage, including people with other serious health issues.

- Few people live for more than a decade on dialysis. And here, again this statistic includes a wide variety of people of various ages and health situations.

- The older dialysis patients are, the lower the survival rate – especially after age 60.

- The five year survival rate for kidney transplant recipients has been about 80%. But the survival rate for a kidney transplant recipients drops the older they get.

  Again, if you are far healthier than most people, including by following a healthy diet, and getting daily exercise, your survival after a transplant is likely to be far longer than average, into the decades.

- Many people on the list for a kidney transplant never get one, and the waiting list is years-long.

- Only about 20% of people on the list get a kidney transplant. With money influencing medicine, people with money can financially maneuver the system to greatly increase their chances of getting a kidney transplant.

- Some people find a match in a living donor, which also has serious complications and risks – both for the donor and the recipient. This includes the possibility of life-long complications for the donor.

- One small risk is the donor can die during the surgery, or because of complications from the surgery.

- Kidney disease can also lead to weakened bones as the kidneys play a role in balancing minerals, and maintaining certain hormone levels. Damaged kidneys can drain too much phosphorus from the blood, leading to the blood to taking calcium from the bones, weakening the bones. This can also trigger the parathyroid glands to release hormones into the blood, also resulting in bone calcium loss.

- Even with a kidney transplant, you are likely to experience cardiovascular disease, and other serious health maladies – especially if you don't significantly clean up your diet, practice daily exercise, and avoid alcohol and tobacco, and other damaging substances, and otherwise take care of yourself. A low-quality diet and unfortunate lifestyle choices can damage the donated kidney.

- Transplant recipients have an increased risk of skin cancer. Skin cancer can also spread more quickly in people taking the anti-rejection medications.

"Studies have shown that only about one-quarter of transplant recipients known they are at increased risk for developing skin cancer.

Organ transplant recipients, including kidney transplant recipients, have more skin cancers than the general population, because the immunosuppressive

47

medications that help to protect their transplanted organ also increase their risk for skin cancer."

– Protect the Skin You're In, by Kara S. Nunley, MD; National Kidney Foundation; 2025

"Posttransplant skin cancer is the most common malignancy after patients have undergone renal transplantation.

A total of 199,564 renal transplants were included. After renal transplantation, 7,334 (3.68%), 6,093 (3.05%), and 936 (0.47%) were diagnosed with squamous cell carcinoma, basal cell carcinoma, and melanoma, respectively."

– Skin cancer outcomes and risk factors in renal transplant recipients: Analysis of organ procurement and transplantation network data from 2000 to 2021; *Frontiers in Oncology* journal; Nov. 2022

In other words, I would likely have been gone many years ago – if I had followed the doctors' advice to go onto dialysis – and chase after getting a kidney transplant.

For those who do go the route of dialysis and a transplant, that's their choice. Maybe they are doing what will be best for them. That's their business. It wasn't my choice, and I now feel it would have been an absolutely ruinous choice – for me. Other people should do what is right for them.

Do your research, and consider your options.

Doctors are not your parents, baby sitters, or rulers

I currently know someone who is on dialysis, and who eats junk food – as he's on the waiting list for a transplant. He says he isn't worried about his diet, as the doctors didn't say he couldn't have that unhealthy stuff. As if someone is supposed to wait until their doctors tell them what to do – every step of the way. He's in terrible health. His horrid diet is likely the main culprit in his health troubles. He's not doing himself any favors by eating the garbage he does.

No matter what information is presented to them, many people will continue to do exactly what is wrong for them. It might be because of addictions, or misinformation, or bad advice, or pressure from others, or low self-esteem, or habit, or some other driving force not in their best favor.

To get, or not to get: dialysis and a transplant

I am not telling you to – or not to – go onto dialysis, or to get – or not get – a kidney transplant.

I'm not your doctor, your healthcare professional, your parent or guardian, boss, parole officer, judge, or jury. I'm a person who experienced horrid kidney health, and, according to doctors, at one point I "died" in the hospital a few days after undergoing kidney surgery. I'm also someone who continues to undergo testing showing my kidney function is considered in the "normal" range – 40 years after being told I needed dialysis I never had, and a transplant I never got.

Do your research, upgrade your nutrition, and do what is right for you

Consider the impact nutrition, exercise, sleep, and "recreational substances" (alcohol and/or drugs) have on your kidney health.

Your unfortunate food choices can be damaging your cardiovascular system, kidneys, liver, spleen, adrenal glands, nerves, and other areas of health as badly as addictive substances – and perhaps worse.

Whether or not you have kidney, cardiovascular, digestive, or other health problems, it is good to follow a kidney-safe, heart-safe, clean, well-rounded, plant-based diet. It is a liver-safe, adrenal-safe, spleen-safe, intestine-safe, colon-safe, bone-safe, brain-safe, and an overall health-safe diet.

What you might find is you will relearn what food is, and what is not food. This means learning about both what nurtures, and what degrades your health.

When you walk into a food store or a restaurant, know what is food, and what is non-food.

Know which dietary choices work to reduce, dull, or even obliterate your health.

Know which dietary choices could help to heal you, nurture a healthy gut biome, and lead to vibrant health.

Look into the information provided by ForksOverKnives, NutritionFacts, and The Physicians Committee for Responsible Medicine.

Consider going through the plant-based nutrition program offered by the T. Colin Campbell Center for Nutrition Studies, or the plant-based nutrition program offered by eCornell of Cornell University.

Pioneer kidney researcher Thomas Addis

Stanford School of Medicine clinical scientist, physician, and professor Thomas Addis (1881-1949) was a pioneer in what is now known as nephrology, the branch of internal medicine focused on the study and treatment of diseases of the kidneys.

After decades of study, in a paper* published in 1948, Addis concluded that a low-animal protein diet rich in plant matter reduces or prevents the progression of kidney disease, and can play a role in reversing some of the damage. (*Protein consumption in glomerulonephritis: Effect on proteinuria and the concentration of serum protein. Edward C. Perside, M.D., Thomas Addis, M.D.; *Archives of Internal Medicine*; May 1948)

Addis identified animal protein specifically as causing "work overload" to the kidneys. He identified a diet heavy in animal protein as being especially harmful to those with kidney disease.

Addis found that restricting animal protein in the diet reduced kidney failure by 33 to 55%.

Addis employed a multidisciplinary approach of doctors, lab technicians, and dieticians to work together on patient care. His was considered to be the first "evidence-based" dietary treatment of kidney disease.

Addis' interests included what was then called Bright's disease, now known as nephritis – or kidney disease.

In addition to the structures and functions of the kidneys, Addis studied blood clotting, the pathogenesis of hemophilia, blood transfusions, and bile metabolism.

Among Addis' discoveries were how to measure the protein, red blood cell, white blood cell, and epithelial cell content of urine. This advanced the ability to diagnose and treat kidney disease.

Addis found that diets with reduced animal protein and more reliant on plant matter resulted in healthier kidney function, and fewer incidents with chronic

49

kidney disease, kidney stones, and renal failure.

Dr. Addis vs. the medical industry

Addis was compassionate to poverty-stricken people. He was an early proponent of a national health insurance plan.

Addis lost his membership in the American Medical Association because, in an act of protest, he didn't pay his dues. He was in disagreement with the AMA refusing to support President Truman's plan to start a national health insurance plan.

Instead of a national health insurance plan, what the U.S. has today is a massively profitable medical system that makes the rich wealthy as the system is about shareholder profit and upper management making enormous salaries, and denies healthcare to the poor who can't afford it.

A lack of access to adequate medical care is also to blame for much of the unhoused population, who are often ruined because of untreated medical issues, mistreated medical issues, medical malpractice, and medical debt throwing them into poverty with chronic and degenerative, and otherwise debilitating health issues.

Kidney- and heart-safe diet

As you age, your kidney function and cardiovascular system will degrade. Through healthful food choices, sleep patterns, exercise, and lifestyle choices you have some control over this.

Luckily, less than a third of your kidney function is needed to keep you healthy, and your vascular system can remain health – IF you make wise dietary and lifestyle choices.

The standard American diet (SAD diet) – which is rich in salt, clarified sugars, and various types of animal protein, and farming, industrial, and artificial chemical residues and additives, and extracted, clarified, and degraded oils – damages the kidneys and cardiovascular system, and the gut biome, and other areas of health.

A diet rich in animal protein increases inflammation and the workload of the kidneys, and leads to renal hypertension in combination with cardiovascular issues.

Renal hypertension is high-blood pressure in the kidneys. Sustained high blood pressure can permanently damage kidney function, and destroy kidney tissue (progressive glomerular sclerosis).

Combined with unhealthful diet, lack of exercise, and substance abuse, it is easy to understand why there are so many people on heart meds and kidney dialysis.

Most people in industrial society are eating toxic garbage that should have never been considered to be food. Many are regularly drinking alcohol, and also using tobacco, and taking addictive "recreational" drugs.

Luckily, a healthy, clean, plant-based diet can help preserve kidney and cardiovascular function. That means, a diet free from meat (mammals, birds, fish, crustaceans, etc.), eggs (bird and fish [caviar]), and dairy (milk, cheese, cream, yogurt, kefir, butter, ghee, whey, and casein), bone broth, and lard. It is wise to avoid fried oils and oil sautéed foods, as well as sugary and salty foods, and all the ultra-processed junk.

Plant-based imitation meat products

As someone with kidney and/or cardiovascular disease, I encourage you to avoid isolated soy protein supplements. Also avoid imitation "vegan" meats made of isolated soy protein (soy dogs, soy sausage, soy burgers), which often also contain other low-grade ingredients, such as canola and other oils, and are ridiculously high in sodium (salt).

Avoid – or greatly limit – other fake meat products meant to smell, taste, feel, and cook like, and otherwise imitate animal meat. These products have grown in popularity, and include everything from breakfast sausages to imitation beef, chicken, turkey, pork, and other meats. They are highly processed, salty, oily, and often protein-rich to the point they can also be problematic. At least don't make them a daily food choice. Mostly, they are good if you are making a dinner for multiple people, and some of them prefer having meat. The products have been successfully produced to the point they can trick someone into thinking they are eating meat. Even regular meat eaters doing taste tests have chosen the vegan meat as the one that is the real meat, and thought the real meat was vegan. (For a humorous video about this, search: "Anti-vegan 'sausage expert' tricked on live TV into saying vegan sausage was 'luscious and lovely.'")

For those with kidney damage, too many beans, lentils, and peas can also be problematically high in protein, as they are about 30% protein per calorie. Limit them to only a few cups pers week, or about half a cup per day. This includes bean soups, spreads, burgers, and hummus.

If you follow a kidney- and heart-safe, clean, plant-based diet, you are also following a nurturing diet beneficial for the other organs, from head to toe, and from the brain and nerves to the bone marrow, to the skin and eyes, and the cardiovascular, lymph, hormonal, thyroid, and digestive systems.

Toxic dietary choices are chasing people into the disease club

With the growth of the kidney and heart disease industries, the horrid food choices people are making, combined with a lack of exercise, and unfortunate lifestyle choices are escorting them into the doorways of the disease industries.

What you do – or don't do – in relation to your health are keys to determining if you end up being a member of the disease club.

What isn't being done enough is people are not learning about – or practicing – healthful nutrition. Instead, they are bombarded with mass marketed food products that are not good for them, and degrade their cardiovascular and kidney health, and everything from their gut biome to their bone, eye, brain, and nerve function, and all tissues, from their skin to their muscles, and all organs and their function.

Be wise, educate yourself, and earn the keys to your health solutions.

Reducing risks of chronic and degenerative diseases

"Chronic kidney disease is one of the top ten leading causes of premature death in the United States, and its incidence is increasing.

Chronic kidney disease affects more than ten percent of the adult population, and each year, more than 100,000 Americans develop end-stage kidney disease, and have to go on dialysis.

What's crazy is that a staggering 96 percent of individuals with mild to moderate decreases in kidney function, and about half of individuals with severely decreased kidney function go undiagnosed. Meaning the vast majority – like 24 out of 25 people with chronic kidney disease – don't even know they have it.

What can we do to maintain our kidney function?

Well, in a study that followed more than a thousand older women for a decade, those consuming a diet that is richer in plant-based protein had a slower decline in kidney function – extending support for the health benefits of plant-rich diets in the general population to maintain kidney health.

Compared with protein from plant sources, animal protein has been associated with increased risk of end-stage kidney disease in several such studies.

Kidney damage from animal protein could result from the dietary acid load, excess phosphorus, or gut microbiome bad bacteria, and the resultant inflammation.

– Plant-based Diet for Minimal Change Disease of the Kidney, by Dr. Michael Greger, NutritionFact.org; DrGreger.org; July 2023

There are many reasons why kidney function is negatively impacted by eating animal protein, including the acids, saturated fat, and cholesterol, and the lack of fiber in meat, dairy, and eggs. More reasons include the types of microorganisms the animal foods establish, nurture, and proliferate in the human gut microbiome that then promote a pro-inflammatory state, and can lead to a leaky gut that then plays into autoimmune disorders. Then there are also the inflammatory and carcinogenic chemicals formed by cooking meat, dairy, and eggs. And the farming chemical, pharmaceutical, and other industrial pollution residues found in meat, dairy, and eggs, which also all play into the incidence of chronic and degenerative diseases.

As is detailed later in the book, what you eat impacts the bacteria and other microorganisms in your digestive tract. There are pro-inflammatory and problematic gut bacteria that produce substances that negate health, and there are helpful gut bacteria that assist in nutrient absorption, form certain vital nutrients, and also break down substances that would otherwise degrade health.

Eating for nutrition, not for luxury

I'm not here to sell you any products. I don't sell pills, potions, or elixirs.

I encourage you to go to the produce section of your grocery store, to go to a local farmers' market selling fresh fruits and vegetables from your region, and to support your local organic vegetable and fruit farmers. Where possible, I encourage you to grow food and learn about harvesting wild foods. And to know how to make a variety of healthy foods from scratch based on nutrition, and not on luxury.

I encourage you to know the difference between what tastes good, and what is good for you. Healthy foods can also taste quite luxurious.

Plant-based diet is nutrient-dense, and protects against disease

Studies reveal how fruits and vegetables not only provide needed nutrients beneficial to health, but they also contain properties that prevent certain ailments, such as diabetes, cancer, Alzheimer's, MS, and heart, liver, and kidney disease, and macular degeneration; limit intestinal exposure to carcinogens; and help the body to contain, transport, and eliminate toxins.

"A number of studies have shown that cancer risk is lower and immune competence is higher in individuals who consume a vegetarian diet. Epidemiological studies almost unanimously report a strong correlation between a diet high in fruits and vegetables, and low cancer risk."
– John Boik, in his book *Cancer & Natural Medicine: A Textbook of Basic Research and Clinical Research*

Eat your greens, and other vegetables

Learn ways of making vegetables raw, or only steamed, or boiled.

Grilling, frying, oil sautéing, roasting, searing, toasting, and other high-heat forms of cooking are not advised for maintaining vibrant health, and especially for those with – or who want to avoid – kidney, heart, digestive tract, neural, and autoimmune issues.

More about heat-generated chemicals is covered later in the book.

Learn about and include a wide variety of greens in your diet. Consider arugula, asparagus, bok choy, broccoli greens, cauliflower greens, celery, cilantro, collards, cucumber, dandelion, fennel, kale, lettuces of all types, wild greens, microgreens, stinging nettle, and sprouts, and herbs like dill, oregano, basil, thyme, rosemary, and others.

Green veggies are some of the keys to everything from bone, brain, nerve, blood, lymph, kidney, liver, lung, heart, teeth, and eye health, to skin, nail, and sexual health, and the health of the gut microbiome and digestive tract.

There are a wide variety of vegetables, including many you likely have never heard of, or have never seen or eaten. It helps to include an assortment of them in your diet.

The antioxidants, anti-inflammatories, amino acids, enzymes, essential fatty acids, fiber, minerals, and variety of vitamins, and other substances in plants are what you need to maintain healthy organs, and vibrant health.

There are ways of making foods that decrease their nutrition, or increase it. Later in the book I go into more detail about this.

Create a healthful body terrain

The best way to prevent disease is to avoid doing things likely to create the terrain for diseases to take hold.

Following a vibrant diet is a major key to maintaining vibrant health.

Foods that damage enzymatic activity within the body include meat, milk, and eggs, and products made with them, which are rich in free radicals that play a role in inflammation. This is especially so with animal protein that has been highly heated, creating heat-generated chemicals that are pro-inflammatory and introduce more free radicals.

Enzyme damaging foods also include those that had been fried and hot oil sautéed, and other foods containing highly heated oils, and foods containing MSG, bleached foods, and artificial sweeteners, dyes, scents, and flavorings, as well as other artificial ingredients. Eating these deadened or chemically-saturated foods clutters and dulls the system, and puts a body out of tune with vibrant health.

The good news is a system damaged by unhealthful eating can be improved by eliminating damaging foods, and by eating a healthful, vibrant diet.

Regional differences in diet and health

Regionally, humans who follow a certain diet experience health conditions at rates not seen in regions where that type of diet is not followed.

Those living in areas of the world where meat and dairy consumption is highest also have the most elevated rates of heart disease, heart attacks, strokes, colon cancer, arthritis, diabetes, certain types of kidney disease, and other maladies not experienced among people living in areas where meat and dairy consumption is lower.

Even within cities, there are areas where fresh food is less common, and unhealthy food is more common, and people rely on fast food joints, liquor stores, and "convenience stores" selling what damages health. Those are referred to as "food deserts." There are other parts of the cities where fresh food is more available, and stores are more likely to sell healthier food.

Isn't it interesting that violent crime might be more common where unhealthy food is common? Food impacts nerve and brain function, stress levels, and hormonal activity. Nutrition plays a role in the ability to learn and cope with life. It is important that all people have access to healthy, fresh foods free of junk ingredients.

It is important for everyone from expectant mothers to infants, toddlers, school children and adults in all situations, including in rehabilitation facilities, to get health-infusing food that gives them the best chance of functioning at a higher level. Otherwise, unhealthy foods can perpetuate low-grade behaviors, societal problems, and debilitating health issues.

People shouldn't wait for some authority figure or government entity to make the decisions about what to eat. Instead, it's helpful to be proactive in learning about nutrition, and in making the most healthy nutritional choices available to you.

National Heart Act and the National Institutes of Health

U.S. President Harry Truman signed the National Heart Act on June 16, 1948, creating the National Advisory Heart Council and the National Heart Institute as part of the National Institutes of Health. At the time, heart disease – and deaths from heart attacks and heart failure – had been identified as an increasingly common cause of disability and death.

As the relatively new inventions of freezers and refrigerators were becoming common in every household, people were eating more meat, dairy, and eggs than humans ever had in history. More people also were suffering the consequences of eating so much animal protein – and consuming newly mass marketed, salty, oily, sugary, chemically-saturated processed foods. This dietary changes played into the disease processes being experienced in society, which increased the need for what were seen as necessities offering solutions – those being doctors, hospitals, surgeries, and prescription drugs.

Sometimes real solutions are overlooked, or pushed aside or quashed, as more profitable "solutions" are promoted because they favor the financial interests of investors. This could mean things not in the best interests of those who need solutions to their problems.

The disease industries

The animal protein-rich diet infused by the increasingly common industrial animal farming industry reliant on massive numbers of overly bred farm animals being slaughtered, "processed," packaged, and refrigerated, and distributed to the new supermarkets and fast foods restaurants helped spur the rise of the heart disease, kidney disease, cancer, arthritis, osteoporosis, diabetes, and other disease industries. It also lead to the rise of the pharmaceutical and surgery industries. And the increasingly common dialysis and kidney transplant industries.

Enormous amounts of private and government money poured into the medical industry. The search was on to "find the cause" and cure for each diseases. At least, that was the narrative. How much of it has been – and is – about money?

Each disease had its own non-profit organization established to raise funds, hire staff, and open offices to headquarter and manage the organizations, and promote themselves as part of the solutions. Yearly charity events, marathons, walks "for a cure," and golf, tennis, and other sporting events became part of their fundraising practices. How much of those funds raised were – and are – going to administrative costs, and not to doing anything about "finding a cure"? How much money was being given to increase tax write-offs with no real concern about what was happening with the donations, and not really to benefit the problem?

Both the cause and cure of increasingly common chronic and degenerative diseases treated by the medical and pharmaceutical industries have been and are on the grocery and snack store shelves. The causes of diseases are sold at fast food and other restaurants, and at "convenience stores," and gas station snack shops. They are also the foods served in school and hospital cafeterias, and the buffets of hotels and cruise ships, and in the dining halls of the military and prison complexes. The foods in the kitchens, and on the plates of everyone either can be health-infusing, or health damaging. Including foods served at the charity events supposedly meant to raise money to go for finding cures for the very same diseases certain foods promote.

There are foods that nurture degenerative and chronic disease processes, and foods that fuel healing and vibrant health. Which foods are you eating?

Consider that at least some of your health problems are directly related to what you have been eating. Perhaps it is time for you to reconsider what food is.

The rise of processed foods, and related diseases

Nutritional ignorance has been as rampant as diets rich in animal protein and junk foods. There has been an increasing dependance on processed foods, fast foods, and those containing a variety of synthetic chemicals.

Since the mid-1900s, toxic, chemically saturated, overly processed, sugary, salty, and oily foods have become common – from birth, through school, and into adulthood.

Medical staff, including doctors and nutritionists, are largely also following the increasingly unhealthful diets rich in processed foods, synthetic chemicals, clarified sugars, salts, damaged oils, and factory farmed animal protein. They also are experiencing the related chronic and degenerative diseases.

Pharmaceutical companies typically send catered meals to the office staffs of doctors who prescribe the drugs made by those companies. The catered meals are from typical restaurants serving foods not based on nutrition, but based on flavor, scent, color, and texture. Interesting that those who work in the medical profession are eating the same foods that promote chronic and degenerative diseases.

Cut and drug away the diseases

Over the past century, an increasing dependance on pharmaceutical drugs and various surgeries has become of the most common treatments for chronic and degenerative disorders largely brought on by bad food, lack of exercise, the rise in modern-day stressors, and unhealthful living.

Depending on your situation, what is considered to be the cure for some people might not your answer.

Nutrition-, activity-, and lifestyle-based health – or sickness

As the popularity and easily availability of chemically-saturated and ultra-processed fast foods, and the animal protein-rich foods continue to increase across the globe, so have debilitating health issues triggered by bad diet.

People experiencing what are diet-related health conditions have explored all sorts of ways to find answers to their health problems. It's like eating fire, and wondering why your mouth is burning. Often, people have become lost in what have not been solutions, but what only worsened their health problems. Many of the products, potions, pills, and procedures promoted as solutions only benefit the pocketbooks of those selling the products, or performing the procedures.

Vegetarianism and veganism have been growing in popularity. Some of it is related to people wanting to reduce their impact on the planet, and to protect the climate and wildlife. While the environmental benefits of a clean, plant-based diet are becoming obvious, more research is revealing the nutritional and preventive benefits of avoiding animal protein and ultra-processed foods.

Nutritional ignorance, misinformation, and irony

Even as the multiple benefits of a clean, plant-based diet continue to be revealed, it remains a target of negative views, ridicule, and ignorant commentary.

Meanwhile, the toxic food industry continues pouring huge amounts of money into global advertising. In addition to commercials, sports team sponsorships, paying celebrities to promote the toxic foods, and getting TV shows and movies to feature the unhealthful foods and drinks, the toxic foods industries have targeted children.

It's no doubt much of the advertising for toxic foods has been styled to attract the attention of children, including through jingles, imagery, and colorization. Toys and other merchandise for children are included in promoting toxic foods. Commercials playing during children's TV shows are often for toxic foods. It should not be a surprise that chronic and degenerative diseases in children have been increasing.

The toxic foods industries advertising to hook children should be viewed as just as bad as it would be if they were to market cigarettes to children.

Ironically, McDonald's has their "Ronald McDonald House Charities" with their mission statement stating they aim to "create, find, and support programs that directly improve the health and well-being of children." If McDonald's wants to improve the health of children, the company should stop selling them toxic foods and drinks, stop using non-compostable packaging that pollutes the planet, stop supporting the factory animal farms, stop supporting the GMO crops industries, and stop selling foods grown using chemicals that poison the land, water, and air, and that kill migrating and other wildlife.

As all of this has been going on, for many people veganism was nearly unheard of. If they do hear about it, it often is in a negative way, through cynical jokes, and views of people considering veganism as absurd.

Without knowing the nutritional and preventive benefits, veganism could be considered outlandish by people who grew up eating meat, dairy, and eggs, and ultra-processed foods. Especially with how veganism has been mentioned as if it is a joke, and for weak and unrealistic people.

The negative views about the plant-based diet have been held and expressed by the same people suffering the health consequences of horrible diets rich in ultra-processed foods, and problematic xenoproteins. (Xenoproteins: Those from a different species: In human food choices, it is usually protein from cows, pigs, goats, chickens, turkeys, and fish. As in: dairy, eggs, and meat.).

I have heard the most blatantly ignorant things about the plant-based diet. Remaining poker-faced usually is my response. If only they knew of the ignorance they spew and agree with. Some of the very same people who have expressed those views to me later have contact me telling me about a health condition they have been diagnosed with, and ask what I would do. I refer them to the ForksOverKnives site, which was put together by doctors and nutritionists. And also to the NutritionFacts site. They need to take the effort to educate themselves about plant-based nutrition, and to make the changes that would help them. Nobody can do it for them. I can now refer people to this book.

Growth of teaching hospitals

The money pouring into the medical industry fueled the construction of large hospitals, and medical schools – including to treat more and more diet- and lifestyle-induced illnesses, and to train more and more doctors, nurses, and other necessary health professionals.

Research and training hospitals became common, including in association with universities. These gained partial government funding, including for being education facilities for the medical students. Some hospitals have been given or granted – or provided with inexpensive – land to build on, and to grow. Other infrastructure needs are provided by city, county, state, and federal governments.

Having a hospital is necessary for a city to also attract other businesses. It's a way to both provide medical care, and employment to local people, and could play into building up a medical school, which brings more tax-paying citizens, and businesses that need real estate, services, and supplies. With more businesses and people, the city, county, and state collects more taxes.

Wealthy and corporate financial donors to the medical facilities get tax write-offs, and they have specialty wings or medical wards named after them. With university medical school hospitals, a donor could be a graduate who made it big in some area of business, and might be someone who helped raise building funds for the hospital. A wealthy person might have also been so impressed by the medical care they received, they can also see their donation as a way to thank the facility – and to gain the tax write-off.

Going into a training hospital means you also are going into a school. Under the supervision of a doctor, patients being treated, cared for, or undergoing procedures is how medical students learn. But then, as a benefit to the patients, university hospitals also typically have the newest equipment. Not always. And the students in those medical school hospitals are supposedly being taught the most advanced healthcare. Not always.

As it is, when you enter a hospital, you are a part of all those layers of things going on. If it is a teaching hospital, students will be involved in part of your care, and participate in, or observe, the tests and procedures, and help to keep your charts.

Hospital food

As the reliance on the surgical and pharmaceutical industries increased, and hospitals became large, and larger, there needed to be kitchens to feed all of the patients, and the hospital office staff, maintenance staff, and medical staff, and the drug and medical technology salespeople. Industrial kitchens were set up in the hospitals, serving food not much better – and perhaps worse – than food people ate at home, in restaurants, and at other industrial food places: schools, business, and other staff cafeterias.

Because of four kidney surgeries, a horrible arm injury and surgery to repair it, and other situations, I've seen what hospital kitchens serve to patients. It is perplexing to see the abysmal quality of hospital food. I learned to bring my own food stuffed into a backpack, and to tell visitors what to bring me.

"Hospital food needs a revolution.

I was surprises to find out most inpatient meals served in hospitals are not required to meet any sort of national nutrition standards for a healthy diet. And indeed, an analysis on the nutritional value of food served to patients in teaching hospitals found many did not meet dietary recommendations.

The presence of foods on the tray sends a message to patients as to what is healthful and acceptable for them to eat. We still can think of no better place or good opportunity to set an example of good nutrition than when patients are in hospitals.

Meals offered to patients may actually contribute to the exacerbation of the very conditions that may have lead them to the hospitalization."

– *Just How Bad Is Hospital Food?*, a video by Dr. Michael Greger, NutritionFacts.org; DrGreger.org; April 2021

Within medical facilities, fast and convenient foods containing ingredients from chemically-treated monocrop farms, and ingredients from the animal factory farms and slaughterhouses are common.

All the unhealthful foods you could get at fast food restaurants and gas station snack shops are common in hospitals – including in the typical type of convenience stores operating in the hospital. That is, salty, oily, sugary, animal-protein heavy, and ultra-processed foods, sweet drinks, and chemically-saturated foods. Many of the convenience stores inside hospitals and medical centers even today – in the year 2025 – also sell cigarettes along with the most toxic snacks containing ingredients that can play into cardiovascular, kidney, and liver disease, autoimmune disorders, gut dysbiosis, and various forms of cancer.

Heart and diet

Studies done as part of the 1940s and 1950s National Heart Institute found fat in food is converted to cholesterol. It is called *dietary cholesterol*, and adds to the necessary cholesterol naturally produced by the liver. The abundance of cholesterol (from eating meat, milk, and eggs), and saturated fat both from animal protein or from bottled oils overloads the cholesterol in the system. This plays a lead role in myocardial infarction (heart attacks), and strokes, and increases health issues like macular (eyes) and brain degeneration. It also plays into men experiencing erectile dysfunction.

Throughout the 1900s, industrial food containing health-dulling substances became both worse (more processed and unnatural) and more common. There have been foods containing more chemicals, less healthful fats, and more toxic oils being sold into the global food market, including in schools. Junk foods that were once most common in industrialized nations are increasingly available in less developed parts of the world. Because of this, chronic and degenerative conditions related to the junk diet are increasing in countries where those same conditions were once not common.

"Global energy imbalances related to obesity levels are rapidly increasing. The world is rapidly shifting from a dietary period in which the higher-income countries are dominated by patterns of degenerative diseases to one in which the world is increasingly being dominated by degenerative diseases."
– Global nutrition dynamics: the world is shifting rapidly toward a diet linked with noncommunicable diseases; *The American Journal of Clinical Nutrition*; Aug. 2006

"Transition from traditional high-fiber to Western diets in urbanizing communities of Sub-Saharan Africa is associated with increased risk of non-communicable diseases, exemplified by colorectal cancer risk."
– Diet changes due to urbanization in South Africa are linked to microbiome and metabolome signatures of Westernization and colorectal cancer; *Nature Communications* journal; April 2024

"A switch of just two weeks from a traditional African diet to a Western diet causes inflammation, reduces the immune response to pathogens, and activates processes associated with lifestyle diseases. Conversely, an African diet rich in

vegetables, fiber, and fermented foods has positive effects."
   – Western diet causes inflammation, traditional African food protects: Study from Tanzania shows major impact of diet on the immune system; Eureka Alert, Radbound University Medical Center; April 2025

Young children are getting kidney, cardiovascular, and autoimmune diseases, with dreadful long-term impacts

"Poor nutrition and physical inactivity increase the risk of chronic conditions like obesity, depression, type 2 diabetes, heart disease, and some cancers – which can lead to disability and premature death.
   Fewer than 1 in 10 children and adults eat their recommended vegetables.
   A quarter of adults and even fewer adolescents (16%) meet U.S. physical activity guidelines.
   As many as 40% of adults and 20% of adolescence have obesity."
   – Nutrition, Physical Activity, and Weight Status; U.S. Centers for Disease Control and Prevention; 2025

As toxic foods have become common, an increasing number of children under age ten in many countries are found to have cardiovascular and renal and reno-vascular disease (kidney disease), and other degenerative and chronic health conditions previously not commonly seen in younger children. This should not be a surprise, considering what more and more children are eating, and how weight issues are now common among the young who spend an increasing amount of time sitting and playing screen games or scrolling social media.

"Regular exercise offers many health benefits, especially for people with kidney disease. It helps people maintain a healthy weight, blood pressure, and cholesterol levels. One study showed that people with advanced kidney disease who exercised regularly had about a 50% lower risk of death compared to those who didn't."
   – 10 Common Habits That May Harm Your Kidneys; National Kidney Foundation; June, 2016

"The most important cardiovascular risk factors in the pediatric age and adolescence are excess weight, arterial hypertension, glucose metabolism, and lipid metabolism alterations.
   An increase in cholesterol and apolipoprotein levels in childhood is associated with an increase in carotid intima-media thickness (cIMT), and a reduction in carotid elasticity, and a compromised brachial endothelial function in adulthood.
   It has been demonstrated that also low fruit and vegetable consumption and poor physical activity are associated with a rapid progression of arterial inflammation and an increase in cIMT during adulthood.
   Continuous exposure to high serum LDL-C levels during adolescence can lead to the accumulation of calcium in the coronary arteries and, consequently, to the development of atherosclerotic plaques in adulthood. This can result in irreversible changes in the coronary arteries and an increased risk of ischemic heart disease in adulthood. Therefore, aiming to low serum LDL-C levels since childhood is fundamental for the prevention of cardiovascular accidents."
   – Cardiovascular risk in children: a burden for future generations; *Italian Journal of Pediatrics*; April 2022

Long-term implications of a junk food and animal-protein heavy diet during childhood play into adult health problems.

It is important to decrease cardiovascular disease and kidney disease risk factors, and to follow a gut-healthy diet starting in childhood.

Among children with end-stage kidney disease, cardiovascular disease is the leading cause of death. What applies to reducing the risk factors in adults also applies to children. These include a clean, plant-based diet, daily exercise, physical activity throughout the day, a regular sleeping pattern, and avoiding addictive substances.

"Over several decades, dietary habits have changed dramatically around the world. Globalization and urbanization have paved the way for a rise in convenience food and drinks products, junk food, and eating out, with fewer people growing or making their food from scratch.

These cheap and ready-to-consume food and drinks products are often ultra-processed and high in calories, fats, salt, and sugar, and low in nutrients. They are produced to be hyper-palatable, and attractive to the consumer, like burgers, crisps [chips], biscuits, confectionery, cereal bars, and sugary drinks.

Ultra-processed foods and drinks typically have a long shelf life, making them appealing for businesses like supermarkets, rather than highly perishable fresh goods. Intensive marketing by the industry – especially to children – has also increased the consumption of these types of goods. Increasingly, these products are displacing fresh, nutritious, and minimally processed goods, shifting population diets and food systems.

Early life nutrition has important impacts on the likelihood of disease and poor health later in life. But childhood malnutrition remains one of the biggest challenges in public health today."
– Unhealthy diets and malnutrition; *NCD Alliance* (Noncommunicable diseases), Geneva; Nov. 2021

It is important for young children to learn how to grow food, and to be taught to make healthy foods from scratch. Check out the plant-based, oil-free recipes on ForksOverKnives. And also the "renal kidney diet recipes" on PlantBasedKidneys.

Diet-heart hypothesis

In 1953, Ancel Keys, a professor of physiology at the University of Minnesota published a piece in *The Journal of the Mount Sinai Hospital* and brought the "diet-heart hypothesis" into the discussion.

Beginning in 1947, Keys started the Minnesota Business and Professional Men's Study which followed 500 men for fifteen years. The goal was to determine why some men developed cardiovascular disease, while others didn't. He found cholesterol appeared to play the key role in the development of cardiovascular plaque, and in the incidence of heart attacks.

The dawning of industrial and "fast" foods

In the 1940s the fast food industry was getting started, with corporations seeking out multiple locations for their restaurants. They also were selling their standardized restaurant concept as franchises to investors who then can run outlets all selling similar packaged items from the same menu with employees all dressed the same, in buildings of the same design, décor, and coloring. The plan was to make it so anyone could stop by for a quick, salty, oily, sugary, chemically-saturated meal meant to satisfy their taste buds and sense of smell. And it had absolutely NOTHING to do with nutrition. Disease prevention was not a consideration. The breads were made from ingredients that were the products of increasingly chemically-treated monocrop fields. The meat, dairy, and eggs were from mass bred, physically altered animals raised in factory containment farms, where they were fed chemically-grown grains not natural to them, and treated with a variety of pharmaceutical drugs, and sprayed with pest control chemicals. The meat was from the noisy slaughterhouses where thousands of animals are killed every day. The "fast food" stuff also contained chemicals used to dye, flavor, scent, preserve, emulsify, and otherwise make the food standard for every outlet of the fast food chain. But the so-called "food" was unhealthful, and addictive in ways humans had never experienced with food throughout previous history. And those who regularly ate the stuff started experiencing similar chronic and degenerative health issues.

The fast food diet is poison.

Corporate food

Since the 1800s, increasingly larger corporations have been taking over the food industry. With this, people rely more on commercial foods, and become less involved with growing their own, and less likely to make food from scratch using natural ingredients.

A benefit of localizing your food choices – especially by growing some of your own food and getting produce from your regional farmers – is you will eat them when they are at – or closer to – their peak ripeness, when they are rich in nutrients and flavor.

The longer your food takes to be processed, packaged, and sit in stores until it is sold, the more likely it is to have chemicals added to it to preserve it, to flavor it, to scent it, to color it, to texturize it, and to make it so it will last months on a store shelf. Corporate food is all about what is marketable, and what will make the most amount of money for the corporation. Mass marketed food is not about what is most healthful.

Multinational corporations limit your nutrition choices

By relying more on locally-grown foods, you reduce your reliance on multinational corporations that can be viewed as destructive to the planet, and that are ruining the possibilities for family farmers to survive.

The mass marketed, industrial food system limits the variety of fruits and vegetables to those fruits and vegetables that are most shippable, least likely to be easily damaged, and more likely to be able to sit on a store shelf until being sold.

That last paragraph is one of the tragedies of the multi-national industrial food industry. For instance, there are thousands of types of apples, but stores usually sell only a few varieties. This limited market availability is similar for everything from tomatoes to melons and other fruit, to greens, squash, grains, nuts, seeds, and beans.

Soil and gut organisms play a role in all life

Soil organisms include everything from worms and bacteria to other bugs and fungus. Each of them play roles in soil production and health, and in the larger plant and animal circle of life. In the long-term, with climate change and the spread of desertification and industrial toxins, which soil organisms survive will help determine which foods will be available to you, and your ability to survive.

It is important for the survival of wildlife that there are the widest varieties of plants growing. This is so not only for birds, mammals, and insects so they have food for survival, but also for soil organisms. Without a healthful, diverse variety of soil organisms, soil and wildlife suffer. With a plunge in the variety of soil organisms, there are fewer plants, water filtration systems within nature decrease, less oxygen is produced, desertification spreads, fewer greenhouse gasses are sequestered, heat increases, weather patterns change, and climate is disrupted, including the ocean climate, as is the life within and around it.

What you consume plays into the health of soil organisms, and the organisms existing in your gastrointestinal tract. For you to survive, you need both the soil organisms and your gut biome organisms to be healthy. You do this by following a clean, plant-based diet, and avoiding foods containing animal proteins, damaged oils, and synthetic chemicals.

"Diet is inextricably linked to human health. Globally, poor diets low in unprocessed, plant-based foods cause more deaths than any other risk factor, with cardiovascular disease, cancers, and type 3 diabetes as the leading causes of diet-related deaths. Unhealthy diets also carry a wide range of negative environmental impacts. Animals-based foods contribute comparably more than plant-based foods to global environmental change through their impact on climate, land, and freshwater use, and biodiversity. Consequently, there is increased interest in diets with higher fractions of plant-based foods that decrease both risk of disease and negative environmental impacts."
– Gut microbiome signatures of vegan, vegetarian, and omnivore diets and associated health outcomes across 21,561 individuals; *Nature Microbiology* journal; Jan. 2025

Wild plant life and its survival plays into your survival

Plants help to build new soil, keep soil healthy, prevent flooding, landslides, and desertification, help to purify water, play a role in forming clouds, sequester greenhouse gasses, stabilize the climate, and provide terrain and food for all forms of wildlife. Plants on the land and in the oceans and lakes create the oxygen we and other animals need to breathe.

The more plant and wild animal life there is, the more soil is built up, the more greenhouse gasses sequestered, the more oxygen produced, the more regular the climate is, and the more water that gets filtered.

Get involved with helping to protect your local environment, plant life, and wildlife. Your food choices and nutrition, and your ability to breathe, depend on it.

Food variety from nature

Each edible plant could have as many as dozens to hundreds to thousands of varieties. If you want to get the varieties of edible plants not available in common stores, you likely will need to grow them yourself, or find your regional family farmers who are intent on bringing more variety to your food choices.

Search, learn, and live:
- rare fruits and vegetables
- rare seeds
- organic home gardening
- wild harvesting
- fruit forest
- permaculture seeds
- native edible plants
- veganic permaculture

Learn to grow fruiting and other trees and fruiting bushes, and plant them in the wilds of your region to help your regional wildlife thrive.

Factory farmed animals

Industrial and fast food meat, dairy, and eggs are from farmed animals kept indoors. Over the past several decades, these animals have been increasingly treated with chemicals, and fed unnatural diets laced with chemicals and pharmaceutical residues. The animals are raised in stressful, crowded conditions that alter their body chemistry, including hormonal balance, ratio of fat and muscle, and type of fat. The drugs get them to grow faster, and they are killed younger – as their stressed and unnaturally heavy bodies become diseased with degenerative and chronic illnesses, and stress disorders.

After World War II, factory animal farming quickly became common – especially to supply the fast food outlets, supermarkets, the increasing number of "convenience" snack stores, and the industrial food systems of the military, travel industry, resorts, amusement parks, school and corporate cafeterias, nursing homes, hospitals, and prisons.

What are the chemically grown, industrialized foods containing toxic residues doing to people's health? Research chemical food additives and farm chemical residues, and you will start to understand.

Fat intake and cardiovascular disease

In 1957, Ancel Keys launched the Seven Countries Study, which analyzed the diets of 12,763 middle-aged men in Greece, Italy, Japan, the Netherlands, the U.S., and Yugoslavia.

Keys' studies revealed the connection between dietary fat intake and cardiovascular disease.

The studies made it clear: fat intake, cardiovascular disease, strokes, and heart attacks were related.

"Dietary fat is the fat that comes from food. The body breaks down dietary fats into parts called fatty acids that can enter the bloodstream. The body can also make fatty acids from carbohydrates in food.

The body uses fatty acids to make the fats it needs. Fats are important for how your body uses many vitamins. And fats play a role in how all cells in the body are made and work.

But all dietary fats are not the same. They have different effects on the body. Some dietary fats are essential. Some increase the risk of disease, and some help prevent disease.

Saturated fats are usually solid at room temperature. The most common sources of saturated fats are meats and dairy products.

Unsaturated fats are usually liquid at room temperature. Vegetable oils, nuts, and fish have mostly unsaturated fats. There are two types of unsaturated fats: monounsaturated and polyunsaturated.

Saturated fat tends to raise levels of cholesterol in the blood. Low-density lipoprotein (LDL) is called 'bad' cholesterol. High-density lipoprotein (HDL) is called 'good' cholesterol. Saturated fats raise the levels of both.

A high level of bad cholesterol in the bloodstream increases the risk of heart and blood vessel disease."

– Dietary fat: know which to choose; MayoClinic.org

Saturated fats from food can lead to plaque in the arteries, veins, and capillaries. The more plaque there is, the more the person is likely to experience things like heart attacks, strokes, and diseases of dementia, including Alzheimer's.

In men, clogged blood vessels cause erectile dysfunction. It is a condition often helping to reveal the man has some level of cardiovascular disease.

Every cell of your body contains fat on the cell wall.

It's best to eat cleaner foods, and not animal fats, which are heavy; or to eat fried or sautéed fats, which contain damaged, sticky oils. Animal fats cooked at high heat also become sticky. If you want to experience the best of health, it is a good idea to avoid foods containing highly heated oils.

Consider the sticky fat left on a pan used to fry or sauté food, and how difficult it is to scrub the pan clean. This isn't the quality of fat you want in your body, or on your cell walls.

Polyunsaturated fats from plants that are NOT heated, and are of the Omega-6 fatty acids beneficial to health. These can help to raise good cholesterol, and to lower bad cholesterol and triglycerides. They also play a role in managing blood sugar levels.

A diet rich in a variety of green leafy and other vegetables, and in unprocessed, whole fruit, and in things like sprouts, seaweeds, and activated nuts, seeds, and grains (activating foods is covered in another chapter of this book), provides for not only the healthy fats you need from food (without added oil), but also includes vitamins, minerals, enzymes, amino acids, fiber, and other nutrition you need to thrive in health.

Search and learn about essential fatty acids

• Partially hydrogenated oils
• Triglycerides
• Omega-6 fatty acids
• Omega-3 fatty acids

- Alpha-linolenic acid (ALA) nutritional benefits
- Docosahexaenoic acid (DHA) nutritional benefits
- Eicosapentaenoic acid (EPA) nutritional benefits
- Algal oil nutritional benefits (only use raw, unheated)
- Perilla oil nutritional benefits (only use raw, unheated)
- Chia seed nutritional benefits
- Flax seed nutritional benefits
- Hemp seed nutritional benefits
- Oregano nutritional benefits
- Walnut nutritional benefits
- Essential fatty acids in microgreens
- Essential fatty acids in sprouts

Sprouts

Mentioning all those problematic foods is important. So is mentioning one of the best foods you can incorporate in your diet to improve your nutrition, and reduce the risks of a variety of illnesses. This food is: sprouts.

You would do yourself a favor by learning about and growing sprouts, and regularly eating them.

Sprouts have a wide variety of beneficial qualities, and can be more nutritious than the adult plant. Those nutrients include anti-inflammatories, antioxidants, enzymes, minerals, vitamins, and fiber.

Sprouts have anti-cancer and antiviral components, and those that help to prevent cardiovascular and kidney disease, and to reduce diabetes and the risks of experiencing other autoimmune disorders.

Regularly including sprouts in your diet can help maintain a healthy gut biome. This can help prevent a wide variety of diseases, including cancer, and immune disorders.

"Non-phenols, such as the saponin component of alfalfa play key biological functions in the body. Saponins and their derivatives such as prosapogenins and sapogenins have been reported to exert a high antimicrobial activity against yeasts and bacterial strains. Studies also reveal that saponins can inhibit cholesterol esterase, acetyl coenzyme, and carboxylase enzymes, thereby preventing fatty acid synthesis in the body. The inhibitory function of the saponins on fatty acids synthesis helps balance the ratio between high-density lipoprotein (HDL) cholesterol and low-density lipoprotein cholesterol."
– Edible Plant Sprouts: Health Benefits, Trends, and Opportunities for Novel Exploration; *Nutrients* journal; Aug. 2021

Sprouts are low cost and easy to grow.

Find a source for organic sprouting seeds, and have a place to keep them dry. Get some sprouting jars with stainless steel screen lids.

Including homegrown sprouts in your diet is a way to lower food costs, to improve nutrition, to reduce risks of experiencing various illnesses, to be more sustainable by reducing your carbon footprint, to reduce pollution and use of resources, and to avoid supporting the multinational corporate food industry that isn't interested in your health, but wants your money.

Greed and the industrial food industry

The food industry does not seem to care about medical studies – unless they can twist the studies into some sort of marketing tool to sell more product.

Greed rules the food industry. Not your health.

What sells is what matters – to them. Not to your health.

What makes stockholders of the multinational food corporations rich is what matters to the companies. Not your health.

Over the past century, the processed food and fast food industries have flourished, as have the factory farmed meat, dairy, and egg industries, and the feed crop industry that is ruinous to the land, water, and climate.

For a better world, we need to change human reliance on industrial foods, and bring about a more sustainable humanity nurturing organically-grown local produce.

Forks Over Knives

The team of doctors and nutritional bioscientists behind the *Forks Over Knives* documentary, website, and recipe books have helped to expand the knowledge of diet-related diseases, and what role plant-based nutrition can play into the solution. Their goal has been to teach people how to prevent and reverse cardiovascular disease, and to lower their risks of experiencing cancer, diabetes, osteoporosis, kidney disease, liver disease, Alzheimer's, lupus, Sjogren's syndrome, and other chronic and degenerative diseases by following a low-fat, plant-based diet, free from clarified sugars, synthetic chemicals, processed junk foods, and garbage snacks.

The medical team behind Forks over Knives is far from alone in concluding the benefits of a plant-based diet in disease prevention and reversal. There are too many studies to mention, detailing research around the world that has made similar conclusions about a plant-based diet and human health.

Two other diseases that can be improved or prevented with a plant-based diet are lupus and Sjogren's syndrome.

"A vegan diet may effectively reduce or even eliminate symptoms of two autoimmune disorders: systemic lupus erythematosus (SLE) and Sjogren's syndrome (SS). A small study followed just three women with SLE and SS who adapted a mostly raw, plant-based diet that focused on leafy greens, cruciferous vegetables, and omega-3 polyunsaturated fatty acids, and found their symptoms resolved after four weeks. Other studies have found similar findings."
– Plant-based diets may reduce or eliminate symptoms of lupus; Physician's Committee for Responsible Medicine; Mar. 2024

"There is a strong body of evidence suggesting that plant-based diets are beneficial for reducing mortality and metabolic risk. Although less studied, plant-based diets may also have great potential for managing symptoms of autoimmune disease, such as systemic lupus erythematosus (SLE)."
– Six Week Raw Vegan Nutrition Protocol Rapidly Reverses Lupus Nephritis: A Case Series; *International Journal of Disease Reversal and Prevention*; March 2019

The biological factory in the body

Because the biological factory within the body functions in a certain way, it will always work better if it is provided the proper fuel in tune with how it functions.

Your body cannot function at its highest level if you are not feeding it what it needs to function at that level. You can change the situation with your food choices.

It's only been until recently that humans started ingesting such a wide variety of synthetic chemicals as food additives, industrial residues, and leached chemicals from food packaging and can linings. And also absorbing chemicals through their skin from toxic cosmetic and cleaning products, and from plastics.

The human species didn't advance by eating chemicals. The species always ate "natural foods." It is only since chemical engineering kicked into gear that humans started putting unnatural things into their bodies. It's also been relatively recently that humans have been collecting microplastics and synthetic chemicals in their bodies, including through polluted air, and through foods, water, clothing, and household items. In the modern worlds, are bombarded with synthetic chemicals, including those that disrupt our hormones, and increased diseases.

One way to protect the biological factory that is your body is to eat more whole, plant-based foods, and to stay away from foods containing synthetic chemicals, and those grown using toxic chemicals.

Search: How to reduce exposure to toxins.

Digestion begins in the mouth

Be sure to chew food. It is part of the digestive process as the salivary glands excrete substances initiating the breakdown of what you eat so you can absorb the nutrients, and your body can breakdown antinutrients, and also metabolize other nutrients.

Saliva contains epidermal growth factor (EGF), a polypeptide found to play a role in the growth of the epithelial cells lining the digestive tract. EGF is particularly important to the replacement of the cells lining the tract, which continually slough off and regenerate.

You may have heard the saying, "Chew your juices and drink your solids." In other words, don't guzzle juices or smoothies. Slow down and savor juices and smoothies. Chew solid food so that it is practically liquid.

Feeding your good gut bacteria

As detailed elsewhere in the book, what you are doing when you eat is you are feeding the helpful bacteria, fungus, viruses, and other microorganisms living in your digestive tract. These organisms are necessary for nutrient absorption, nutrient production, toxin breakdown, and brain, heart, liver, pancreas, spleen, kidney and other organ function, and for your survival.

Your gut bacteria need the substances making up the components of the plants, including the fiber, enzymes, amino acids, vitamins, and minerals, as these components and others often also work as antioxidants, anti-inflammatories and/or contain what the gut bacteria can turn into other substances beneficial you.

Whole plant foods are important to health, as they contain a variety of substances. Instead of having fruit juice, eat whole fruit. Instead of juiced veggies, dice them, and use them in various dishes – from bowls and salads to wraps and soups, and mix them with beans and avocado, or with oil-free hummus.

This isn't to say I always avoid juices, but I prefer to make my own vegetable juices, rather than to buy juice from a store.

When we make juice at home, we use organic fruits and vegetables. We don't strain the juices to make them completely free of pulp, as it contains nutrients.

Improve your nutrition

Make a conscious decision to select and eat foods of high quality, and preferably largely consisting of raw, unheated, organically grown fruits, vegetables, sprouts, seaweeds, and herbs, and activated nuts, seeds, and grains, and fermented foods.

Some foods, such as hard vegetables, and things like beans, breads, soups, chilis, and stews will be cooked. There are healthier ways to cook, and then there are types of cooking that create problematic, inflammatory, and otherwise unhealthful chemicals. There are also helpful ways to prepare foods, before you cook them. (See the information about soaking beans, legumes, and grains.)

"May the food we are eating make us aware of the interconnections between the universe and us, Earth and us, and all other living species and us. Because each bite contains in itself the life of Sun and Earth, may we see the meaning and value of life from these precious morsels of food."
– Thich Nhat Hanh

Fiber is a key to – and absolute necessity for – good health

One way of damaging the digestive tract is by following a diet low in fiber.

Low fiber diets are found to **increase** permeability of the intestinal tract, which is not good. It is the problematic condition called leaky gut.

High fiber, low-fat diets increase the variety of microorganisms in the intestines, and **decrease** intestinal permeability, which is good.

As mentioned, meat, dairy, and eggs do not contain fiber. Plant matter contains fiber.

By eliminating the non-fiber items while increasing the fiber in the diet, the digestive tract will function better, and the gut microbiota will be both more diverse and populated by more helpful varieties of bacteria. (This is explained later in the book.)

A diet rich in fiber decreases inflammation, which is protective of all tissues, from the kidneys and intestines, to the heart, lungs, muscles, joints, bones, eyes, nerves, and brain.

A plant-based diet is rich in soluble fiber. This fiber is beneficial in that it doesn't hold onto iron and some other nutrients like non-soluble fiber. Both soluble and non-soluble fiber are beneficial.

"According to the results of the multiple-linear regression in our study, the higher dietary fiber consumption of vegetarians may contribute to better renal function. Chronic kidney disease is often accompanied by a chronic inflammatory state characterized by elevated serum C-reactive protein, IL-6, and TNF-alpha levels. High fiber intake has been proven to reduce oxidative stress status by affecting bacterial fermentation of proteins in the colon. Some small scale studies have reported that increasing fiber intake in CKD patients may reduce serum creatinine levels and improve the eGFR. A study among 110 community-dwelling male participants aged 70-71 years from Sweden demonstrated that high dietary fiber intake was associated with better kidney function and lower inflammation."

    – Healthy adult vegetarians have better renal function than matched omnivores: a cross-sectional study in China; *BMC Nephrology* journal; July 2020

Vegans get plenty of fiber

While some people concern themselves with getting enough fiber, going so far as trying to calculate how much fiber they get at each meal – such as aiming for the suggested 14 grams of fiber for every 1,000 calories – I don't concern myself with those numbers. Everything I eat consists of plants, and all plants contain fiber. There is no way I'm *not* getting enough fiber.

It is the meat, dairy, and egg diet that lack fiber – because, meat, dairy, and eggs don't contain any fiber.

A vegan diet rich in fruits, vegetables, sprouts, nuts, seeds, beans, grains, and seaweeds contains plenty of fiber.

"There are many types of 'extracted' fiber products on the market, including tablets and powders that can be mixed with water and taken as a drink.

Most health care professionals would advise a healthy adult to eat a pear, or a handful of raisins, instead of turning to a supplement.

Satisfying your daily fiber needs with food is the best way to get a healthful balance of soluble and insoluble fiber. It's also a great way to improve the overall quality of your diet, since fiber-rich foods tend to be rich in vitamins, minerals, and disease-fighting phytochemicals."

    – Nancy D. Berkoff, RD, EdD, Ask the Nutritionist: How much fiber do I really need?; VegetarianTimes.com

Fiber from plants nurtures healthy gut bacteria

A diet rich in fiber is essential to vibrant health. Without adequate fiber, your digestive tract does not function at its best. This includes because fiber helps nurture the good gut microorganisms you need for maintaining a healthy digestive tract, and to also metabolize substances you rely on for health. Yes, the microorganisms in your gut create some of the nutrients you need for experiencing vibrant health.

"Aberrant gut microbiota profiles have been associated with obesity, type 1 and type 2 diabetes, and non-alcoholic fatty liver disease. Transfer of microbiota from obese animals induces metabolic diseases and obesity in germ-free animals. Conversely, transfer of pathogen-free microbiota from lean, healthy human donors to patients with metabolic disease can increase insulin sensitivity. Not only are aberrant microbiota profiles associated with metabolic disease, but the flux of metabolites derived from gut microbial metabolism of choline, phosphatidylcholine, and l-carnitine has been shown to contribute directly to cardiovascular disease pathology, providing one explanation for increased disease risk of eating too much red meat. Diet, especially high intake of fermentable fibers and plant polyphenols, appears to regulate microbial activities within the gut, supporting regulatory guidelines encouraging increased consumption of whole-plant foods (fruit, vegetables, and whole-grain cereals), and providing the scientific rationale for the design of efficacious prebiotics. Similarly, recent human studies with carefully selected probiotic strains show that ingestion of viable microorganisms with the ability to hydrolyze bile salts can lower blood cholesterol, a recognized risk factor in cardiovascular disease. Taken together such observations raise the intriguing possibility that gut microbiome modulation by whole-plant foods, probiotics, and prebiotics may be at the base of healthy eating pyramids advised by regulatory agencies across the globe.

Dietary strategies which modulate the gut microbiota or their metabolic activities are emerging as efficacious tolls for reducing cardiovascular disease risks and indicate that indeed, the way to a healthy heart may be through a healthy gut microbiota."

– The way to a man's heart is through his gut microbiota – dietary pro- and prebiotics for the management of cardiovascular risk, by Karen M. Tuohy, Francesca Fava, and Roberto Viola; *Proceedings of the Nutrition Society* journal; Feb. 2014

Following a **low**-fiber diet increases your chances of experiencing hemorrhoids, varicose veins, vision problems, hiatal hernia, cardiovascular disease, a stroke, a heart attack, kidney disease, liver malfunction, and cancers, especially cancer of the colon and rectum, and a variety of autoimmune disorders. For men, a low-fiber diet increases their chances of experiencing E.D.

"Fiber, found only in plant foods, has many health-promoting qualities. It binds with carcinogens, fats, and cholesterol, and eliminates them in the feces. By eliminating carcinogens, it reduces your risk of developing cancer, and by eliminating fat and cholesterol, it reduces your risk of heart disease, atherosclerosis, and obesity. Fiber also improves the efficiency of insulin, so that we need less of it to maintain appropriate blood-sugar levels."

– Dr. John McDougall, author of *The Starch Solution*

Fiber helps to remove toxins from the system, reduces cholesterol, improves digestion, and liver and kidney function, and helps with weight and blood sugar maintenance.

Meat, dairy, and eggs don't contain fiber

Meat (including the tissues of mammals, fish, crustaceans, birds, reptiles, and amphibians), dairy (milk and milk products: cheese, kefir, yogurt, cream, ice cream, sour cream, cream cheese, butter, whey, and casein), and eggs (from birds or fish [roe and caviar]) are all void of fiber.

Following a diet rich in animal protein increases the chance of experiencing a variety of health problems.

Especially with those who have kidney issues – or want to avoid them – dairy is not something you want to put in your body.

Eggs also increase a variety of health risks, and especially the more you eat eggs.

The same with meat.

There are many issues related to dairy, eggs, and meat containing residues of farming chemicals. They likely are saturated with industrial chemicals, including pharmaceutical drug residues.

Probiotics and intestinal flora

You likely will benefit by adding vegan probiotics to your foods, or taking a vegan probiotic supplement. This is especially so if you are transitioning from an unhealthful diet.

An unhealthful diet of junk foods, fried things, oil sautéed foods, bottled oils, processed sugars, and bleached grains, and animal protein bring about an abundance of problematic intestinal bacteria, including candida, Citrobacter, clostridium difficile (also known as C.diff, and which can cause chronic and severe diarrhea), and hafnia. These bacteria can contribute to leaky gut syndrome, and interfere with both nutrient production and nutrient absorption.

Following a gluten-free, low-fat vegan diet while also taking a vegan probiotic supplement can eliminate the dysbiosis (microorganism imbalance in the digestive tract), restoring balance to the intestinal flora, helping to heal the digestive tract.

The intestinal microorganism imbalance that is dysbiosis contributes to everything from inflammation, metabolic diseases, intestinal diseases, autoimmune diseases, cardiovascular diseases, pulmonary diseases, blood disorders,, and diseases of dementia, and liver disease, kidney disease, skin disorders, vision degradation, and bone issues, and cancer.

It is important to follow a diet that nurtures a healthy gut biome, and to stay away from what harms the gut biome (a diet that is high-fat, and rich with clarified sugars, animal proteins, processed foods, chemical food additives, and industrial toxins).

Beneficial strains of bacteria include Bifidobacterium, lactobacillus, and saccharomyces boulardii. There are many, many other varieties of helpful gut bacteria, each nurtured by eating a variety of fruits, vegetables, sprouts, beans, legumes, nuts, seeds, and seaweeds, and fermented foods.

(Do a search for: vegan probiotics Bifidobacterium, lactobacillus, and saccharomyces boulardii.)

Because beneficial intestinal bacteria are necessary for the immune system to function, a healthful digestive tract will result in a stronger immune system, lowering disease risk.

Not only will a clean diet improve the immune system, but also other systems and organs will function better, including the liver, bile ducts, pancreas, and kidneys, and the lymph and blood systems, as they will have fewer toxins flowing through them, will be less susceptible to inflammation, and not cluttered with problematic substances – including TMAO.

TMAO and cardiovascular disease

Once you learn about TMAO, and how it negatively impacts health, including how it increases kidney disease, and cardiovascular disease, and the risk of stroke and heart attack, know it is easy to reduce it in your system: by following a clean, plant-based diet. This is so because eating animal protein increases TMAO.

"Trimethylamine N-oxide (TMAO) is a small, colorless amine oxide generated from choline, betaine, and carnitine by gut microbial metabolism.

Plasma level of TMAO is determined by a number of factors, including diet, gut microbial flora, and liver flavin monooxygenase activity. In humans, a positive correlation between elevated plasma levels of TMAO and an increased risk for major adverse cardiovascular events and death is reported. The atherogenic effect of TMAO is attributed to alterations in cholesterol and bile acid metabolism, activation of inflammatory pathways, and promotion foam cell formation. TMAO levels increase with decreasing levels of kidney function, and is associated with mortality in patients with chronic kidney disease."

– Trimethylamine N-Oxide: The Good, the Bad, and the Unknown; *Toxins* journal; Nov. 2016

"It is fairly well known that artery-clogging saturated fat and cholesterol are bad for your heart, but the picture of our heart health is every-expanding. Red meat, processed meat, and animal fats are the primary sources of L-carnitine; egg yolks are the primary sources of choline in our diet. In and of themselves, L-carnitine and choline have important roles in our health. But the trouble comes when these substances are metabolized in our intestines by gut bacteria to produce a chemical called TMA, which subsequently converts to TMAO. High levels of TMAO are associated with an increased risk of cardiovascular disease and cardiac events, such as heart attacks.

This is where things get interesting. It appears that the type of bacteria we have in our gut determines whether we produce harmful TMAO from L-carnitine and choline. Long-term vegans and vegetarians do not convert L-carnitine and choline to TMAO at the same rate as omnivores. (In fact, vegans produce a negligible amount of TMAO). And heavy meat eaters have a different mix of bacteria than those who eat little or no meat and more carbohydrates, particularly vegetables and fiber.

An individual's microbiome enterotype depends on many factors, but a major factor is long-term food intake. The Bacteroid enterotype is associated with diets that are high in animal protein and fats; the Prevotella enterotype is associated with carbohydrates as well as plant-based diets. It is more of a spectrum than a distinct category. It appears that people who have more heart disease, diabetes, and metabolic syndrome tend toward the Bacteroid enterotype. Differences in these microbial communities may also be responsible for digestive disorders, skin diseases, gum disease, and even obesity."

– Eating Less Meat May Help Your Gut, by Becky Ramsing; Johns Hopkins Center for a Livable Future; July 2016

"Another possible beneficial linkage observed in these intervention studies was the correlation of TMAO measurement with the relative abundance of specific microbes. [Researchers] observed a significant correlation between the genus Bifidobacterium and several species of Lachnospiraceae and Ruminococcaceae. They also observed a reduction in the plasma L-carnitine (a metabolite found in red meat) among subjects with ischemic heart disease who adhered to the vegan diet intervention. Red meat consumption has been associated with inflammatory bowel disease. The study suggests cardiometabolic benefits (reduced oxidized LDL-C, TC, and body weight) in vegetarian diet interventions, supporting the beneficial role of gut microbiota in modulating the biochemical parameters associated with CVD (cardiovascular disease) risk.

Research suggests that switching to a plant-based diet may help increase the diversity of health-promoting bacteria in the gut."

– Effect of Plant-Based Diets on Gut Microbiota: A Systematic Review of Interventional Studies; *Nutrients* journal; Mar. 2023

Bacteria more commonly found in the intestines of those who consumer meat, dairy, and eggs and that are associated with increased levels of TMAO include: Anaerococcus hydrogenalis, Colostridium asparagiforme, C. hathewayi, C. sporogenes, Edwardsiella tarda, Escherichia fergusonii, Proteus penneri, and Providencia rettgeri. Follow a pure, clean, plant-based diet, and your levels of those bacteria will plunge, as will the TMAO in your system. This will decrease a variety of health risks, including of cardiovascular disease and vascular dysfunction, cancer, autoimmune disorders, inflammatory bowel issues, leaky gut, metabolic syndrome, and kidney disease.

Dysbiosis and symbiosis in the gut

The helpful microorganisms naturally existing in your digestive tract are central to your health. There are ways to nurture the gut microbiota to nurture better health.

The microorganisms in your digestive tract play a role in all areas of your physical function, including everything from your brain, heart, kidneys, liver, adrenal glands, and other organs, and your blood, bones, muscles, and eyes. Your gut microbiota also plays a role in your energy and mood.

"The gut microbiota affects numerous biological functions throughout the body, and its characterization has become a major research area of biomedicine. Recent studies have suggested that gut bacteria play a fundamental role in diseases such as obesity, diabetes, and cardiovascular disease. Data are accumulating in animal models and humans suggesting that obesity and type 2 diabetes are associated with a profound dysbiosis. First human metagenome-wide association studies demonstrated highly significant correlations of specific intestinal bacteria, certain bacterial genes, and respective metabolic pathways with type 2 diabetes. Importantly, especially butyrate-producing bacteria such as Roseburia intestinalis and Faecalibacterium prausnitzii concentrations were lower in type 2 diabetes subjects. This supports the increasing evidence, that butyrate and other short-chain fatty acids are able to exert profound immunometabolic effects."

– Microbiota and diabetes: an evolving relationship; *Gut* journal; Sept. 2014

Pathobionts and dysbiosis

A diet rich in animal protein increases the problematic gut bacteria, known as pathobionts. A diet rich in animal protein also *decreases* the variety of microorganisms in the tract, which is dysbiosis. This includes a reduction in the firmicute bacteria that metabolize beneficial plant polysaccharides.

A state of dysbiosis weakens the immune system, can damage the intestinal lining, increases both the likelihood of leaky gut syndrome, and the chance for harmful pathogens to take hold and cause illness.

Dysbiosis disrupts the homeostasis, increases the risk of experiencing inflammation, urinary tract infections, kidney infections and kidney disease, yeast infections, constipation, bloating, irritable or inflammatory bowel issues, colitis, celiac disease, cardiovascular disease, heart attack, stroke, colon and rectum cancer, liver disease, other organ dysfunction, polycystic ovary syndrome, Parkinson's disease, and dementia.

Dysbiosis increases the likelihood of experiencing a host of autoimmune disorders like arthritis, diabetes, lupus, asthma, and others.

Dysbiosis can also lead to weight gain, and difficulty losing unwanted weight.

Inflammation of the bowel

There are certain foods that can cause bowel issues in some people. Switching to a clean diet helps. For some time they might find they can't eat certain fruits, vegetables, nuts, beans, legumes, and seeds. The longer they follow a clean diet, they may find formerly irritating foods will no longer be a problem. Consulting with a gastroenterologist and dietitian can help with these matters.

"Researchers found that those who adhered to a healthy plant-based diet had a lower risk of IBD, whereas those eating an unhealthy plant-based diet (high in processed plant foods) showed an increased risk of the conditions."
 – Diets filled with nutrient-dense plant foods tied to lower IBD risk, by Katharine Lang; *Medical News Today*; March 2025

"In the UKB (UK Biobank), higher adherence to health PDI (plant-based diet indexes) was associated with a lower IBD risk, while higher alignment to an unhealthy PDI associated with an increased risk when comparing extreme quintiles of PDIs. Among individuals with established IBD, healthy PDI was inversely associated and unhealthy PDI was positively associated with need for IBD-related surgery.
 In our sensitivity analyses, we observed a consistently protective potential of a plant-based diet, independent of ultra-processed food intake."
 – Composition of plant-based diets and the incidence and prognosis of inflammatory bowel disease: a multinational retrospective cohort study; *The Lancet* European medical journal; May 2025

Unhealthful plant-based foods include those that are fried or oil-sautéed, to those containing rancid oils, high salt, and sugar extracts. Unhealthful plant-based foods also include meat substitutes, snack bars, and others foods containing questionable substances, such as industrial farming chemicals, and synthetic chemical dyes, flavors, scents, emulsifiers, and preservatives. These unhealthy foods can irritate the gastrointestinal tract, and contribute to nutritional deficiencies, anemia, autoimmune disorders, thyroid issues, muscle weakness, bone loss, neural problems, and kidney, liver, and heart disease.

"Avoidance of certain food additives, in particular emulsifiers, is increasingly considered important for the prevention and treatment of IBD do to their ability to promote intestinal inflammation, alter gut permeability, and the negative impact on gut microbiota. These compounds are found predominantly in ultra-processed foods, both animal-and plant-based products. Thus diet quality when adopting a plant-based diet remains paramount. Some plant-based dairy alternatives also contain emulsifiers and caution with these products I the setting of IBD may be a sensible approach."

> – A Whole Food Plant-Based Approach to Ulcerative Colitis: A Case Series; *Sage Journals*; Nov. 2023

A person can drink beer, eat fried chips, and salty, oily microwavable foods, and snack on vegan cake and candy all day, and call themselves "plant-based." They are eating a vegan diet, but it is toxic junk. Their health, including their gut biome and intestinal tract, kidneys, and cardiovascular system will suffer from consuming such unhealthful foods.

- **Inflammatory Bowel Disease [IBD]** symptoms include anemia because of low iron, belly pain for a day, or more (especially at night), fever, diarrhea, intestinal inflammation, nausea, rectal bleeding, and weight loss.

  Underlying disease can include Crohn's and colitis.

  Ulcerative colitis can lead to blood in the stool, and often watery stool as the inflamed intestines have difficulty absorbing fluids.

  Seek treatment, as this can quickly get serious, including because it can lead to dehydration, an imbalance of electrolytes.

  IBD can be diagnosed by a gastroenterologist who may do blood testing, similar to what is done for irritable bowel syndrome (IBS).

  Things that can also be an issue causing IBD-like symptoms include bacterial overgrowth in the intestines, bile acid malabsorption, gastrointestinal tract infection, dairy intolerance, and side effects of medications. Aspirin, ibuprofen, and antibiotics can cause irritation.

  Foods that can be more irritating for people with IBD include clarified sugars (corn syrup, rice syrup, cane sugar, beet sugar, etc.), and coffee, colas, sodas, and carbonated drinks, dairy products, fried and oil-sauteed foods, synthetic/artificial sweeteners, and also alcohol.

- **Irritable Bowel Syndrome [IBS]** symptoms include bloating, constipation, distension, gas, and stomach pain. They often occur after a meal, and/or because of stress, and are likely to be temporary.

  Irritants include large meals, and also alcohol, carbonated drinks, chocolate, coffee, dairy, fried foods, gluten, oil sautéed foods, oily foods, and wheat.

  Smoking and trigger flareups, and worsen symptoms.

  Like IBD, a gastroenterologist may perform a colonoscopy exam, and take a CT scan and possibly x-rays of the abdomen and pelvis. An upper endoscopy via the throat and esophagus may be performed, including to take a tissue sample, and a fluid same to test for bacterial overgrowth. These may also be done in relation to celiac disease. A breath test that checks for bacterial overgrowth can be performed. A stool test will be done to check for parasites, examine the bacteria, and check for bile acids.

Foods you may be advised to eliminate include all dairy products, gluten, and fried and oil-sauteed food. In combination with seeing a dietitian, you may be put through the FODMAPs testing, which is avoiding certain fruits, grains, and vegetables, as well as dairy products.

Inflammatory arthritis and other rheumatic diseases

People with inflammatory arthritis are often found to have inflamed and otherwise damaged intestinal walls. They are often given pharmaceutical drugs which carry the risks of also damaging the intestinal walls, including by forming ulcers, making the patient's condition chronically worse (especially if they are eating a terrible diet). The patient may be treated with immunosuppression drugs that carry a number of risks. The patient also might take common over-the-counter anti-inflammatory drugs, which can also damage the intestines, increasing permeability, which is "leaky gut syndrome" – which increases the passage of antigens and bacteria into the blood, and this situation increases the possibility of arthritis, kidney disease, vision and joint degeneration, and damage to other areas with smaller blood passageways consisting of capillaries and other microvascular structures. The drugs can also increase the possibility of other health problems, including osteoporosis – leading people to reason they need to increase their calcium and vitamin D intake, and this may lead them to drink more milk with the belief milk contains what they need. Increasing their milk intake could magnify their health problems, including the risk of experiencing leaky gut, arthritis, and osteoporosis... and macular degenerations, lupus, and cardiovascular and kidney disease, strokes, heart attacks, and cancers.

Sufferers of rheumatic diseases could benefit by cleaning up their diet, including by eliminating all synthetic chemicals, clarified sugars, highly heated or otherwise damaged oils, and animal protein from their food choices.

Tendinitis, periostitis, and bone and joint lesions

People with other inflammatory conditions, including tendinitis, periostitis, and granulomatous bone and joint lesions, also benefit from a low-fat vegan diet containing absolutely no heated oils, but rich in raw fruits and vegetables, and what improves the gut microbiome. They may then experience a halt to the immunopathogenesis of their ailment. This is especially so if the diet is geared toward alkaline foods, including green vegetables, but excludes gluten and bleached grains (and bread and other flour foods containing potassium bromate, and other additives).

Taking a vegan probiotic supplement, on top of following a clean, low-fat diet free of animal protein, aids in the healing of the intestines.

Lymphoid tissue

"The largest amount of lymphoid tissue in the body is associated with the gut. This tissue protects the body from antigens that do get through the intestinal barrier. Unfortunately, an unhealthy diet – too high in fat, cholesterol, and animal protein – can compromise the capacities of the lymphoid tissue to destroy invading antigens that make it through the intestinal wall.

Fasting is known to decrease intestinal permeability, thus making the gut 'less leaky.' This may be one of the reasons fasting has been shown to dramatically benefit patients with rheumatoid arthritis. When patients return after the fast to a diet with dairy products, the gut becomes more permeable and the arthritis returns."

– Diet: Only Hope for Arthritis, by Dr. John McDougall, author of *The Starch Solution*; DrMcDougall.com

Intestinal damage from anti-inflammatory drugs

Anti-inflammatory drugs carry the side effect of causing intestinal damage. Consuming animal protein and taking drugs that increase the possibility of damaging the intestinal barrier when it is already damaged increases the possibility of undigested proteins and bacteria passing through the intestinal walls and entering into the bloodstream – landing in the soft tissues. The antigens then would be attacked by the immune system. The scenario increases the likelihood of an "autoimmune disorder diagnosis" – for which pharmacology medications would be prescribed. And round and round the disease game goes.

Inflammatory arthritis

With an understanding of the situation leading to inflammatory arthritis, it should be no surprise so many sports stars end up with arthritis. They often spend years eating pro-inflammatory, high-protein diets, and taking anti-inflammatory drugs, and painkillers. It is the perfect scenario for creating leaky gut syndrome, and triggering their chronic and degenerative health conditions.

The low-fat, plant-based diet advocated in this book specifically encourages alkaline foods rich in omega-3 fatty acids, which are important for those experiencing inflammatory and autoimmune ailments, including celiac, Crohn's, leaking gut, ulcers, tendinitis, arthritis, and other conditions.

Gut bacteria help to prevent kidney stones

A healthy base of bacteria in the digestive tract is also needed for the prevention of kidney stones.

"Oxalate degradation by the anaerobic bacterium Oxalobacter formigenes is important for human health, helping to prevent hyperoxaluria and disorders such as the development of kidney stones.

Oxalate is formed in the liver by amino acid catabolism. It is also present in a wide range of food and drinks, including tea, coffee, chocolate, and fruits and vegetables. The concentration of oxalate voided in the urine plays an important role in urolithiasis, the formation of calcium oxalate kidney stones. The main known bacterial species involved in oxalate degradation in the gut is the anaerobe Oxalobacter formigenes.

It remains questionable whether O. formigens is the only, or most-important, species involved in oxalate degradation in the human gut. Other oxalate-degrading bacteria that have been isolated from human stool samples include Eubacterium lentum WYH-1 and Enterococcus faecalis. "

– Oxalobacter formigenes and Its Potential Role in Human Health; *Applied and Environmental Microbiology* journal; Aug. 2002

"An analysis of fecal samples showed that patients with recurrent idiopathic calcium stones exhibited lower fecal microbial diversity than controls. In particular, these samples were characterized by low levels of bacteria capable of oxalate degradation. Therefore, previous studies have suggested that probiotic bacteria, especially O. formigenes, Lactobacillus spp., and Bifidobacterium spp., which can degrade dietary oxalate in the gastrointestinal tract allowing it to be absorbed, may help reduce urinary oxalate levels."
– Probiotics in the Prevention of the Calcium Oxalate Urolithiasis; Cells journal; Jan. 2022

Besides a meat-based diet, other things that can cause a reduction of good bacteria, and an increase in bad bacteria include infection, antibiotics and certain other pharmaceutical drugs, bad dental hygiene, having numerous sexual partners, alcohol consumption, stress and anxiety, synthetic food additives, industrial farming chemical residues, and a diet high in clarified sugars, and high in fat, including fried oils, sautéed oils, and other damaged oils.

"Good bacteria, those that live in symbiosis with us, are nourished by fruits and veggies, grains, and beans – whereas dysbiosis, bad bacteria that may contribute to disease, are fed by meat, junk food, fast food, seafood, dairy, and eggs. Typical western diets can decimate our good gut flora. We live with trillions of symbionts, good bacteria that live in symbiosis with us. We help them, they help us, and a month on a plant-based diet results in an increase of the good guys, and a decreased in the bad, the so-called pathobionts, the disease-causing bugs."
– Dr. Michael Greger, in the video *Microbiome: We Are What They Eat*; NutritionFacts.org; DrGreger.org

Dysbiosis can also involve the skin, and increase the likelihood of experiencing skin infections, rashes, acne, eczema, and genital infections.

Dysbiosis testing

A test for dysbiosis – or overgrowth, imbalance, or presence of harmful intestinal microorganisms – can include taking a feces and/or urine sample to check for abnormal acid levels in the urine, and for certain bacteria, fungi, and yeast in the stool – and testing for faecal lipocalin-2, which is more present in cases of digestive tract inflammation. A special type of breath test and/or a swab sample taken from the throat can also detect an imbalance of gut bacteria.

Plant-based diet improves symbiosis

A plant-based diet *increases* the population of good, anti-inflammatory microorganisms in the digestive tract. A plant-based diet also increases the varieties of bacteria in a beneficial relationship between the host human and the bacteria, which is a state of symbiosis. This decreases inflammation, and improves the intestinal lining, nutrient absorption, the metabolic state, and the immune system, and cardiovascular, liver, and kidney, and other organ function.

As explained later, a healthy gut microbiota protects the brain, and improves the function of the nerve system.

"Overall, westernized diets tend to **decrease** microbial diversity [dysbiosis] and plant-based diets (PBD) tend to **increase** microbial diversity. This difference in microbiota results in differences in microbial metabolites. Westernized diets result in increased production of ammonia, indoles, phenols, and sulphide that may be detrimental to our health. In addition, they result in decreased production of short-chain fatty acids like butyrate. These metabolites have diverse beneficial effects in nutrition, immunity, and epithelial barrier. PBD result in increased production of short-chain fatty acids.

Altogether, westernized diets are pro-inflammatory and PBD are anti-inflammatory. These observations indicate that westernized diets increase susceptibility to not only irritable bowel syndrome (IBD), but also other chronic diseases. The above phenomena associated with westernized diets are observed in IBD. Based upon the changes in the intestinal microbiota and metabolites, dietary intervention is justifiable in the treatment in IBD.

Based on the rationale of the diet, gut microbiota, and health consequences and excellent outcomes with therapy incorporating PDB, PBD is unreservedly recommended for IBD."

– Recommendation of plant-based diets for inflammatory bowel disease; *Translational Pediatrics* journal; Jan. 2019

Purple and phenol nutrition

You may have heard people advise eating five colors of fruits and vegetables every day. This is good advice.

Many people don't eat a spectrum of colors, and often lack one important plant color: purple.

It is wise to include foods rich in anthocyanins, which are the colors in red, blue, and purple fruits, berries, veggies, and legumes.

By including five colors of fruits and vegetables in your daily diet, such as from purple, yellow, red, brown, green, and orange, you will get such a wide variety of nutrients your health will benefit.

Anthocyanins and mitochondrial nutrition

Anthocyanins are anti-inflammatories and antioxidants. They provide a number of health benefits – including to the mitochondria in every one of your cells.

Each cell contains hundreds to thousands of mitochondria that exist within the fluid of the cell surrounding the cell nucleus. Mitochondria are structures that convert food energy into a form used by cells.

Common anthocyanins in fruits, vegetables, sprouts, and other edible plants include cyanidin, delphinidin, malvidin, peonidin, petunidin, and pelargonidin. However, there are thousands of varieties of anthocyanins.

In plants, anthocyanins help protect the plant from stressors, including cold and heat.

Anthocyanins are *neuroprotective*, which means they are protective of the brain and nerves.

Anthocyanins have been shown to aid in memory and speech, to reduce dementia, and to protect the eyes.

Anthocyanins aid in kidney function, and have been shown to be beneficial for diabetics.

Anthocyanins help to regulate amino acid metabolism. (Amino acids are the components of protein.)

Anthocyanins protect DNA. They prevent tumor growth, reduce the progression of tumors into malignant growths, and they inhibit cancer metastasis.

Anthocyanins have been shown to reverse multidrug resistance, improving the effectiveness of chemotherapy. (By saying this, I'm not advocating – nor am I discouraging – chemotherapy. It is up to the individual to research and choose which treatments they undergo.)

Anthocyanins help to reduce blood pressure and hypertension. They reduce cholesterol and inflammation of the cardiovascular system, helping to prevent heart disease, heart attacks, and strokes. What helps to protect the heart helps to protect the kidneys.

Which foods contain anthocyanins?

Black elderberries and Aronia berries are particularly rich in anthocyanins.

Other berries also contain significant amounts of anthocyanins, including acai, blueberries, blackberries, hawthorn berries, logan berries, raspberries, and strawberries.

Bananas also contain anthocyanins, with darker-colored bananas containing more anthocyanins than yellow bananas. Most people are familiar with yellow bananas, but bananas grow in a variety of colors, and sizes.

Dark grapes, cranberries, currants, pomegranates, plums and prunes, blood oranges, and dark cherries also contain anthocyanins.

Raisins are a source of anthocyanins.

Among wines, Cabernet-Sauvignon contains the most anthocyanins. (Not that I advocate for the use of alcohol, as some people need to stay away from it.)

Vegetables containing anthocyanins include purple broccoli, purple cabbage, purple cauliflower, purple corn, purple eggplant, red radishes, and red spinach.

Beets get their color from betalain pigments, and not from anthocyanins.

Black and purple carrots contain significant amounts of anthocyanins.

Purple potatoes and purple sweet potatoes are sources of anthocyanins.

Black beans, black rice, and black soybeans contain anthocyanins.

Chocolate contains anthocyanins. This does not mean you should eat low-quality chocolate. Most chocolate products are a mix of all sorts of health-dulling ingredients, including clarified sugars, and dairy. Get raw, organic, pure chocolate powder. Learn about using it in smoothies or in coffee, or in a dandelion root latte, or mixed in with overnight oats, and only in the first few hours of your day. Chocolate later in the day can interfere with sleep. To get the nutrients from pure, raw chocolate powder, you can also simply mix it into water and drink it. This is eating for nutrition, and not for luxury.

Anthocyanins are also in turmeric, which is a strong anti-inflammatory containing a variety of other beneficial substances.

Anthocyanin supplements, or from food

Get anthocyanins from food, not from supplement pills.

To get the most anthocyanins, aim to eat some or most of the fruits and vegetables raw, as anthocyanins are damaged by heat. Boiling and steaming does the least amount of damage, while baking, frying, broiling, and other high-heat methods of cooking do the most damage to anthocyanins.

For potatoes and carrots, to preserve the anthocyanins, instead of frying, baking, or other high-heat ways of cooking, choose to cut them thin or in chunks, soak them in water for a half hour, rinse, and then boil or steam them, or use them in soups or stews.

Polyphenols

One of the benefits of following a diet rich in anthocyanins is that it will automatically make your diet rich in a type of anthocyanins called polyphenols. These antioxidants and anti-inflammatories are neuroprotective, help balance blood sugar levels, and protect against type-2 diabetes. They protect the heart, brain, and other organs from damage by free radicals that can damage tissues, including the nerves.

Polyphenols are mitochondrial nutrients.

Polyphenols also protect against cancer (especially of the breasts, colon, prostate, skin, and uterus), cardiovascular disease, diabetes, and diseases of dementia (including Alzheimer's, and other neurodegenerative diseases).

Where do you get polyphenols?

Polyphenols are compounds in berries, fruits, vegetables, nuts, seeds, and legumes.

There are thousands of types of polyphenols, including ellagitannins, epigallocatechin gallate, flavonoids (including flavan-3-ols, flavones, flavonones, and flavonols), lignans, stilbenes, and phenolic acids, including hydroxybenzoic acid, and hydroxycinnamic acid, including tannic acid.

"Flavan-3-ols have been reported to exhibit several health beneficial effects by acting as antioxidant, anticarcinogen, cardioprotective, antimicrobial, anti-viral, and neuroprotective agents."
– Flavan-3-ols: nature, occurrence, and biological activity; *Molecular Nutrition & Food Research* journal; Jan. 2008

"There is a growing body of research that suggests that certain bioactives – specific food components beyond those needed to maintain basic human nutrition – may also play an important role in lowering the risk of cardiometabolic disease.

Among these health-promoting bioactives are flavan-3-ols, the most highly consumed subclass of flavonoids. Flavan-3-ols are commonly found in tea, apples, pears, berries, chocolate, and cocoa products."
– Are You Getting Enough Flavan-3-ols? by Eric Graber; *American Society for Nutrition* journal; Jan. 2023

Notice flavan-3-ols are in plants, you aren't going to get them from eating meat, dairy, or eggs. Flavan-3-ols are in apples, blackberries, blueberries, chocolate, citrus, cranberries, grapes, green tea, kale, onions, parsley, red cabbage, red peppers, and soybeans.

"Dietary flavan-3-ols can help improve blood pressure, cholesterol

concentrations, and blood sugar. Strength of evidence was strongest for some biomarkers (i.e., systolic blood pressure, total cholesterol, HDL cholesterol, and insulin/glucose dynamics). It should be noted that this is a food-based guideline, and not a recommendation for flavan-3-ol supplements..”
– Flavan-3-ols and Cardiometabolic Health: First Ever Dietary Bioactive Guideline; *Elsevier Advances in Nutrition* journal; Oct. 2022

Notice the study above mentions the flavan-3-ols should be from foods, not from supplements. In other words, eat your fruits and vegetables. By eating the whole foods, you will get the undamaged nutrients accompanied by a host of other beneficial components.

Foods higher in polyphenols include apricots, artichokes, asparagus, berries, blueberries, broccoli, carrots, cherries, chia, chocolate, cranberries, garlic, grapes (including raisins and red wine), nectarines, nuts (including raw/unheated/untoasted almonds, chestnuts, hazelnuts, and pecans), olives, onions, peaches, peanuts, pears, plums, peppers, pomegranates, red lettuce, shallots, spinach, and whole grains. Green tea, black tea, and coffee are also sources of polyphenols.

Herbs and spices for polyphenols

Herbs and spices including anise, basil, cinnamon, cloves, cumin, curry, ginger, lemon verbena, marjoram, oregano, parsley, peppermint, rosemary, sage, and turmeric are often noted as being good sources of polyphenols.

The ellagic acid polyphenol is found in berries, and in the skin of tree nuts.

The polyphenol in turmeric is called curcumin. It is beneficial to have whole turmeric, rather than to have an extract. There are a variety of beneficial substances in turmeric.

Capsaicinoids

The heat of hot peppers comes from a polyphenolic amide called capsaicinoids. Capsaicinoids also exist in cilantro, cinnamon, and oregano. They have been revealed as cardioprotective, as in: good for the cardiovascular system. They also can protect against cancer, diabetes, and fibrosis of the liver.

“Capsaicin in cayenne pepper actually stimulate the nerves in your stomach that produce digestive fluids, which helps your digestion. Research shows it may even help prevent the most common type of stomach ulcers, which are caused by the H. pylori bacteria.”
– Health Benefits of Cayenne Pepper; WebMD, 2023

Capsaicin can increase the metabolism while also reducing hunger, and plays a role in weight loss.

Those with high blood pressure might want to avoid hot, spicey peppers, as these can increase blood pressure.

People with bleeding disorders, and those who are planning to undergo – or who have recently undergone –surgery, including any kind of recent transplant or tissue graft, should avoid hot peppers.

Women who are breastfeeding should avoid hot peppers.

People who have an allergic reaction to avocado, bananas, chestnuts, kiwi, or latex might also have a reaction to hot peppers.

"Capsaicinoids are a group of compounds responsible for the spicy, pungent taste of hot chili peppers (Capsicum annuum, and Capsicum frutescens). The family of capsaicinoids is primarily comprised of capsaicin, dihydrocapsaicin, nondihydrocapsaicin, homohydrocapsaicin, homodihydrocapsaicin, and nonivamide."
– Bioavailability of capsaicin and its implications for drug delivery, by William D. Rolyson; Science Direct; 2014

Polyphenolic amides

Among the beneficial substances in plants are polyphenolic amides. These are antioxidants that protect against oxidative stress. It is the kind of stress that causes premature aging, plays a role in chronic and degenerative conditions, increases the risk of sprains and fractures, and damages cells, reducing their lifespan by also reducing the presence of the telomerase enzyme.

Inflammation plays a role in many health conditions, including autoimmune disorders like arthritis, asthma, diabetes, and lupus. It also worsens conditions like cancer, cardiovascular disease, kidney disease, and neurodegenerative disorders like Alzheimer's and Parkinson's.

"Dietary polyphenols have received tremendous attention among nutritionists, food scientists, and consumers due to their roles in human health. Research strongly supports a role for polyphenols in the prevention of degenerative diseases, particularly cancers, cardiovascular diseases, and neurodegenerative diseases. Polyphenols are strong antioxidants that compliment and add to the functions of antioxidant vitamins and enzymes as a defense against oxidative stress caused by excess reactive oxygen species (ROS).

Dietary phenolics or polyphenols constitute one of the most numerous and widely distributed groups of natural products in the plant kingdom. More than 8,000 phenolic structures are currently known, and among them over 4,000 flavonoids have been identified. Although polyphenols are chemically characterized as compounds with phenolic structural features, this group of natural products is highly diverse and contains several sub-groups of phenolic compounds. Fruits, vegetables, whole grains, and other types of foods and beverages such as tea, chocolate, and wine are rich sources of polyphenols."
– Chemistry and biochemistry of dietary polyphenols; *Nutrients* journal; Dec. 2010

People see chocolate and wine listed as containing polyphenols, and think they should have more of those. But there are things to know about them, before considering those choices.

Research: chocolate polyphenols.

As far as wine, many people have an addictive issue with alcohol and should stay away from it. Alcohol also is not great for the brain or nerves, and can increase cancer risk.

Instead of drinking wine, eat grapes. Find a source of organically grown, seeded grapes – instead of "seedless." Where possible, grow your own.

A diet rich in polyphenolic amides by way of a variety of colors in fruits, vegetables, sprouts, and activated grains, beans, and seeds benefits cardiovascular health, improves blood pressure, protects the endothelium cells of the cardiovascular and lymph systems, reduces atherosclerosis, and lowers the risk of everything from diabetes to cancer, and diseases of the liver and kidneys.

To learn more about flavones, research:
- Anthocyanidins
- Chalcones
- Ellagic acid
- Flavanones
- Flavanonols
- Flavones
- Flavonoids
- Flavonols
- Hydrolysable tannins
- Isoflavones
- Lignans
- Neoflavanoids
- Phenolic acids: non-flavonoid polyphenolic compounds
- Proanthocyanidins
- Resveratrol
- Rosmarinic acid

Avenanthramides: a group of polyphenolic acids

Avenanthramides are polyphenolic amide compounds found in oats and white cabbage. They are anti-inflammatory, and help balance the low-density lipoproteins ("bad" cholesterol) of the blood.

"Oat is a cereal known since antiquity as a useful grain with abundant nutritional and health benefits. It contains distinct molecular components with high antioxidant activity, such as tocopherol, tocotrienols, and flavonoids. In addition, it is a unique source of avenanthramides, phenolic amides containing anthranilic acid and hydroxycinnamic acid moieties, and endowed with major beneficial health properties because of their antioxidant, anti-inflammatory, and antiproliferative effects."
 – Biological Activities, Health Benefits, and Therapeutic Properties of Avenanthramides: From Skin Protection to Prevention and Treatment of Cerebrovascular Diseases; *Oxidative Medicine and Cellular Longevity* journal; Aug. 2018

Oats

The nutrients in oats include oleic and linoleic acids, amino acids, and fiber with a high content of beta-glucan.

The beta-glucan soluble fiber in oats may help to lower blood pressure, to reduce blood glucose, and work as a prebiotic that benefits good bacteria in the digestive tract.

"The high levels of beta-glucan present in oats have been shown to contribute in reducing total plasma concentrations of cholesterol and low-density lipoprotein (LDL) cholesterol, the main risk factors for coronary heart disease.

A growing body of evidence suggests that oats contain other important bioactive compounds, such as phenolic compounds, which exert protective effects against the development of various pathologies, including cardiovascular disease, diabetes, inflammatory bowel disease, cancer, obesity, and celiac disease, acting synergistically with dietary fibers"

– Biological Activities, Health Benefits, and Therapeutic Properties of Avenanthramides: From Skin Protection to Prevention and Treatment of Cerebrovascular Diseases; *Oxidative Medicine and Cellular Longevity* journal; Aug. 2018

Beta-glucan also helps the gut to release the YY peptide hormone. This satiety hormone gives the satisfying feeling of being full. This can lead to reducing hunger, and lowering calorie intake. This is why oats are often part of a weight-loss diet.

Because oats are rich in fiber, protein, vitamins and minerals, and contain anti-atherosclerotic, anti-inflammatory, and antioxidant properties, people concerned with cardiovascular health include oats in their food choices.

Oats both protect against oxidative stress and increase the production of nitric oxide. It is nitric oxide that helps the flow of both blood and lymph fluid. This is an excellent benefit combined with the way oats help to reduce LDL cholesterol.

Oats have origins in the Middle East or Mediterranean region. They have been farmed in Europe and Asia, and were brought with early travelers, including Europeans who settled in what became the U.S. and Canada.

Starting in the 1500s, the use of oats as a food for humans and farmed animals soon spread throughout the world.

Simply because oats contain beneficial nutrients doesn't mean you should eat anything containing oats. There are many products sold containing oats as an ingredient, like sugary cookies, ice cream sandwiches, low-quality cereals, and other mass marketed, ultra-processed products.

Find a source for organic, raw, untoasted oats.

I don't cook oats. I soak them in water with some chia seeds, or mix them with coconut yogurt to soften them.

"Overnight oats" have become popular with people wanting the benefits of eating raw oats. This means unheated oats with their nutrients undamaged by heat.

With their soluble fiber that forms a gel, oats work as a binder agent in recipes. Oats are often used as an ingredient in vegan bean burgers. Soaked oats can be made into oat milk, and used to thicken smoothies.

The oat milk products sold in stores might contain some additives not so beneficial to health. They also might contain chemicals leached from the lining of the container. It is easy enough to inexpensively make your own oat milk, rather than to pay several times more to purchase oat milk.

Soaked oats blended with water and a date and/or a banana might be the flavor you like, without the food additives of commercially-sold oat milk. Experiment with different ways of making oat milk from scratch, and find a flavor that works for you. These might include maca powder, lucuma fruit powder, monk fruit powder. (See oat milk recipes online.)

Flax seed

Flax seeds are often mentioned as a good source of polyphenols. This is because they contain about 1,528 milligrams of polyphenols per 100 grams, including lignans.

Flax seeds should be raw, untoasted, unheated, and organic. You can grind them in a coffee grinder to make the nutrients more available. Also, it is better if you soak the flax seeds for several hours, then spread them thinly in a glass casserole to dry them – or use a food dehydrator to dry them. You can keep those dried "activated" or "germinated" seeds in a jar stored in the fridge or a cool area for when you use them.

Flax seeds can be quite stubborn to get off what they have dried on. Some people will use a very light coat of raw coconut oil on the glass or on a bamboo cutting board before spreading the wet flax seeds to dry them. If you dry them on parchment paper, make sure the parchment paper is non-toxic, and not coated with petroleum chemical wax.

In addition to flax seeds, lignans are also in nuts and sesame seeds, and whole grains (including barley, buckwheat, millet, oats, rye, and wheat, particularly in the bran).

Polyphenols are mitochondrial and digestive nutrients

Polyphenols help to feed the good bacteria of the gut, aiding in digestion and nutrient absorption, and assisting both the immune system and production of messenger molecules. Polyphenols also inhibit the growth of bad gut bacteria.

Supplemental polyphenols

It's best to get polyphenols from food, and not from supplements or extracts. If you are on certain medications, there can be interactions with certain supplements.

Supplements aren't regulated by the Food and Drug Administration, so be careful if you choose to take polyphenol supplements. Research the source.

This book couldn't possibly include all of the helpful information on anthocyanins, including polyphenols, and about other nutrients. For more information, check sites like NutritionFacts.org and ForksOverKnives.com.

Enzymes

"What is the great secret that has been eluding the investigations of scientists and lives of laypersons for centuries? Enzymes. You are only alive because thousands of enzymes make it possible. Every breath you take, thought you think, or sentence you read, is a result of thousands of complex enzyme systems and their functions operating simultaneously."
– Ann Wigmore, author of *The Hippocrates Diet*

Enzymes aren't the only reason you are alive, but they do play key roles in the function of every part of you. They work in combination with everything else consisting of your structures, including the dependance on nutrients from a healthy diet, as well as hydration, breathing, and movement.

"Enzymes are substances that make life possible. They are needed for every chemical reaction that takes place in the human body. No mineral, vitamin, or hormone can do any work without enzymes. Our bodies, all our organs, tissues, and cells are run by metabolic enzymes."
– Dr. Edward Howell, *Enzyme Nutrition*

"Through years of research Dr. Ann Wigmore discovered that all the enzymes, vitamins, and minerals the body needs are found within the foods we eat – if these foods are prepared in such a way as to maintain or unlock their life-giving nutrients."
– Creative Health Institute

There is more about enzymes in the following pages.

Blood sugar, digestive upset, allergies, pancreatic function

Those with health issues relating to blood sugar balance, digestive upset, allergies, or problems related to pancreatic function would benefit by consuming raw nuts, beans, seeds, and grains that have been activated through soaking and/or fermenting. Know which beans are not good for sprouting. This is part of learning to include living foods in your diet.

There is more about this topic is in the following pages.

Avoiding allergens through living foods

As mentioned elsewhere, those with allergies and troublesome reactions to various plant-based foods may want to research how to follow a more "living foods" diet, and prepare ingredients like beans, legumes, rices, grains, and nuts by first soaking them to rid them of problematic natural substances – before using them in foods.

People experiencing serious health problems may especially benefit from following this sort of diet consisting of enlivened, germinated, sprouted, activated, blossomed, or otherwise clean, whole, and richly nutritious foods.

It was common for ancient people to soak things like beans, legumes, rices, seeds, and grains, including to help soften the foods. Doing so reduces both cooking times and the amount of wood and/or other materials needed for cooking. Little did the ancient people know they were also increasing the nutrient value of their foods, while also ridding the foods of antinutrients and allergens, and improving their gut biome, digestion, and nutrient absorption.

There is more information about activating and enlivening foods is in the following pages.

Eating disorders, reflux, food allergies, skin issues, and inflammatory diseases

Those with a history of anorexia or bulimia, reflux, heartburn, food allergies, skin disorders, acne, arthritis, osteoporosis, bloating, leaking gut syndrome, Crohn's, or irritable bowel issues, and other disorders may find they do better on a diet of activated nuts, seeds, beans, legumes, and fermented nongluten grains, in combination with a low-fat diet rich in raw fruits, vegetables, and sprouts, and including some boiled and steamed foods.

Certain inflammatory conditions of the bowels in combination with issues like anemia, belly pain, diarrhea, fever, nausea, rectal bleeding, and weight loss may result in a person being advised to avoid gluten, nuts, certain seeds, fruits, and vegetables, oily foods, and fried or heavily heated oils, as well as all dairy products. A gastroenterologist and dietitian can advise you on these matters.

The SAD diet lacks vibrancy

The standard American diet ("SAD" diet) is lacking in useful enzymes. This is because high heat and intense processing of food damages enzymes, which are key to a diet fueling vibrant health.

Life-force energy

This term *life-force energy* might seem hippy-dippy to some people, but there is an energy in raw fruits, vegetables, and sprouts that isn't in cooked food.

You may hear some health food proponents claim enzymes contain the life-force energy of the plant. Well, the plant would not have life if you took away any of a number of components making up the plant, such as the minerals, the water, the biophotons, or one of the varieties of amino acids, and other substances of the plant.

Enzymes are protein, and proteins are composed of amino acids.

Electrical charges, biophotons, antioxidants, omega-3 fatty acids, certain vitamins, minerals, and other nutrients are present in raw plant matter. These are beneficial to human health.

Cooked, damaged, extracted, and processed foods

Food that has been cooked at high temperatures, had materials extracted, or is an extract, or otherwise been altered will not contain all of the substances found in the unprocessed plant matter. In plants, the components work in combination with each other. Undamaged enzymes, amino acids, essential fatty acids, vitamins, and other substances and structures in edible plants provide health benefits for humans.

"The act of cooking – and the resultant loss of nutrients, enzymes, and oxygen – impairs our digestion and elimination, which are the two most controlling factors of nutrient absorption that regulate our metabolism."
– Dr. Brian Clement, HippocratesInst.org

Experience vibrant health

The more your diet consists of a variety of enzyme- and vitamin-rich, raw plant matter, and the less you eat processed, deadened, or otherwise degenerated foods, and the problematic substances found in meat, dairy, and eggs, the more likely you are to experience vibrant health.

When I hear someone say unheated fruits and vegetables contain "life-force energy," I don't simply consider the enzymes. I think of the whole variety of nutrients, electrical charges, and other components needed for the plants to be alive.

Those promoting a living foods diet do have a point in saying that if you want to have a lively, healthy, vibrant body, you increase your chances of experiencing this by following a diet rich in living, vibrant foods from nature. This is, vibrantly alive plant substances not degraded by chemicals, or genetic engineering, saturated with industrial food processing ingredients, or containing what is truly dead: meat, bone marrow, and gelatin.

Later in the book I detail certain heat-generated chemicals formed when foods are cooked. These can play a role in degraded health, including by causing inflammation, damaging the gut biome and lining of the intestines, and playing a role in everything from autoimmune disorders, cancers, and cardiovascular, liver, and kidney disease.

Biophotons, Dugald Semple, galama, and sunfoods

Biophotons are specs of light that disappear when a plant is cooked.

In his 1956 book, *The Sunfood Way to Health*, Dugald Semple provided his level of understanding of nutrition. He wrote, "Cooking devitalizes food, as when we kill seeds by boiling them, and this causes the sun energy – or galama in the plant cells – to be dissipated."

Semple was using the words of George Julius Drews who wrote about galama in his 1912 book *Unfired Foods and Tropho-Therapy*.

Perhaps the modern-day term both Drews and Semple would have used for the sun energy *galama* they spoke of is *biophotons*. Or simply *photons*. Those early plant-based nutrition proponents understood what many people still today don't seem to understand: unheated edible plants contain a nutrient cooked foods do not: that is the biophotons.

Photoreceptor proteins

The tissues of the body, including the brain, contain photoreceptor proteins that interact with light. It's part of how your body knows to shut down for sleep when it is dark, which also plays into hormonal balance, and many other matters going on inside your cells. It is also why it is good to sleep in a dark room.

We are meant to eat unheated plant matter, which contains the microscopic biophoton specs of light. Enzymes also contain both biophotons and electrical charges.

Enzymes are necessary for life. All living things form and contain enzymes made of amino acids, which make up proteins.

Thousands of types of enzymes

There are thousands of types of enzymes in the body. They are made up of protein molecules and are paramount to all chemical reactions within the body. They act along with minerals, fats, carbohydrates, vitamins, and all other necessary components of the body tissues to produce living functions. Enzymes are central to the formation, repair, restoration, and revitalization of all tissues.

If you do not have a healthy bank of enzymes, and don't continue to get them from a healthful diet, your health degrades.

In other words, do eat some raw, unheated fruits, vegetables, and sprouts – preferably every day. If they aren't available, the next better choice would be quality, unheated, truly raw, fermented foods kept in glass or ceramic containers. Then, fresh frozen fruits and vegetables, and then raw juices. There are also low-heat dehydrated foods, which helps to preserve nutrients.

Three classes of enzymes: metabolic, digestive, food/dietary

There are three classes of enzymes: metabolic enzymes, digestive enzymes, and food or dietary enzymes.

The first class, metabolic enzymes, are within the cells of the body tissues. They are essential to all cellular activity, including breathing, healing, and movement.

The second-class, digestive enzymes, are produced by all areas of the alimentary tract, from the mouth through the stomach and intestines to the colon.

The third class, which are essential to the formation of both metabolic and digestive enzymes, are the dietary enzymes from food.

Amylase, lipase, and protease enzymes

Amylase enzymes are essential to the digestion of carbohydrates.
Lipase enzymes are essential to the digestion of fats.
Protease enzymes are essential to the digestion of proteins.

Enzymes are essential nutrients

Enzymes exist in all plant life. They also are essential to the ripening of food.

There are some plants native to regions where temperatures might go above 120 degrees, including some types of cacti, palm trees, and other desert plants. In large measure, most plants perish (because their enzymes are greatly damaged) at temperatures above 120 degrees. Freezing food may degrade enzymes. Some plants exist in areas where temperatures drop well below freezing. Most plants on the planet die when temperatures drop below freezing.

Fermented foods and enzymes

Because fermenting of raw foods, such as sauerkraut, kimchi, coconut yogurt, and seed and nut cheeses, increases enzymatic activity, some people encourage the use of fermented foods for healing.

The late Dr. Ann Wigmore advocated the use of fermented foods in healing. As mentioned, her health retreat continues to operate in Puerto Rico, where people can follow a raw, living diet, do yoga, and participate in other health and outdoor activities.

Soaking raw nuts and seeds activates the enzymes while increasing both the digestibility, and the nutrient content.

Soaking seeds, beans, legumes, nuts, and grains

Substances called tannins, lectins, phytates, and complex sugars are contained in seeds, beans, nuts, legumes, and grains. Some people call these substances antinutrients because they can interfere with certain types of nutrient (copper, iron, zinc) absorption, inhibit digestive enzymes, alter the ability of the digestive system to break down certain substances, impact the function of the pancreas, play some role in autoimmune and allergic reactions, and may contribute to degenerative and chronic health conditions, such as bone loss and joint pain. However, there is the other side of the story as the substances can also work as anticarcinogens (anti-cancer), antioxidants, and be cardioprotective, neuroprotective, and benefit the immune system.

"While antinutrients are often regarded as inhibitors of nutrient absorption with potential adverse health effects, emerging evidence suggests they may also confer neuroprotective benefits under specific conditions. These protective roles are largely attributed to their antioxidant and anti-inflammatory properties, which may play a crucial role in safeguarding neural tissues from damage associated with oxidative stress and chronic inflammation. Phytates are a notable example of antinutrients with neuroprotective potential. These compounds act as potential antioxidants by chelating pro-oxidant metals such as iron and copper, which catalyze the formation of reactive oxygen species. By reducing the availability of these metals for ROS generation, phytates help mitigate oxidative stress. Additionally, phytates may inhibit lipid peroxidation, a process in which free radicals attack neural cell membranes, further contributing to their neuroprotective role. Similarly, polyphenolic compounds like tannins demonstrate significant neuroprotective properties. Furthermore, their anti-inflammatory effects may counteract chronic low-grade neuroinflammation, which is implicated in cognitive disorders such as mild cognitive impairment and dementia. Also, improving cerebral blood flow and oxygenation is critical for maintaining cognitive function. This duel role of antinutrients remains an areas of active research. While their negative effects on nutrient bioavailability are well documented, their capacity to reduce oxidative stress and inflammation poses a new paradigm."

– Impact of Vegan and Vegetarian Diets on Neurological Health: A Critical Review; *MDPI* journal of the Multidisciplinary Digital Publishing Institute; Feb. 2025

By following a diet consisting of a variety of fruits, vegetables, sprouts, nuts, legumes, and other edibles, you are unlikely to have to concern yourself with tannins, and other "antinutrients," nor should you focus on eliminating all of them from your diet – because they carry health benefits.

Lectins

Also known as hemagglutinins. Hundreds of lectins have been identified. They are carbohydrate-binding proteins that form in plants, microorganisms, and animals.

In plants, lectins are part of their defense against fungi, diseases, and wounds, and against certain birds, insects, worms, slugs, and other animals.

Lectins are found in a wide variety of foods, including fruits, vegetables, sprouts, nuts, legumes, seeds, and whole grains. Lectins are more present and otherwise bioavailable in raw legumes, and in grains. The soil in which – and region where – the plants were grown plays a role in their lectin content.

Lectins show some health benefits, including as anti-cancer agents. It is unlikely you will eliminate all lectins from the diet – nor should you attempt to. But steps can be taken to avoid large doses of them – which is done by the way beans and grains and other foods containing them are prepared.

Because lectins are in fruits, vegetables, sprouts, nuts, and seaweeds, which all are foods containing fiber, antioxidants, anti-inflammatories, vitamins, minerals, amino acids, and other beneficial components, it is not wise to try eliminating lectins from the diet.

Food poisoning can occur after consumption of undercooked legumes or bean flours overload the system with lectins. Large amounts of lectins can impair the gut flora, leading to – or playing a role in – altered nutrient absorption, and in leaky gut, and contributing to autoimmune disorders. These are some of the reasons why properly preparing and cooking beans is important for maintaining health in immunocompromised, pregnant, and elderly people, and those with certain health conditions, including kidney, cardiovascular, and intestinal issues.

Soaking, steaming, and boiling beans and grains helps to greatly reduce or eliminate their lectin content. Fermentation also greatly decreases lectin content. Wetting bean flours, and letting them sit for an hour or more before using in recipes to be cooked can reduce or eliminate lectins in bean flours.

Phytates

Phytate – or phytic acid – is a naturally occurring protective substance bound with phosphorus in nuts, beans, legumes, seeds, and grains, and prevents the embryo of the seed from damage.

Phytates can interfere with nutrient absorption, including of calcium, copper, iron, magnesium, and zinc.

Using Alliums (onions, garlic, shallots, leeks, scallions, chives, or green onions) with beans helps the digestive system absorb minerals.

"Phytic acid is a substance found in many plant-based foods. It is also called inositol hexaphosphate and IP6. This acid is the primary way phosphorus is stored in many plants, including beans, seeds, and nuts.

When phytic acid is consumed, it binds to other minerals to create phytates. Because you don't have any enzymes that can break phytates down, their nutrients cannot be absorbed into your body.

Most beans and legumes contain a high amount of phytic acid. However, studies have shown that soaking beans before [cooking and] eating them significantly reduces their phytate levels. When a plant is ripening, phytate rapidly accumulates in its seeds."
– Foods High in Phytic Acid; WebMD; Sept. 2024

One enzyme produced when seeds germinate is phytase, which neutralizes phytic acid (see the phytate section of this book, describing why phytates are an important nutrient). This is one reason why people soak nuts, beans, legumes, and seeds before consuming, including before boiling or any type of cooking. It is also why it is good to soak and/or ferment grains before consuming. Be sure to drain the soak water.

"There are several methods of decreasing the inhibitory effect of phytic acid on mineral absorption (cooking, germination, fermentation, soaking, autolysis). Nevertheless, inositol hexaphosphate is receiving increased attention owing to its role in cancer prevention and/or therapy and its hypocholesterolaemic [cholesterol-lowering] effect."
– The role of phytic acid in legumes: antinutrient or beneficial function?; *Journal of Physiology Biochemistry*; Sept. 2000

As mentioned, it is not necessary to try to follow a diet free of all phytic acid, as there are nutritional benefits associated with phytic acid, including for cardiovascular health, and cancer prevention. More focus should be on a low-fat diet, especially free from damaged – highly heated or rancid - oils.

Raw vegans calling themselves "living foodists" aim to consume only raw, soaked, germinated, bloomed, or otherwise "activated" nuts, seeds, and certain legumes. This is in addition to consuming raw fruits and vegetables, sprouts, and seaweeds, and foods consisting only of those ingredients without being heated.

Whether it is pumpkin seeds, sunflower seeds, chia seeds, garbanzo beans (chickpeas), black beans, hazelnuts, walnuts, almonds, pine nuts (pignolis), or other nuts, seeds, or beans, there is nutritional benefit in getting them raw, unheated, unpasteurized, and viable, and activating them before consumption by soaking them. Certain ones, including nuts, legumes, pumpkin seeds, and beans can then be dried for use in coming weeks or months, such as by placing them in a dehydrator at low temperature to dry them, and then storing them for later use.

It is best to store them in a cool, dry place, or in a container in the refrigerator. (Glass jars work well: If you buy the large, glass jars of sauerkraut, save the jars and lids for food storage.) To prevent mold, make sure they are dry.

Some natural foods stores sell activated seeds and nuts that have been dried. The label might say "sprouted" – even though they were not sprouted to the point of forming a leaf or root. (Understand which beans should NOT be eaten after they reach the stage of a leaf or root forming.)

Zinc

Zinc is one mineral those with kidney disease should take note of when their blood is tested for nutrient levels. Damaged kidneys can play a role in a zinc deficiency as they can excrete zinc.

Zinc is important for a wide variety of tissue functions, from the eyes and brain, the immune system, hair follicles, and the senses of smell and taste. Zinc also is important for wound healing, bone health, and the production of certain hormones, including insulin and testosterone.

Foods containing high levels of zinc are also foods best to get raw (untoasted, unheated), and soak them before using, which makes the zinc more accessible. These include: almonds, adzuki beans, black beans, Brazil nuts*, buckwheat, chia seeds, chickpeas, flaxseeds, lentils, oats, pecans, pine nuts, pinto beans, pumpkin seeds, sesame seeds, sunflower seeds, walnuts, and wild rice. (*Brazil nuts are high in the trace element selenium. 3-4 Brazil nuts contain your daily maximum of selenium. Use Brazil nuts sparingly.)

Other foods high in zinc include asparagus, avocado, cashews, chocolate*, green peas, hemp seeds, miso paste, peanuts, tahini, tempeh, and tofu. (*Refrain from eating most commercial chocolate, as it likely contains less healthful ingredients, including sugar and dairy. If you use chocolate, get pure, organic chocolate powder, and used it earlier in the day.)

The way sourdough bread is made, as it is essentially a fermented food, also breaks down the protective coating of the grain, and results in better zinc absorption. (Avoid breads containing potassium bromate or potassium bromide.)

Quinoa contains zinc, but is also high in oxalates*, and is therefore a food restricted in the diets of those who are likely to form kidney stones. If you do eat quinoa, soak it first, discard the water, then add new water before boiling. Soaking quinoa for a few hours breaks down the anti-nutrients, reduces the oxalate content, increases the amino acids, and makes the zinc more easily absorbable.

Considering oxalates

*Whenever oxalates are considered, it should be understood that the gut microorganisms Bifidobacterium spp, Oxalobacter formigenes, and Lactobacillus spp – which are probiotics – break down some of the dietary oxalates [oxalates from food] and use them as an energy source. Another intestinal microorganisms that may help to reduce the formation of oxalate stones is Eubacterium. These are more reasons to follow a diet that nurtures a healthy gut biome, which is a clean, low-fat, plant-based diet.

The body doesn't absorb many of the dietary oxalates, and other oxalates are naturally produced by the body.

A diet completely free of oxalates isn't realistic, and would also be avoiding many beneficial nutrients. Be sure to drink plenty of water, and also know that avoiding oils and damaged oils also helps to reduce kidney stone formation.

"Previous analyses have shown that up to 40% of the oxalate present in the urine may come from the intestines. These results suggest that limiting the absorption of oxalate in the gut may be important for minimizing the risk of developing or recurring urolithiasis. O. formigenes regulates intraluminal oxalate availability by degrading dietary oxalate, using oxalate as an obligatory energy source, thereby reducing intestinal oxalate absorption and urinary excretion. Consequently, oxalate degradable O. formigenes limits the availability of oxalate for intestinal absorption. However, the intestinal colonization by O. formigenes does not affect other factors related to the development of urolithiasis, such as concentration of calcium, uric acid, sodium, citrate, and magnesium in the urine. Hatch et al. suggested that O. formigenes may also interact physiologically with the colonic mucous membrane by inducing enteric oxalate secretion, leading to additional reduction of urinary oxalate excretion."
– Probiotics in the Prevention of the Calcium Oxalate Urolithiasis; *Cells* journal; Jan. 2022

Sauerkraut for intestinal health

Some mention sauerkraut as a source of zinc in the vegan diet. But sauerkraut only has trace amounts of zinc, as well as boron, choline, cobalt, copper, fluorine, phosphorus, selenium, silicon, and sulfur. It has higher amounts of calcium, iodine, iron, magnesium, manganese, potassium, and sodium. (Those watching their sodium intake will need to be aware of the salt in sauerkraut. Make your own sauerkraut, and use less salt.)

Vitamins in sauerkraut include A, Bs, C, K1, and U.

It is good to include fermented foods in the diet, as they can improve the gut biome, and this boosts immunity, including by improving or enhancing nutrient absorption, as well as the metabolization of other nutrients. It also helps to protect the gut lining, preventing leaky gut syndrome.

Sauerkraut is both easy to make, and an excellent choice for quality nutrition.

If you purchase sauerkraut, make sure it is raw, not in a can, not heated, and has not been heated (pasteurized), which damages some nutrients.

People taking monoamine oxidase inhibitors [MAOIs] for anxiety, depression, or Parkinson's should discuss with their healthcare provider if sauerkraut is okay for them to eat.

Tannins

Tannins are part of a plant's defense system. They are polyphenol compounds in plants, and can be what gives them an astringent taste.

There are two classifications of tannins: condensed (proanthocyanidins, including catechin, epicatechin, epigallocatechin, epicatechin 3-gallate, and epigallocatechin-3-gallate) and hydrolysable (including ellagitannins and gallotannins).

People often mention the benefits of the polyphenols in certain foods, including those found in applies, apricots, beans, black grapes, cherries, cocoa beans, cranberries, grains, nuts, pears, plums, pomegranates, raspberries, strawberries, tea, whole grains, wine, and varieties of other fruits, vegetables, and sprouts. Part of the benefit is the tannins are accompanied by other components of the plants, including thousands of bioactive substances that help advance the nutrient use of tannins, and others that work against the tannins from interfering with processes like mineral absorption.

The benefits of polyphenols include protecting against atherosclerosis, heart attack, stroke, insulin resistance, memory loss, metabolic syndrome, neurodegenerative diseases, type 2 diabetes, vision loss, and other health issues.

Flavanols, which are condensed tannins, work as prebiotics boosting healthful gut flora, including Bifidobacterium and Lactobacilli – which then plays into a healthy gut lining, a reduction of inflammation, some protection against autoimmune disorders, a reduction in C-reactive protein and plasma triacylglycerol, and the production of helpful substances like serotonin, benefiting mood, energy, sleep, and otherwise brain, muscle, and organ function. This is one reason people include pure cocoa powder in a smoothie or early day meal, or simply mix with water and drink, as cocoa is rich in flavanols.

A person may say they have been eating seeds, beans, legumes, nuts, and grains their entire life, and they are fine. Of course, but there are ways to improve nutrition. Including by increasing the nutrients in beans, grains, nuts, legumes, and seeds – by enlivening them: soaking some, sprouting others. Learn which ones are better to not sprout, and which ones are good to sprout.

Allergies, sinus issues, stomach upset, stress

Maybe some of the health problems you have experienced, including allergies, sinus issues, stomach upset, stress injuries, sleep disorders, delayed healing of wounds, and other maladies have been related to substances you have consumed in common foods. Some of the substances are destroyed by heat, which is why you may not have experienced their effects. (Also see: the section of the book about avoiding the potassium bromate that is added to commercial breads and other flour-containing foods.)

This book isn't about saying you are going to get sick, it is about improving nutrition, and reducing disease risk. It is also about getting more vibrant, nutrient-rich foods into your diet, and helping you to get the full nutritional value from your foods. It's about being more likely to experience a higher level of health in which you can thrive.

Some of the chemicals produced by plants are part of their defense mechanism, meant to protect the plant, seed, bean, legume, grain, or nut from fungi, bacteria, viruses, and insects and other animals, and exposure to sun radiation, and extreme temperatures.

The presence of the defensive substances in plants is why some seeds can remain viable for many years. When the conditions are right, with the temperatures and moisture ideal for the seed to germinate and sprout, certain inhibitors are no longer needed, the coat or skin of protection will break down, fall from, or peel from the seed, or become a nutrient base, and enzymes will enliven as the seed turns on its nutrition factory, and the plant grows.

Enzyme inhibitors

As described, enzyme inhibitors in nuts, seeds, beans, legumes, and grains can interfere with digestive and other enzymes in our system, and play a role in nutrient absorption, in the gut microbiome, and in bodily functions, including the cardiovascular and immune system. While heat can destroy some of these substances, the enzyme inhibitors are also neutralized by soaking raw, unheated nuts, seeds, beans, legumes, and grains before use. Some of those natural plant chemicals work as nutrients.

Soaking breaks down complex sugars, phytates, tannins, and other components, and triggers the production of beneficial enzymes rich in the amino acids we need for forming various proteins.

Soaking makes nuts, seeds, beans, legumes*, and grains more digestible and nutritious. (*Beans are legumes, but not all legumes are beans.)

Fermenting certain beans, legumes seeds, and grains can also help disable, disband, or otherwise neutralize certain potentially problem substances, and make food more nutrient-dense.

Trypsin

Trypsin is an enzyme produced in the small intestine from trypsinogen secreted by the pancreas. It is important in the digestion of protein as it breaks down protein molecules into amino acids and peptides. Its function can be limited by trypsin inhibitors in some beans, legumes, and grains. This is another reason why soaking these foods can improve digestion.

Wild animals have been known to avoid eating plants containing trypsin inhibitors.

People who have difficulty with digestion (malabsorption) – or who have certain inflammatory conditions – are sometimes given a trypsin supplement. Trypsin may also be given to people who have anemia. Often this supplement is of trypsin taken from the pancreas of a slaughtered cow (bovine trypsin) or pig (porcine trypsin). However, there are vegan sources of trypsin produced by bacteria, or fungus.

Diets rich in trypsin inhibitors can alter the function of the pancreas, and trigger the hypersecretion of pancreatic enzymes. This can inflame the pancreas

97

and interfere with insulin resistance, alter the immune system, and make the person more susceptible to allergy issues.

Some people who have had experiences with digestive upset, bloating, and gas, food allergies, and asthma, say they have favorable experiences with soaking beans, legumes, grains, and seeds before use. Perhaps this is partially related to reducing or eliminating trypsin inhibitors.

Taking vegan probiotics for a month while following a clean diet can also help reduce digestive issues, increase nutrient absorption, and help to build a healthy gut lining. (Also see: information about avoiding flours containing the potassium bromide additive.)

Fermented and activated foods

You may benefit by learning about fermented foods made of activated seeds and/or activated nuts, including activated, fermented, raw vegan seed and nut cheeses. These are rich in a variety of nutrients, including probiotics – especially if probiotics were used as one of the ingredients.

Primates don't typically consume seeds or legumes, and humans appear to have only done so at an increasing rate mostly with the start of agricultural practices that developed over thousands of years into modern-day crop farming techniques.

One reason for the lack of seeds or grains in the human diet previous to about 10,000 or so years ago is that they are too not so easy on digestion – unless they are soaked, soaked and boiled or steamed, soaked and dried, or soaked and made into a powder, and/or boiled, roasted, or otherwise cooked – including then pulverizing them into bean paste or hummus. Even today there are those who avoid eating nuts, beans, legumes, and seeds, and they find their health is perfectly fine on a diet consisting of some combination of fruits, vegetables, and sprouts, including in juices, smoothies, salads, fermented foods, and other concoctions.

Soaking was an ancient food prep practice

Ancient peoples may not have known about the reactions that could result when eating unsoaked grains, beans, legumes, seeds, and nuts. One reason they soaked them is it makes them easier to chew, and, as mentioned earlier, because soaking makes them softer, which resulted in less fuel (wood, or other matter) to cook them into a more easily chewed state. They didn't know soaking and fermenting also helped to deactivate and break down what we now both accurately and inaccurately call antinutrients, including phytates, complex sugars, tannins, certain enzyme inhibitors, and so forth.

Activating raw nuts, seeds, beans, legumes, and grains by soaking them makes them more nutrient dense, and the nutrients more bioavailable. It triggers them to begin producing more nutrients in the form of antioxidants, vitamins, and amino acids needed for the seed to grow into a plant.

Use glass, ceramic, or stone containers for soaking. Don't use aluminum, plastic, or wax-, silicon-, or Teflon-coated containers.

Beans and oligosaccharides

Hard beans, including adzuki, black beans, kidney beans, mung beans, navy beans, and pinto beans, contain complex sugars called oligosaccharides. These substances are not broken down by the digestive system. Instead, oligosaccharides can ferment in the digestive tract, resulting in gas. This is another reason why it is good to get your beans raw, then soak them in water for a few hours before rinsing, and then boiling or compression steaming them.

Soak water: dispose of it

Be sure to dispose of the soak water. Do not use it to boil the beans, legumes, rice, or grains. Do not use it in recipes.

The soak water is good for watering plants, and putting in your compost bin.

Chickpea germinating

Chickpeas that have been soaked to soften them are often eaten by those who follow a "living foods" diet. Anyone following the diet avoids anything that had been cooked, baked, steamed, boiled, toasted, grilled, or otherwise flamed.

It is good to soak chickpeas before steaming, boiling, or otherwise cooking. One reason is it rids them of enzyme inhibitors, making the beans easier to digest. Another is to increase the nutrient content.

Use about three times more water in volume than the amount of chickpeas = one cup of dried chickpeas and three cups of water. The beans will become plump as they absorb water. As they soak, the peal will making snapping noises.

Chickpeas that have been soaked can be used to blend into raw hummus.

Change the water after about 10 to 12 hours – which might be all you need to soak them… depending on how warm the day is. If it is a hot day, you might find it is best to soak them for no more than ten hours – so they don't get to the rooting stage.

As with other beans, don't use the soak water to boil or steam* the beans. Use a fresh pot of water for boiling. (*While it is okay to steam chickpeas, other beans, including – kidney beans – should be boiled so the temperature gets hot enough to eliminate the phytohemagglutinin toxins.)

Some people add a little baking soda and/or salt to the soak water as it helps to break down the coating or peal.

"Milan-Noris, et. Al. discovered that germinated chickpeas possessed a great potential to exert anti-inflammatory effects in the lower gut which enhanced the prevention of bowel inflammatory diseases. According to the researchers, sprouted chickpeas are abundant in peptides, proteins, and isoflavones which have beneficial effects in the gut health. In pardine lentils and green peas, sprouting was reported to reduce gas production by the gut microbiome, thereby reducing flatulence caused when raw seeds are consumed. Therefore, consuming sprouted seeds could improve the gut function and reduce negative outcomes associated with raw seed meals. In general, sprouting is marked by synthesis of bioactive molecules which may possess great benefits to the gut health."
    – Edible Plant Sprouts: Health Benefits, Trends, and Opportunities for Novel Exploration; *Nutrients* journal; Aug. 2021

Beans to NOT root or sprout: know your beans

Do not soak these beans to the point of them having a root: Adzuki beans, black beans, black eyed peas, cannellini beans, great northern beans, lentils, lima beans, navy beans, peas, pinto beans, red kidney beans, white kidney beans, or white butter beans.

If the bean is broadly- or flat-shaped, avoid eating it raw. Do not eat them germinated and uncooked (soaked in water and unheated). Do not eat them as sprouts (raw or cooked). Sprouted means if they have begun to grow a root, and/or have begun splitting to form a leaf.

Phytohaemagglutinin and linamarin

Certain beans form phytohaemagglutinin. When eaten raw, they can cause gastroenteritis.

Some beans also form linamarin that breaks down into cyanide in the digestive tract.

"Among the lectins known to have toxic effects is phytohemagglutinin, which occurs at relatively high levels in the seeds of legumes (i.e. beans). Phytohemagglutinin is involved in defense against plant pests and pathogens.

Phytohemagglutinin, as its name implies, can agglutinate many mammalian red blood cells, and interfere with cellular metabolism. Moreover, phytohemagglutinin is an antinutrient, which can interfere with the absorption of minerals, particularly calcium, iron, phosphorus, and zinc.

Phytohemagglutinin is found in many beans, but the level varies among different species of beans. The concentration of phytohemagglutinin is the highest in red kidney beans. White kidney beans (Phaseolus vulgaris), another variety of P. vulgaris, contain about one-third the amount of toxin as does the red variety.
– Phytohemagglutinin poisoning, by Dr. Jon Lum; Centre for Food Safety; Nov. 2023

Hemagglutinins (haemagglutinins)

Red kidney beans have been identified as having the highest amount of hemagglutinins.

Hemagglutinins are substances that cause the agglutination of red blood cells, and also interfere with cellular metabolism processes.

Small doses of ricin, the toxic hemmagglutinin lectin extract of the castor bean, can kill a human.

Kidney beans should be boiled until soft using high heat.

If soaked kidney beans get beyond the activated stage, and turn into germinates – with a root, a stem, or a sprout (with leaves), they should NOT be eaten, even if cooked, as they can sicken you. Toss them into the compost.

Phytohemagglutinins

Phytohemagglutinins in germinated or sprouted adzuki beans, black beans, black eyed peas, lentils, lima beans, peas, and white butter beans can be problematic. Soak them for fewer than three hours, and boil them at high heat until soft.

In other words, hemagglutinins are toxic. Because cooking destroys the hemagglutinins, these foods should be consumed only in a well-boiled stage. Steaming them may not get them hot enough to destroy the toxin. So, boil them.

"Although lectins are fairly resistance to enzymatic digestion in the gastrointestinal tract, they can be removed from foods by various processes. For example, soaking, autoclaving (pressurized steaming), and boiling causes irreversible lectin degeneration. Boiling legumes for one hour reduced hemagglutinating activity by 93.77 - 99.81%. Adeparusi et al. found that autoclaving lima beans for 20 minutes eliminated all anti-nutrients except tannins. Boiling of red and white kidney beans, notoriously rich in phytohemagglutinin (PHA), also resulted in complete elimination of lectins. Microwave ovens on the other hand, are not an effective method for lectin deactivation. Though microwaving destroyed hemagglutinins in most legume seeds, it did not significantly affect lectins in common beans. Additionally, fermentation over 72 hours has been demonstrated to destroy almost all lectins in lentils.

The safety and overall health effects of dietary lectins has long been a topic of concern among researchers, with some suggesting that they are harmful to health, hence the term 'anti-nutrients.' Cases of food poisoning involving raw or inadequately cooked legumes are well documented. For example, in the UK between 1976 and 1989, 50 cases of food poisoning were suspected to be caused by inadequately prepared kidney beans. PHA toxicity, caused by consumption of fresh kidney beans, is also common in China, and affected over 7,000 individuals between 2004 and 2013. In all cases, beans were either consumed raw, soaked, or cooked using temperatures inadequate to destroy PHA. Nonetheless, PHA toxin appears to be eliminated by 10 minutes of boiling. Mechanistically, lectins and hemagglutinins are resistant to digestion by both host enzymes and bacteria, and therefore pass through the gastrointestinal tract functionally and immunologically intact. Upon arrival into the small intestine, lectins can bind to glycan receptors and glycoconjugates on the luminal surface of enterocytes.

Overall, research does demonstrate that lectin-rich foods, if not prepared properly, can lead to food poisoning. However, traditional processes such as soaking, sprouting, fermenting, boiling, and autoclaving care all methods that can significantly reduce lectin content. In the case of high-lectin legumes, such as soybeans and kidney beans, boiling or autoclaving is required to eliminate lectins, as reduced cooking temperatures do not significantly affect lectin content."
– Is There Such a Thing as "Anti-Nutrients"? A Narrative Review of Perceived Problematic Plant Compounds; *Nutrients Journal*; Sept. 2020

In other words, thoroughly boil beans until they are soft.

Soak kidney beans, white beans, and larger – flat or broad – beans for only up to a few hours, then boil.

Lentils, garbanzo beans/chickpeas, black beans, and pinto beans can be soaked for longer – 10 to 12 hours.

When in doubt of which beans can be soaked for longer, simply only soak the for fewer than four hours, then boil thoroughly.

Also, if you are using purchased bean powders, consider soaking them for a couple of hours before cooking, to make sure they are also free of the anti-nutrients, and thoroughly cooked.

Lentils and peas

People often make lentils and split peas without soaking them. Like other legumes, it is good to activate lentils and split peas before using. That is, soaking in water for a few hours.

What to put in the soak water

Some people use a little salt or baking soda in the soak water when soaking legumes as these help to disable the enzyme inhibitors. Others say you should skip the salt or baking soda, because it makes it take longer to cook the beans. Instead, add a little apple cider vinegar, or freshly squeezed lemon or lime juice to the soak water. Or, first add salt and baking soda, soak for an hour, then rinse. Then do the water with the lemon or lime juice for a couple of hours.

Changing the soak water after a couple hours can help in the activation process.

Experiment and learn for yourself. You will figure out your own way.

You might be one who doesn't add anything to the soak water. Know why, or why not.

Soaking nuts and seeds

When soaking raw nuts, including almonds, Brazil nuts, hazelnuts, macadamia, pecans, pine nuts, pistachio, and walnuts, and also seeds like pumpkin, fenugreek, and sesame, use one-quarter teaspoon of natural, unprocessed sea salt, pink salt, or other natural salt in the water per cup of nuts or seeds.

Cashews are not truly raw, even if they are labeled as "raw," and there is no need for soaking to activate cashews. Living foodists might not use cashews. Soaking does soften them, if you need them to be that way for certain recipes.

The Aztecs traditionally soaked pumpkin seeds in salt water.

After an hour or two, you may want to strain the water and add more, and let them soak for another few hours. If you are in warm climate (soak for less time), or longer for a cold climate.

When done soaking, strain and spread the nuts or seeds on a ceramic platter and put them in a barely warm (not hot) oven, or briefly in the sun, or on a dehydrator sheet and dehydrate on low heat to fully dry. Or on a bamboo or other untreated wood board, or a clean, natural fiber cloth (not synthetic).

If you are going to store the activated nuts or seeds, make sure they are well dried. Keep them in a sealed container in the refrigerator or other cool storage. Glass containers work well.

Phytates / phytic acid

Phytic acid (myo-inositol hexakisphosphate, or InsP6) in grains, beans, legumes, nuts, and seeds stores phosphorus, which is used as the seeds sprout and grow.

Phytic acid binds with minerals in food to form phytate. The minerals include calcium, chromium, iron, magnesium, manganese, and zinc.

As a beneficial nutrient, phytate is a substance that is an antioxidant and anti-inflammatory, antimicrobial, anti-diabetic, an anti-carcinogen, and is neuroprotective (including against Alzheimer's), and it is protective of the bones and against bone loss. Phytate is protective of the macro- and microvascular systems – including in the kidneys. And phytate helps to prevent formation of calcium oxalate kidney stones.

While some people call phytate an "antinutrient," it both is and is not quite that, as it both apparently can interfere with mineral absorption, but also absolutely does have nutritional benefits. A well-rounded diet with foods that have phytic acid and foods that do not will provide adequate mineral content, and a person is unlikely to be bothered by the phytate content of their foods.

There is a mix of information to know about phytate. Do some research and discover it for yourself, including how phytates protect health – including everything from the bones, to the brain and nerves, and the kidneys to the eyes and cardiovascular system.

A meal high in phytic acid can reduce the mineral absorption for that meal as it binds with minerals. This is one of the reasons why people get raw, uncooked, untoasted, viable nuts, grains, beans, legumes, and seeds, and soak them before use. The soaking, sprouting, and fermentation breaks down the phytic acid. This includes sourdough bread, which is fermented. The process of yeast leavening bread also breaks down phytic acid. (As always, avoid breads containing potassium bromate or potassium bromide.)

To improve mineral ingestion, eat more green leafy vegetables, including adding pinches of nori (seaweed) powder or nori flakes to your smoothies, salads, soups, bowls, and other dishes.

Onions, garlic, chives, leeks, shallots, and green onions in bean dishes help with the absorption of minerals, including iron and zinc.

While it is good to enliven – soak, blossom, sprout, germinate, and ferment – foods, you likely are not going to get rid of all phytic acid from your diet. Nor should you aim to eliminate phytic acid from your diet, because, as mentioned, the resulting phytate is a nutrient.

Sometimes you'd have a low-phytate meal, and other meals with phytates. But, don't be so focused on it. Simply eat a variety of foods throughout a week, and you will benefit by the variety of nutrients.

"Phytic acid can affect how the body absorbs some minerals, including iron. It may contribute to mineral deficiencies over time, but this is rarely a concern for people who eat well-balanced diets."
– Phytic Acid 101: Everything You Need to Know; Healthline; Nov. 2023

"Phytate (myo-inositol hexakisphosphate or Insp6) is the main phosphorus reservoir that is present in almost all whole grains, legumes, and oilseeds. It is a major component of the Mediterranean and Dietary Approaches to Stop Hypertension (DASH) diets. Phytate is recognized as a nutraceutical and is classified by the Food and Drug Administration as Generally Recognized As Safe (GRAS). Phytate has been shown to be effective in treating or preventing certain

103

diseases. Phytate has been shown to inhibit calcium salt crystallization and, therefore, to reduce vascular calcifications, calcium renal calculi, and soft tissue calcifications. Moreover, the absorption of phytate to the crystal faces can inhibit hydroxyapatite dissolution and bone resorption, thereby playing a role in the treatment/prevention of bone mass loss. Phytate has a potent antioxidation and anti-inflammatory action. It is capable of inhibiting lipid peroxidation through iron chelation, reducing iron-related free radical generation. As this has the effect of mitigating neuronal damage and loss, phytate shows promise in the treatment/prevention of neurodegenerative disease. It is reported that phytate improves lipid and carbohydrate metabolism, increases adiponectin, decreases leptin, and reduces protein glycation, which is linked with macrovascular and microvascular diabetes complications.

When phytate is consumed in large amounts, by itself and without being processed/cooked, it can reduce the absorption of some minerals. This has led to phytate being classified by some authors as an antinutrient. Nevertheless, this effect is only seen in laboratory conditions, and real-world data in humans do not demonstrate mineral deficiencies induced by phytate intake. Phytate is instead considered a nutraceutical: a compound that could threat or prevent disease or disorders through a variety of bioactive (e.g., antioxidant, immunomodulatory, lipid lowering) functions. These properties and multiple health benefits have been repeatedly seen in the scientific literature."
– Phytate Intake, Health and Disease; *Antioxidants* journal; Jan. 2023

Coconuts

Like other nuts and seeds, coconuts contain phytic acid – however, they contain lower amounts than other nuts.

The phytate content in coconut is why some living foodists will ferment coconut meat into raw vegan yogurt – in a sanitary process that can take days – by blending or mashing the coconut meat. With that, they add vegan probiotics, and let it sit at room temperature in a bowl covered with a <u>clean</u> cloth for a day, or two. (Don't add salt.)

People who have had stomach or intestinal upset often find fermented coconut yogurt rich in probiotics to be soothing.

I have never had a bad reaction to coconut.

The phytate content in coconut is one reason why people who are otherwise raw vegans may eat coconut that has been heated or steamed, or dehydrated, which are processes that can reduce the phytates.

If someone were to heat coconut, the young coconut meat is somewhat liquid, or gel-like, and would need to be heated in a double boiler. The harder coconut meat can be steamed in a vegetable steamer.

I don't typically eat heated coconut. I do eat raw coconut, and drink coconut water (or make a chia seed pudding with coconut water or mashed young coconut meat). I also sometimes have fermented coconut yogurt we make at home. Or, I purchase GTs coconut yogurt (sold in many natural foods stores in the U.S.), as he uses high quality probiotics.

Chia, flax, and buckwheat seeds

Chia seeds, flax seeds, and buckwheat can quickly become mucilaginous (coated with a gel) when soaking, so it can be a bit difficult to strain them. This gel is rich in enzymes.

Chia seeds quickly germinate, and are pretty much impossible to dry out, so they need to be used within minutes, hours, or a day of soaking. They can also be added to coconut yogurt, and to overnight (soaked) oats.

Flax seeds that are wet tend to stick to anything, and need to be used in recipes soon after soaking. They also can be dried in a dehydrator or through other drying means – including to turn them into crackers. (On YouTube: See videos about how to make flax crackers.)

Buckwheat can be strained and rinsed in a mesh strainer and kept in the fridge for use within coming days, and can also be dried, such as in a dehydrator. They can be one of the ingredients in crust, in a breakfast dish, or in fermented vegan cheese. Buckwheat can also be ground into flour, then mixed with water and used to make buckwheat bread.

Rejuvelac

Buckwheat water can be fermented – in a container covered with a paper or tight, clean cloth, and kept at room temperature. If it turns black, or smells badly, toss it – or use it to water plants.

First, rinse the buckwheat in a strainer, moving them around to rid them of dust.

Then, put them in a ceramic, glass, or stainless steel container, and add filtered water. Soak them for a day. Strain the water into another clean container, cover with a clean cloth, and keep at room temperature in a dry room free of dust, mold, and mildew. After a day to three you will notice the water has fermented.

Fermented buckwheat water should be clear and have a nice, fermented scent. Some describe it as a sweet scent, and which might have a sort of light sting when tasted.

This fermented buckwheat water is called rejuvelac, which some people drink as it is a "fermented food." Some stores sell rejuvelac.

The fermented buckwheat water – rejuvelac – can be used as soak water to make fermented nut and seed cheeses blended with vegan probiotics. One of these cheeses involves soaking raw/untoasted pine nuts in rejuvelac for a day, then blending. Place in a covered bowl, and then stir in nutritional yeast and herbs. Let it sit in the covered bowl for one more day. It can be used as a soft, spreadable cheese, or dehydrated into a flaky cheese for salads.

Bean powders

If you purchase bean powders, "instant beans," and "instant falafel" products that you add water to before eating, and other such processed and "instant" foods, you may want to consider how you feel after consuming them. If you experience digestive upset, the beans may not have been cooked thoroughly enough to rid them of hemagglutinins. Some people discourage the use of these "instant" bean products, including because they can be high in salt, and may contain low-quality ingredients.

People might also discourage eating canned beans – which may not have been soaked before cooking, and may not have been thoroughly cooked (and can contain a variety of toxins leached from the chemicals in the lining of the can). I almost completely avoid canned foods. Including because they typically have high salt content.

Lentils and hemagglutinin

You may say you consume germinated or sprouted lentils all the time in your salad. Pay attention, and consider how you feel after eating soaked, germinated, or sprouted lentils. If you feel they are giving you intestinal discomfort, discontinue eating them raw.

Hemagglutinin poisoning may include digestive upset, cramping, abdominal pain, headache, nausea, and diarrhea. You may want to stick to well-boiled lentils.

Amaranth and rices, millet, quinoa, and oats

Amaranth, brown rice, buckwheat, millet, quinoa, wild rice, and steel cut oats can all be soaked for two to several hours before use in various recipes, including those for breakfast cereals, cobbler, granola, and pie crusts. Rinse them in a screen strainer to rid them of dust before soaking. It can also be helpful to add a little bit (a tablespoon per cup of grain) of an acidic ingredient to the soaking water, such as apple cider vinegar, or freshly squeezed lemon or lime juice. Do not use salt when soaking grains. After soaking for two to several hours (fewer hours if it is a warm day), strain out the soak water.

Raw grain flours can also be mixed with water several hours before use. Obviously, flours can't be strained. Simply then use the wet flour in recipes. Those who do soak their flours have found the subsequent food to be lighter, fluffier, and might have a more pleasing taste. Some call this "blossoming" the flour. (Avoid flours that have had potassium bromate added.)

Bread: gluten free sourdough

Read up about how sourdough bread is made in a traditional manner, by fermenting the flour. The fermenting process and soaking gluten grains (wheat, rye, barley, bulgur, durum, kamut, semolina, spelt, triticale) can help to break down gluten. But there may still be some reaction in people sensitive to gluten.

Brown rice flour, psyllium, and ground flax can be used to make fermented sourdough bread so there is no concern about reactions to gluten. The sourdough starter also needs to be gluten free.

Some use buckwheat flour in gluten free sourdough. Buckwheat isn't "wheat," or even officially a grain, but can be used like one. It is a pseudograin, is gluten free, and contains anti-inflammatory properties. Buckwheat flour is also known as kasha flour or beech wheat flour. You might notice those listed as ingredients on gluten free sourdough bread labels.

Can bread give you cancer? Potassium bromate and potassium iodate: the flour additives to avoid

Many of the food additives in processed foods have specific negative impacts on the kidneys.

Potassium bromate and potassium iodate are two ingredients people with kidney issues should know about – and watch out for – when purchasing bread, and other baked items containing flour.

"For over nine decades, potassium bromate has been widely used as a flour additive because it is an excellent dough improver and a maturing agent. In the late dough stage, potassium bromate oxidizes the sulphydryl groups of flour's gluten protein, making the dough less extensible and more elastic such that it can retain the carbon dioxide gas produced by the yeast used in leavening. It also bleaches the dough, increases loaf volume, and improves bread texture. Moreover, potassium bromate is probably the cheapest and most effective oxidizer used in bread production, and bakeries exploit these beneficial properties for profit. During baking, heat catalyzes the conversion of potassium bromate into a less toxic substance (potassium bromide). However, excessive use of potassium bromate results in residual concentrations in bread having potentially harmful effects.

Free radicals of potassium bromate in the human blood result in nephrotoxicity and cancer. It also induces renal cell tumors, mesotheliomas, and thyroid follicular cell tumors in rats. In addition, it exerts mutagenic effects and causes injury to the tissues of the central nervous system and kidneys."
– Potassium bromate in bread, health risks to bread consumers and toxicity symptoms amongst bakers in Bamenda, North West Region of Cameroon; *Heliyon*; Jan. 2023

Potassium bromate, which is often added to flour as a bleaching agent, and to improve the texture and volume of baked goods has been identified in animal studies as damaging to DNA, and increasing the risks of experiencing gastrointestinal, kidney, and thyroid cancers. Potassium bromate has been classified as a possible carcinogen by the International Agency for Research on Cancer.

"Potassium iodate is sometimes used as a dough strengthener in bread and rolls. Some bakers may switch to this ingredient when they stop using its chemical cousin potassium bromate, which poses a small cancer risk. However, potassium iodate, too, is not well tested, and may also pose a slight cancer risk.

A committee of the World Health Organization concluded that use of potassium iodate as a flour treatment agent was unacceptable because it could result in excessive intake of iodine."
– Potassium iodate; Center for Science in the Public Interest; Feb. 2022

Potassium iodate may increase blood potassium levels, and cause retinal pigmentary abnormalities, and impair retinal function.

People with cardiovascular or kidney disease, and diabetes and other autoimmune disorders – and anyone wanting to protect their vision – should avoid foods containing this additive.

"The European Union banned it [potassium bromate] in 1990. Canada and Nigeria followed shortly after. Over the last 30 years, various countries such as Brazil, Columbia, Sri Lanka, India, Saudi Arabia, Egypt, China, South Korea, Australia, and New Zealand have prohibited the use of potassium bromate and iodate in baked goods."

– Beyond Bromate: Healthier & More Sustainable Baked Goods; Novonesis.com; Jan. 2025

"Potassium bromate can affect you when breathed in and by passing through your skin.

Potassium bromate should be handled as a carcinogen – with extreme caution.

Contact can irritate and burn the skin and eyes.

Breathing potassium can irritate the nose, throat, and lungs, causing coughing, wheezing, and/or shortness of breath.

Repeated exposure to potassium bromate may affect the nervous system, causing headache, irritability, impaired thinking, and personality changes.

Potassium bromate may damage the kidneys.

This chemical is on the *Special Health Hazard Substance List* because it is a carcinogen."

– Hazardous Substance Fact Sheet, New Jersey Department of Health and Senior Services; July 2005

People who work in bakeries using potassium bromate have experienced symptoms identified as potassium bromate toxicity, including respiratory issues, sore throats, eye pain, abdominal pain, and diarrhea. This includes because the additive ends up in the vapor emitted by the baking bread.

"EWF has identified over 200 products that contain potassium bromate, including Gomez flour tortillas, Hy Vee blueberry crisp, and Hanover baked sourdough soft pretzels, among others. The use of this additive in the U.S. is widespread and legal, even though it's been banned in other countries because of health concerns.

In 1999, the World Health Organization's cancer arm, the International Agency for Research on Cancer, echoing the findings of several studies, determined potassium bromate may cause cancer in humans.

In lab tests, animals exposed to potassium bromate had increased incidence of both benign and malignant tumors in the thyroid and peritoneum, the membrane lining the abdominal cavity. Later research found that ingesting the additive increased cancer of the animals' thyroid, kidneys, and other organs.

The food industry has long argued that potassium bromate isn't a concern in baked products, because in theory the baking process fully converts it into potassium bromide, which is similar but does not cause cancer. But tests in the U.K. found that potassium bromate remains detectable after baking, with all six unwrapped breads and seven out of 22 packaged breads tested found to have measurable levels."

– This cancer-causing chemical may be lurking in your bread; Environmental Working Group; May 2022

Those are some of the risks associated with only one of the many additives used in processed foods.

Because additives in the foods you eat eventually make it into your blood system, and go through your kidneys, it is a good idea to follow a diet free from ultra-processed foods and the chemicals they contain. Especially if you already have kidney issues.

Some U.S. states, including California, are taking actions to ban the sale of foods containing potassium bromate. Because the California economy is so large, some large food companies will stop adding potassium bromate to the foods they sell in all U.S. states.

Read food labels. If a food ingredient label lists potassium bromate or potassium bromide, don't buy it.

Learn to make sourdough bread from scratch. Don't use cookware coated with toxic non-stick chemical surfaces. You don't need a bread making machine. People have been making fermented bread for thousands of years using the most basic tools made of stone and/or ceramics.

Advanced glycation end products: AGEs, inflammation, and disease

I've known of advanced glycation end products (AGEs) for decades. I learned about them while recovering from kidney failure, and as I was working to improve my diet to be kidney safe.

I'm amazed by how most people STILL don't know about AGEs. It's perplexing that doctors aren't telling their patients to follow a low-AGEs diet to prevent and reduce intestinal issues, inflammation, and chronic and degenerative diseases. But then, look at hospital foods, rich in exactly the substances that increase the risks of experiencing intestinal issues, inflammation, and chronic and degenerative diseases. Many people working in the healthcare field also regularly eat foods rich in AGEs.

"Over the past two decades there has been increasing evidence supporting an important contribution from food-derived advanced glycation end products (AGEs) to the body pool of AGEs and therefore increased oxidative stress and inflammation, processes that play a major role in the causation of chronic diseases.

AGEs are important in clinical science because they are associated with oxidative stress and inflammation, processes that eventually cause most chronic diseases, including cardiovascular disease, diabetes, chronic kidney disease, and neurodegenerative disease. Of note, AGEs cause oxidative stress, but oxidative stress leads to AGE formation [formed within the body = endogenous AGEs].

AGEs were first recognized as endogenous compounds that formed in excess in diabetes due to hyperglycemia. It is now clear that they can also be generated in conditions of increased oxidative stress, even in the absence of hyperglycemia. Moreover, increasing evidence points to exogenous AGEs (derived mostly from food and tobacco) as important contributors to the body's AGE pool, where they become indistinguishable from endogenous AGEs, both in structure and function.

The main factors determining the rate of AGE formation in food include nutrient composition (protein > fat > carbohydrate), temperature, and duration of heat application, humidity, pH, and the presence of trace metals."

– Dietary Advanced Glycation End Products and Their Role in Health and Disease; *Advances in Nutrition* journal; July 2015

"AGEs form when sugar interacts with proteins or fats in the bloodstream. The process is called glycation.

High levels of AGEs have been linked to inflammation, oxidative stress, Alzheimer's, diabetes, heart disease, and renal failure.

Overeating and obesity are known to cause serious health problems. They increase your risk of developing insulin resistance, diabetes, and heart disease.

However, studies have found that harmful compounds called advanced end products (AGEs) may also have a powerful effect on your metabolic health – regardless of your weight.

AGEs accumulate naturally as you age, and are created when certain foods are cooked at high temperatures.

Diet is the biggest contributor of AGEs.

While low levels are generally nothing to worry about, high levels have been shown to cause oxidative stress and inflammation. In fact, high levels have been linked to the development of many diseases, including diabetes, heart disease, kidney failure, and Alzheimer's, as well as premature aging."

– What Are Advanced Glycation End Products (AGEs)?; Healthline.com

Learning about AGEs

When learning about advanced glycation end products (AGEs), keep in mind that your body can form AGEs, especially when certain diseases are in play, which can then also advance chronic and degenerative conditions, including cardiovascular, liver, and kidney disease, autoimmune issues, and neurodegenerative disorders like Alzheimer's, Parkinson's, and ALS. You can trigger the body to form more AGEs by eating an unhealthful diet.

You ingest AGEs when you are eating low-quality foods, and especially those cooked at high temperatures, and also by eating meat, dairy, and eggs, because of their protein and fat mix.

"One study examined a group of 559 older women and found those with the highest blood levels of AGEs were almost twice as likely to die from heart disease than those with the lowest levels. [citing: Advanced glycation end products and their circulating receptors predict cardiovascular disease mortality in older community-dwelling women; *Aging Clinical and Experimental Research* journal; April 2009]

Another study found that among a group of individuals with obesity, those with metabolic syndrome had higher blood levels of AGEs than those who were otherwise healthy. [citing: Elevated serum advanced glycation end products in obese indicate risk for the metabolic syndrome: a link between health and unhealthy obesity?; *Journal of Clinical Endocrinology & Metabolism*; Feb. 2015]

Women with polycystic ovary syndrome, a hormonal condition in which levels of estrogen and progesterone are unbalance, have been shown to have higher levels of AGEs than women without the condition. [citing: Increased levels of serum advanced glycation end products in women with polycystic ovary syndrome; *Clinical Endocrinology* journal; Jan. 2005]"

– What Are Advanced Glycation End Products?: When AGEs accumulate, they can seriously damage health, by Mary Jane Brown, Pd.D., RD; Healthline.com; Oct. 2019

AGEs can bind with receptors on cell membranes, increasing inflammation, oxidative stress, and other adverse health responses. Even the presence of AGEs in the body increases oxidative stress, raises the risk of experiencing diabetes, and the risks of tissue injury, including of the cardiovascular system, brain, nerves, digestive tract, kidneys, and other organs.

AGEs increase the risk of experiencing chronic and degenerative conditions, including metabolic disease, renal dysfunction, and neurodegenerative diseases like Alzheimer's, Parkinson's, and amyotrophic lateral sclerosis (ALS).

AGEs increase the risks of experiencing various types of cancer.

All of the types of glycoxidative damage, biochemical abnormalities, and/or instabilities, or otherwise tissue degradation from AGEs are encouraged through a diet rich in AGEs.

AGEs break down in the body, and are eliminated through the kidneys.

A key to better health is to ingest fewer AGEs, this means doing so through a plant-based diet rich in raw fruits, vegetables, and sprouts, and other plant matter, and staying away from highly processed foods. This will reduce your AGEs intake, and also prevent conditions that could lead your system to produce more AGEs.

Phytochemicals (substances in plants) have been identified as helping to prevent AGE formation within the body. These substances include flavonoids (including quercetin), phenolic acids, and stilbenes, which are all polyphenols. Vitamin C also helps prevent internal formation of AGEs. (Research: polyphenols and polyphenol-rich foods.)

Reducing and inhibiting AGEs formation in the body

Plants and plant-derived substances that help inhibit the formation of advanced glycation end products include:
- Anti-inflammatories found in plants.
- Antioxidants found in plants.
- Green tea.
- Padma 28 and Padma Circosan herb mixes.
- Polyphenols. Many types of these are found in fruits, vegetables, sprouts, nuts, seeds, grains, beans, legumes, and seaweeds. They work as anti-inflammatories and antioxidants.
- Quercetin. One of the polyphenols classified as a flavonoid and identified as a strong antioxidant.
- Vitamin C. Better to obtain by eating raw fruits and vegetables, and not through vitamin pills.

The low-AGE diet

Basically, a low-AGE diet is a plant-based diet rich in raw fruits, vegetables, and sprouts, but that avoids processed foods, synthetic food chemicals, and highly heated foods.

It is foods that have been grilled, griddled, fried, broiled, roasted, seared, toasted, or otherwise cooked at high heat that contain AGEs. Meat, dairy, and eggs – and especially processed meats – can be especially rich in AGE content.

Boiling, stewing, and steaming don't result in the abundance of heat-generated chemicals that other types of cooking create.

Heat-generated substances impacting health

The mitochondria located in each of our cells are damaged by the oxidative free radicals in meat, milk, and eggs, and highly heated oils. They are also damaged by the heat-generated substances called AGEs, and that have been identified as being genotoxic and carcinogenic. The heat-generated chemicals effect the nerve and brain function, and fertility, make allergies worse, and increase tissue inflammation – worsening arthritis, diabetes, lupus, asthma, and other autoimmune disorders.

The heat-generated substances include heterocyclic aromatic amines, c-monochloropropane-1-diol esters, glycidyl esters, acrylamides, furan, polycyclic aromatic hydrocarbons, and ethyl carbamate.

All sorts of highly-heated foods contain heat-generated chemicals. This includes everything from fried and oil sautéed foods to roasted foods (including coffee and nuts), and grilled, baked, smoked, toasted, torched, seared, griddled, and broiled foods. These are all: highly heated foods.

"What are heterocyclic amines and polycyclic aromatic hydrocarbons, and how are they formed in cooked meats?

Heterocyclic amines (HCAs), and polycyclic aromatic hydrocarbons (PAHs) are chemicals formed when meat – including beef, pork, fish, or poultry – is cooked using high-temperature methods, such as pan frying or grilling directly over an open flame. In laboratory experiments, HCAs and PAHs have been found to be mutagenic – that is, they cause changes in DNA that may increase risk of cancer.

HCAs are formed when amino acids (the building blocks of proteins), sugars, and creatine or creatinine (substances found in muscle) react at high temperatures. PAHs are formed when fat and juice from meat grilled directly over a heated surface or open fire drip onto the surface or fire, causing flames and smoke. The smoke contains PAHs that then adhere to the surface of the meat. PAHs can also be formed during other food preparation processes, such as smoking meats.

HCAs are not found in significant amounts in foods other than meat cooked at high temperatures. PAHs can be found in other smoked foods, as well as in cigarette smoke and car exhaust fumes.

Well-done, grilled, or barbequed chicken and steak all have high concentrations of HCAs. Cooking methods that expose meat to smoke contribute to PAH formation.

HCAs and PAHs become capable of damaging DNA only after they are metabolized by specific enzymes in the body, a process called 'bioactivation.' Studies have found that the activity of these enzymes, which can differ among people, may be relevant to the cancer risks associated with exposure to these compounds.

Studies have shown that exposure to HCAs and PAHs can cause cancer in animal models. In many experiments, rodents fed a diet supplemented with HCAs developed tumors of the breast, colon, liver, skin, lung, prostate, and other organs. Rodents fed PAHs also developed cancers, including leukemia and tumors of the gastrointestinal tract and lungs."

– National Cancer Institute; Chemicals in Meat Cooked at High Temperatures and Cancer Risk; July 2017

Heterocyclic aromatic amines

Heterocyclic aromatic amines are carcinogenic, pro-inflammatory substances formed when meat is exposed to high heat.

"Heterocyclic aromatic amines (HAAs) form when meat, poultry, and seafood are cooked at a high temperature. Frying, broiling, and grilling produce the largest amounts of HAAs, and polycyclic aromatic hydrocarbons."

– What are heterocyclic aromatic amines?; USDA; Feb. 2024

"Heterocyclic aromatic amines (HAAs) are types of poisonous compounds, which form during long-term cooking of protein-rich foods, such as meat and fish. Several studies have revealed that when meat-based foods are cooked with different cooking procedures, including roasting, grilling, barbecuing, frying, and smoking, the high temperature of these heating methods contributes to the formation of HAAs.

Several types of HAAs are reported as possible human carcinogens by the International Agency for Research on Cancer.

The trace amount of HAAs in cooked food can cause serious illness in human organs in the long term, and can finally bring about various types of cancers."

– Heterocyclic aromatic amines in cooked food: A review on formation, health risk-toxicology, and their analytical techniques; Science Direct; Dec. 2018

C-monochloropropane-1-diol esters

C-monochloropropane-1-diol esters have been classified as carcinogenic by the International Agency for Research on Cancer. The substances are a concern with extracted oils.

As this book suggests, greatly reduce or eliminate extracted oils, including olive oil, coconut oil, and any bottled oils, and foods containing them. Learn how to make foods from scratch without using bottled oils (Access: ForksOverKnives).

"3-monochloropropane-1, 2-diol esters (3-MCPDE) and glycidyl esters (GE) are contaminants that can occur in edible oils, such as vegetable oils, and foods made with these oils. Both food manufacturers and consumers use edible oils as an ingredient in foods and for cooking. During industrial refining, 3-MCPDE and GE can form in edible oils when the oils are heated at very high temperatures to remove unwanted tastes, colors, or odors. The highest concentrations typically occur in refined palm oil and palm olein oil, but 3-MCPDE and GE also are found in other refined vegetables oils (such as safflower, coconut, sunflower, and soybean oils) and refined marine oils (such as fish oils).

113

During digestion, 3-MCPDE and GE break down to the organic chemicals 3-monochloropropane-1, 2-diol (3-MCPD) and glycidol. In studies of rodents, 3-MCPD and glycidol caused cancer [of the kidneys and testes]."

— 3-Monochloropropane-1,2-diol (MDPD) Esters and Glycidyl Esters: Process contaminants in food; U.S. Food and Drug Administration; 2025

"Chloropropanols are foodborne contaminants that can be formed during the processing of various foodstuffs. This class of food contaminant was first recognized at the Institute of Chemical Technology in Prague in acid-hydrolyzed vegetable protein (HVP), a seasoning ingredient widely used in a variety of processed and prepared foods, such as soups, sauces, bouillon cubes, and soya sauce. 3-MCPD is the most abundant chloropropanol found in foodstuff, while 1.3-DCP generally occurs at lower levels.

During the last decade, renewed interest in chloropropanols and the development of analytical methods of their presence in food matrices other than acid-HVP was triggered by the detection of 3-MCPD in a wide range of foods and food ingredients, notably in thermally processed foods such as malts, cereal products, and meat. In addition, domestic processing (e.g. grilling and toasting) can produce substantial increases in the 3-MCPD content of bread or cheese.

Although the overall levels of 3-MCPD in bakery products are relatively low, the high level of consumption of bread, and its additional formation from toasting, indicate that this staple food alone can be a significant dietary source of 3-MCPD.

Concentrations of 3-MCPD above 0.02 mg/kg were recently found in smoked fermented sausages and smoked ham, and the smoking process was identified as a major source."

— 3-monochloro-1,2-propanediol; National Library of Medicine; 2010

"3-monochloropropan-1,2-diol is in vivo carcinogenic, and in vitro genotoxic. Glycidyl esters are suggested to be formed through an intermediate stage during 3-MCDP ester formation via monoacylglycerol-derived acyloxonium ion pathway. The free form of glycidyl is carcinogenic directly acting multisite mutagen in animal studies that reacts readily with cellular nucleophiles.

Frying oils that are transferred into the fried potatoes can be the main sources of 3-MCPD esters in fried potatoes. A potato, which contains carbohydrates, protein, fat, vitamins, and other minor constituents, can undergo a very complex chemical reaction with salt under prolonged high-temperature deep frying."

— Monitoring of heat-induced carcinogenic compounds (3-monochloropropane-1,2-diol esters and glycidyl esters) in fries; *Scientific Reports*; Sept. 2020

When I learned how toasting bread could increase the acrylamides and the 3-MCPD substances that are harsh on the kidneys, and doctors advised me to avoid toast, we got rid of the toaster. I have almost completely not had toast in decades.

Acrylamides

Acrylamides are in some cooked foods, and can be especially harsh for those who have kidney and cardiovascular disease, and autoimmune disorders.

Acrylamides form in vegetables containing the amino acid asparagine, including potatoes, and especially starches that have been browned to a crisp.

Acrylamides are in bread (especially toast and crust), crackers, cookies, cereals, canned black olives, coffee, French fries, and chips.

Acrylamides also are in tobacco smoke.

The amount of heat applied to the foods, and the length of time they are cooked plays a role in how much the acrylamides form.

Acrylamides are considered a nephrotoxin, meaning they can cause damage to the kidneys.

"Wet cooking," as in steaming, stewing, and boiling foods is safer for kidney patients.

Dry cooking includes baking, browning, frying, grilling, searing, broiling, griddling, and microwaving.

"Animal studies of the effects of acrylamides on kidney tissue have determined that degeneration in tubule and glomerular cells is caused by acrylamide-induced oxidative stress."
– Oleuropein Mitigates Acrylamide-Induced Nephrotoxicity by Affecting Placental Growth Factor Immunoactivity in the Rat Kidney; *Eurasian Journal of Medicine*; Oct. 2023

"Studies in rodent models have found that acrylamide exposure increases the risk for several types of cancer. In the body, acrylamide is converted to a compound called glycidamide, which causes mutations in and damage to DNA. However, a large number of epidemiologic studies in humans have found no consistent evidence that dietary acrylamide exposure is associated with the risk of any type of cancer. One reason for the inconsistent findings from human studies may be the difficulty in determining a person's acrylamide intake based on their reported diet.

The National Toxicology Program's Report on Carcinogens considers acrylamide to be reasonably anticipated to be a human carcinogen, based on studies in laboratory animals given acrylamide in drinking water. However, toxicology studies have shown that humans and rodents no only absorb acrylamide at different rates, they metabolize it differently as well."
– Acrylamide and Cancer Risk; National Cancer Institute; Dec. 2017

Ethyl carbamate

Ethyl carbamate is mostly a concern with alcoholic beverages.

It is good to mostly or completely stay away from alcoholic beverages.

Especially if a person has addiction issues: completely eliminate all distilled, brewed, and fermented alcohol drinks.

Alcohol is a leading cause of cancer

According to a 2025 U.S. Surgeon General advisory, alcohol is the third-leading preventable cause of cancer in the U.S. It is right behind tobacco and obesity.

Alcohol depletes folate and other B vitamins, which are keys in the immune system.

Alcohol forms unstable molecules known as free radicals, which can damage DNA. Also, alcohol is metabolized into acetaldehyde, which can then damage DNA, increasing the risk of uncontrolled cell division, which is cancer.

Cancers associated with alcohol consumption include those of the lips, mouth, throat, voice box, esophagus, stomach, liver, kidneys, bladder, colon, rectum, breast, and prostate.

Alcohol damages the gut microbiota and intestinal lining

Part of your defense against cancer, liver disease, and inflammation is a healthy gut microbiome, and a healthy gut lining. Alcohol damages the microbiome and intestinal lining, causes inflammation, and can damage the liver so badly a person can die.

"Studies highlight the importance of changes in the intestinal microbiota in alcohol-related disorders. Alcohol-induced changes in the gastrointestinal tract microbiota composition and metabolic function may contribute to the well-established link between alcohol-induced oxidative stress, intestinal hyperpermeability to liminal bacterial products, and the subsequent development of alcoholic liver disease, as well as other diseases. In addition, clinical and preclinical data suggest that alcohol-related disorders are associated with quantitative and qualitative dysbiotic changes in the intestinal microbiota, and may be associated with increases gastrointestinal tract inflammation, intestinal hyperpermeability resulting in endotoxemia, systemic inflammation, and tissue damage/organ pathologies, including alcoholic liver disease."
– The Gastrointestinal Microbiome: Alcohol Effects on the Composition of Intestinal Microbiota; *Alcohol Research* journal; 2015

"Alcohol is one of the many factors that disrupt the proper functioning of the gut, leading to a disruption of the intestinal barrier integrity that increases the permeability of the mucosa, with the final result of a disrupted mucosal immunity. This damage to the permeability of the intestinal membrane allows bacteria and their components to enter the blood, reaching other organs, such as the liver of the brain."
– The Immune System through the Lens of Alcohol Intake and Gut Microbiota; *International Journal of Molecular Science*; July 2021

Alcohol and a diet rich in animal protein

Alcohol can play a role in hypertension, stroke, and heart attack. The hypertension alone is enough to damage the kidneys. Magnify that if a person is consuming a diet rich in animal protein, which increases the risks of experiencing – among other things – hypertension, heart attack, stroke, cancer, and kidney damage. Magnify the risk factors more if the person is eating a diet rich in processed foods, fried foods, and a diet lacking fruits and vegetables.

Alcohol and smoking

Alcohol consumption among people who use tobacco products increases their risks of lip, mouth, tongue, throat, voice box, and lung cancers. This is because alcohol increases the absorption of carcinogens, magnifying risks.

Because what enters the body, is then worked by the system to get rid of toxins and waste, the alcohol and tobacco residue goes through the cardiovascular system, lymph system, liver, intestines, kidneys, and bladder, increasing the risks of damaging and causing problems with them.

Tobacco

Of course smoking is a trigger for lung and cardiovascular disease, and is harmful to the brain, nerves, liver, and kidneys.

Smoking not only increases the risk of lung diseases, but also can play a role in cancers of the mouth, throat, breasts, bladder, kidneys, uterus, and other organs, and of the blood, and the lymph system.

"Did you know that smoking could also harm your kidneys? People who smoke are more likely to have protein in the urine – a sign of kidney damage."
– 10 Common Habits That May Harm Your Kidneys; National Kidney Foundation; June, 2016

If you also follow an unhealthful diet, smoking cigarettes can magnify the health problems caused by bad diet.

I've known people who smoke cigarettes and have claimed their diet is so healthy it counteracts the problems cigarettes cause. That is wishful thinking. Even if they smoke "natural" cigarettes, they are still inhaling toxic gasses, which harm the lungs, and cause other damage throughout the body. Chemicals absorbed into the lungs also make their way into the kidneys.

Smoking can complicate pregnancy, and harm the fetus.

Smoking increases inflammation, and alter both the heart rate and blood pressure, playing a role in hypertension, including in the kidneys.

Smoking also can play a role in diabetes. This is especially so in those who already have compromised kidney function.

The fine blood passageways in the kidneys can become narrower from smoking, also interfering with kidney function and blood pressure, and causing renal hypertension.

If you want long-term good health – including healthy kidneys – don't smoke.

Alcohol altering hormone levels increases cancer risk

Women have a higher risk of cancer from alcohol consumption, including because one drink for the average-size women is stronger per body weight than the same drink for an average-size man.

Alcohol alters the levels of a variety of hormones, increasing the risk of cancer in the hormone-sensitive tissues of the breasts and prostate.

Alcohol is a preventable cause of cancer, and of other diseases

"Alcohol is a well-established, preventable cause of cancer responsible for about 100,000 cases of cancer, and 20,000 cancer deaths annually in the United States – greater than the 13,500 alcohol-associated traffic crash fatalities per year in the U.S. – yet the majority of Americans are unaware of the risks."
– Dr. Vivek Murthy, U.S. Surgeon General; Jan. 2025

Anyone with kidney, liver, bladder, nerve, cardiovascular, inflammatory, and autoimmune issues would be wise to avoid drinking alcoholic beverages.

Non-alcoholic "mocktails" are an option. Be careful of the sugar content. They should be the size of regular cocktails, and not big, and rich in calories.

Polycyclic aromatic hydrocarbons

"Polycyclic aromatic hydrocarbons (PAHs) are a group of contaminants produced by burning of carbon-based materials. They can get into food either from the environment or during food processing. Some PAHs are known to cause cancer because they can damage DNA."
– Polycyclic aromatic hydrocarbons; Food Standards Agency; Feb. 2024

"Polycyclic aromatic hydrocarbons are made whenever substances are burned. PAHs are also found at former coal-gasification sites. Breathing smoke or coming into contact with contaminated soil exposes people to PAHs. Some PAHs may cause cancer, and may affect the eyes, kidneys, and liver.
Barbecuing, smoking, or charring food over a fire greatly increases the amount of PAHs in food."
– Polycyclic Aromatic Hydrocarbons; Illinois Department of Health

"They can get into food either from the environment or during food processing. Some PAHs are known to cause cancer because they can damage DNA. It is therefore important that levels present in food are as low as reasonably achievable.
The following foods could contain PAHs:
• Bivalve shellfish accumulate PAHs from seawater and sediment. Limits are therefore applied to ensure that excessively-contaminated mussels or oysters do not enter the food chain.
• Smoked products
• Certain cooked meat products such as flame-grilled burgers
• Certain types of dried foods, including spices and plant or algae-based supplements can be susceptible to PAH contamination if not dried correctly."
– Polycyclic aromatic hydrocarbons; Food Standards Agency; Food.Gov.UK; Feb. 2024

"PAHs are a class of complex chemicals that are formed and released during incomplete combustion or pyrolysis (burning) of organic matter such as waste or food, during industrial processes and other human activities. PAHs are also formed in natural processes such as carbonization. Studies on individual PAHs in animals, mainly on the PAH benzo[a]pyrene, have shown various toxilogical effects, such as haematoxicity (effects on the blood), reproductive and developmental toxicity, and immunotoxicity. A number of PAHs have shown carcinogenic effects in experimental animals, and it has been concluded that benzo[a]pyrene is carcinogenic to humans.
There is concern therefore, about their formation and presence in food.
In food, PAHs may be formed during industrial processing and domestic food preparation, such as barbecuing, smoking, drying, roasting, baking, frying, or grilling. Direct fire-drying and heating processes used during the production of some oils of plant origin and in particular olive pomace oil (oil extracted from olive pulp after the first press) can result in high levels of PAHs.
The World Health Organization/Food and Agricultural Organization's Joint Expert Committee on Food Additives and Contaminants also concluded that PAHs are clearly genotoxic and carcinogenic."
– Polycyclic Aromatic Hydrocarbons in Food; Food Safety Authority of Ireland; June 2015

Furan

"Furan is a volatile compound formed mostly during the thermal processing of foods. The toxicity of furan has been well documented previously, and it was classified as 'possible human carcinogen' by the International Agency for Research on Cancer. Various pathways have been reported for the formation of furan, that is, thermal degradation and/or thermal rearrangement of carbohydrates in the presence of amino acids, thermal degradation of certain amino acids, including aspartic acid, threonine, a-alanine, serine, and cysteine, oxidation of ascorbic acid at higher temperatures. And oxidation of polyunsaturated fatty acids and carotenoids.

Furan is a colorless heterocyclic compound with high volatility, consisting of a five-membered aromatic ring with four carbon atoms and one oxygen atom. It has been reported that thermal processing is a main cause of furan formation. Thermal processing such as cooking, roasting, baking, pasteurization, and sterilization is involved in many food preparing processes, from the home kitchen to industrial food processing facilities, and it ensures the microbiological safety of the food for preservation and maintains particular sensory features. One of the known reactions during thermal processing is the Maillard reaction. This is a non-enzymatic browning reaction, which involves the reaction of amino acids, peptides, and proteins with reducing sugars and vitamin C."
– Furan in Thermally Processed Foods – A Review; *Toxicology Research* journal; Sept. 2015

Obesogens

Obesogens are chemicals and heavy metals that can alter lipid metabolism and the hormones. Obesogens can interfere with fat metabolism, and trigger the production of new fat cells.

The growing prevalence of these chemicals and heavy metals in food, water, and the general environment are among reasons why more people are classified as obese. A diet rich in obesogens and AGEs magnifies the problems.

"Because many known obesogens activate PPARy (peroxisome proliferator-activated receptor gamma plays a role in fatty acid uptake, fat storage, insulin sensitivity, glucose metabolism, and anti-inflammation) and induce adipogenesis (formation of adipose/fat tissue), PPARy activation is widely believed to be a major mechanism through which obesogens can contribute to obesity. PPARy continues to be the receptor most commonly targeted in screening assays for obesogens. However, recent studies have demonstrated alternative and novel mechanisms of obesogen action. These include activation of RXR to induce adipocyte lineage commitment and impair adipocyte health, activation of multiple other nuclear receptors, induction of epigenetic modifications in fat tissue, alteration of chromatin accessibility or architecture, and induction of gut microbiome dysbiosis. Thus, obesogens have a broad and diverse spectrum of actions."
– Environmental Obesogens and Their Impact on Susceptibility to Obesity: New Mechanisms and Chemicals, by Riann Jenay Eguquiza, and Bruce Bumberg; *Endocrinology Journal*; March 2020

Obesogens can bind with our cell receptors

Obesogens can bind with various receptors on our cells, including receptors for androgen (male hormone), estrogen (female hormone), and glucocorticoid (glucocorticoid plays a role in metabolism, the immune system, and functions as an anti-inflammatory).

Exposure to obesogens – and tissue reactions to them – can start in the womb as they are from what the mother eats, including processed and unhealthful foods, and from what she is exposed to, including pharmaceuticals, household cleaning products, laundry products, cosmetic, skin, and hair products, and environmental toxins.

"Obesogens are a type of endocrine-disrupting chemical.

Your endocrine system is made up of glands that make hormones. To put it simply, those hormones serve as your body's 'chemical messengers' that control many important parts and functions of your body.

Obesogens, as endocrine-disrupting chemicals, hijack that messenger system and can wreak havoc on your health in a variety of ways."
– Obesogens: Chemicals that cause weight gain: It's not all diet and exercise, by Gwen Ranniger; *Environmental Health News*; Dec. 2022

People exposed to obesogens in the womb might have health issues later in life relating to the early exposure.

"Virtually every country in the world has shown a dramatic increase in the prevalence of overweight and obesity since the 1980s. Rapidly changing dietary patterns, reductions in physical activity, and increased sedentary behavior are assumed to be the main drivers of this rising trend, but there is increasing concern that they do not adequately explain the epidemic levels of obesity.

Another suspect has emerged in the past decade, namely human exposure to endocrine disrupting chemicals (EDCs), also referred to as chemical obesogens. There are multiple sources of EDCs, from agricultural chemicals and cosmetic products to plastic particles and plasticizers used in the building trade, furniture, electronics, children's toys, and food packaging.

The plastic additive bisphenol A (BPA) is one of the most often cited potential obesogenic EDCs, and a meta-analysis of epidemiological surveys found that for every 1ng/mL increase in the concentration of urinary BPA, the odds of obesity rose by 15% for adults, and 17% for children. U.S. Centers for Disease Control and Prevention surveys show that the U.S. population typically has a concentration range from less than 1ng/mL to greater than 10ng/mL. In a 2013 study, children with the lowest quartile of urinary BPA concentration showed obesity prevalence of 10%, while children in the upper three quartiles showed obesity prevalence of 17-23%."
– Environmental chemical obesogens, what can we do?, *The Lancet: Diabetes and Endocrinology*; May 2024

"Adult and childhood obesity have reached pandemic level proportions. The idea that calorie excess and insufficient levels of physical activity leads to obesity is a commonly accepted answer for unwanted weight gain. This paradigm offers and inconclusive explanation as the world continually moves towards an unhealthier and heavier existence irrespective of energy balance. Endocrine disrupting chemicals (EDCs) are chemicals that resemble natural hormones and disrupt endocrine function by interfering with the body's endogenous hormones. A subset of EDCs called obesogens have been found to cause metabolic disruptions such as increased fat storage, in vivo. Obesogens act on the metabolic system through multiple avenues and have been found to affect the homeostasis of a variety of systems such as the gut microbiome and adipose tissue functioning. Obesogenic compounds have been shown to cause metabolic disturbances later in life that can even pass into multiple future generations, post exposure. The rising rates of obesity and related metabolic disease are demanding increasing attention on chemical screening efforts and worldwide prevention strategies to keep the public and future generations safe.

Obesity has become a present-day pandemic affecting people of all ages across the world. According to the World Health Organization, the prevalence of global obesity has nearly tripled since 1975 with a continued upward trajectory. In 2016, the WHO reported more than 1.9 billion adults as overweight, with 650 million of those adults as obese."

– Obesogens: How they are identified and molecular mechanisms underlying their action; *Frontiers of Endocrinology*; Nov. 2021

Obesogens can include, or be in:

- **Acrylamide**: As an industrial chemical, acrylamide is used in the manufacture of dyes, paper, cardboard, and other materials.

  Acrylamide is also formed in highly heated carbohydrates, including carbohydrates that are baked, fried, roasted, seared, grilled, and toasted. It is a pro-inflammatory, and can be rough on the cardiovascular and immune systems, and the kidneys. It is the first heat-generated chemical doctors told me to avoid.

- **Artificial sweeteners**: These include acesulfame potassium (Ace-K), saccharin, and sucralose.

  It is wise to avoid artificial sweeteners.

- **Bisphenol A** (BPA): Commonly in plastics, epoxy, and resins, and also in the lining canned foods and food packaging.

  Look for foods in containers and packaging free of BPA, but that might only mean that another bisphenol was used so the packaging could say "BPA free."

- **Bisphenol F** (BPF) **and Bisphenol S** (BPS): These are bisphenol A analogs that are also used in plastics. They also have endocrine disrupting properties.

- **Cadmium**: A heavy metal found in certain types of plastic, and also in tobacco smoke, and in higher rates than natural in polluted water, air, and land.

- **Carbendazim**: Used as a fungicide with uses as wide as in industrial farming, forestry, veterinary and medicine. It is an endocrine disrupter, and a carcinogen. In animal testing, it has been identified as toxic to the liver, and can play a role in diabetes.

- **Chlorpyrifos**: Pesticide used on produce. Read up about this pesticide, and it may help you decide to follow an organic diet.

- **Concentrated foods**: Especially those grown using synthetic farm chemicals. Concentrating the foods also concentrates the industrial chemical residues in them.

   Concentrated foods include sugar extracts, including fructose, and oils extracted from plants, including canola, corn, olive, sunflower, and other oils.

   Veggie broth is a concentrated food because it involves cooking down various herbs, and green leafy vegetables, and fruits like tomatoes and peppers, and root vegetables. Be sure to use organic ingredients.

   Concentrated or dehydrated foods made from chemically-grown and/or treated fruits, vegetables, nuts, seeds, beans, grains, and seaweeds contain more farming chemicals per weight than the same weight of fresh plant material.

   Concentrated foods also can include various forms of animal protein. Examples of concentrated animal protein includes cheeses, spreads, bone broth, meat broth, cartilage broth, gelatin (which is made from bones), gravy, jerky, and lard. As farmed animals bioaccumulate industrial pollutants, including agrichemicals used on feed crops, and the pharmaceuticals, bug sprays, and other chemicals used on or around the farmed animals, anything from the animals that is concentrated or dehydrated would then contain more of the chemicals per weight than those animal-derived substances that had not been concentrated or dehydrated.

- **Corn syrup**: Because of GMO crops and the industrial farming chemicals used on the fields, corn syrup can contain residues of the chemicals that are also obesogens.

- **Dibutyltin** (DBT): In polyvinyl chloride (PVC) plastics, including in PVC pipes used in many homes and other buildings where people drink the tap water.

- **Emulsifiers**: Chemical emulsifiers used in processed foods include carboxymethylcellulose, dioctyl sodium sulfosuccinate (DOSS), and sorbitan monooleate (Span-80). These stabilize foods, including for longer shelf life.

- **Flame retardants**: Often found in certain brands of furniture, clothing, household items, carpeting, tablecloths, drapes, pillows, mattresses, electronics, and paints and finishes.

- **Food additives**: As in synthetic dyes, emulsifiers, flavorings, preservatives, scents, sweeteners, and texturizing agents.

   The chemical emulsifiers carboxylmethylcellulos and P-80 can cause inflammation of the digestive tract, alter the gut microbiome, and play a role in other tissue inflammation, in autoimmune disorders, and in weight gain.

- **Forever chemicals**: These include the chemicals used in plastics, paints, industrial solvents, and food packaging, and food additives, and in nonstick cookware.

- **Fragrances**: Those containing synthetic chemicals. Including perfumes, colognes, body scents, and scents in cosmetics, foods, soaps, cleansers, detergents, furniture polish, and those toxic sprays ironically sold as "air freshener."

- **Fructose**: Found in natural balance in fruits and vegetables, but also extracted and used as a so-called "natural ingredient" in foods and beverages. It is best to avoid foods containing added fructose.

- **Landscape and farming chemicals**: This can include synthetic chemical fertilizers, fungicides, insecticides, miticides, pesticides, and rodenticides.

- **Monosodium glutamate** (MSG): This can interfere with or impair the secretion of glucagon-like peptide-1 hormone that plays a role in the regulation of the appetite. MSG can also alter androgen receptors, and a play a role in metabolic disorders and inflammation.

  Because it has been classified as a neurotoxin that can interfere with energy, and brain, neuron, and muscle function, professional athletes often seek to avoid foods containing MSG.

  MSG can also alter glucose tolerance, and should be avoided by those with blood sugar issues.

  There are so many health issues MSG can alter, it is has been the topic of multiple studies.

  MSG is often in products like Soy Sauce, instant noodle cups, some brands of bouillon and broth, other processed foods, and some Asian foods. It's especially used to provide a savory or umami flavor and/or aroma. Some call it *China salt*.

  Read food labels to avoid MSG. It can be listed under various names. Research MSG.

- **Nonstick cookware**: Instead of nonstick cookware, use cast iron, ceramic, stone, or stainless steel cookware.

  Nonstick cookware typically has PFAS, PTFE, and other chemicals. These can play a role in a variety of health problems, including everything from respiratory issues to hormonal imbalances, to autoimmune disorders, fibrosis, obesity, and cancers.

  Also avoid silicone cookware, as those products have a whole other set of chemicals with related health issues.

- **Perfluorinated chemicals**, including perfluorooctanoic acid (PFOA) and perfluorooctane sulfonate (PFOS): This includes thousands of man-made chemicals containing carbon chains attached with fluorine. These chemicals are found in products including detergents, soaps, dishwashing rinse chemicals, and laundry products, including dryer sheets, and products treated with flame retardants and/or stain-resistant chemicals, including backpacks, luggage, umbrellas, tents, lawn furniture, awnings, and carpeting, and also jackets, shoes, and other clothing, and mattresses. The chemicals are also in nonstick cookware, some brands of dental floss, toilet paper, and disposable diapers.

  Foods more likely to contain PFAS include everything from certain brands of tea bags to various types of processed foods, including "microwave popcorn," processed meats (including jerky, sausages, pizza meats, and sandwich cold cuts), and eggs. More than half of the bottled waters on the market have detectable PFAS.

Choosing organically grown foods is a way to reduce your exposure to PFAS, and a variety of industrial and otherwise synthetic, health-negating chemicals.

In addition to altering lipids and hormones, PFAS chemicals can play a role in autoimmune disorders, cancer, cardiovascular disease, kidney disease, insulin dysregulation, liver disease, reproductive issues, and thyroid function.

"People with the highest blood levels of perfluorinated chemicals had lower resting metabolic rates and regained weight faster after dieting than those with the lowest levels.

Humans with the highest blood levels of perfluoroalkyl compounds had lower bone mineral density at baseline and lost bone mineral density faster in a weight-loss trial.

Similar obesogenic effects have been observed with other environmental chemicals, such as phthalates, persistent organic pollutants, and components of plastics and epoxy resins."
– Environmental Obesogens and Their Impact on Susceptibility to Obesity: New Mechanisms and Chemicals, by Riann Jenay Eguquiza, and Bruce Bumberg; *Endocrinology Journal*; March 2020

- **Pesticides and herbicides** of a wide variety, and the substances left from their breakdown. These include "forever chemicals" like the herbicide glyphosate, and the neonicotinoid insecticide. The mostly banned chemical DDT still persists in the environment, as does it's breakdown product DDE.

  The herbicide quizalofop-p-ethyl is another that has been identified as an endocrine disruptor, and that can play a role in weight gain, and how the body deals with fat.

  These substances are labeled as "forever chemicals" because they persist in the environment, and gather in the tissues of animals, including humans.

- **Phthalates**: Often found in plastics, and in certain products from cosmetics to sunscreens, and hair products, to household cleansers, detergents, and laundry products, to food packaging and storage containers made of plastics.

- **Plastics** and the breakdown substances of them, microplastics and nanoplastics.

  Plastics include a variety of pollutants. Microplastic and nanoplastic pollution is found in everything from ocean water and mist, to lakes, rivers, clouds, fog, the air, and the tissues of animals, including the human animal.

  It is better to use glass, ceramic, metal, natural cloth, or paper to store food, rather than to store food in plastic. Whatever protects your foods from the elements, and from creatures you don't want to give access to your food storage.

  Don't heat your food in plastic. Doing so spreads the chemicals from the plastics into your food. This includes "microwavable" packaging.

- **Polluted air and water, and food containing chemical residues.** This includes meat, milk, and eggs, as animals can collect toxins from the chemically-grown foods they eat, the insecticides and other chemicals they might have been sprayed with, and pharmaceuticals they are treated with, or fed.

  "Forever chemicals" continue existing for many years without breaking down into other substances. They are persistent. It is why some chemicals no longer made remain as contaminants in the environment, and show up on human tissue tests. Not only humans, but animals in remote locations, like Antarctica. For instance, research Medium Chain Chlorinated Paraffins (MCCPs), which are only one of many manmade "forever chemicals" polluting Earth. Companies continue making toxic chemicals, without knowing – or considering – what the toxins will be doing to wildlife around the world, including everything from soil organisms to marine plants and animals, to the live on land, from the grasslands, meadows, and forests, to the streams, rivers, and lakes, and all life.

Animal fat collects toxins. The fat in meat, milk, and eggs can contain residues of chemicals the animal was exposed to. Fish liver oil can contain industrial and pharmaceutical chemical toxins and heavy metals from the environment where the fish lived.

- **Polychlorinated biphenyls** (PCBs): A pollutant formerly commonly found in coolant and dielectric fluids. It is now found as a "forever chemical" residue in chicken, seafood, turkey, and other meats, and in dairy, eggs, broth, and gelatin.

- **Preservatives**: Chemical preservatives used in processed foods are problematic for a number of reasons, including because they can also work as obesogens. The chemicals include 3-tert-butyl-4-hydroxyanisole (3-BHA).

  If difficult to understand words are listed on ingredient labels, the substance likely isn't something you want in your food, or in your body. You can easily research each ingredient on food labels, and find if it is problematic to your health.

- **Processed and non-organic foods**: These are hosts to what could be a variety of obesogens. This includes synthetic dyes, flavors, preservatives, scents, sweeteners, and texturing agents. This is also because of the obesogens found in certain types of food packaging, including cans containing toxic chemical liner.

- **Surfactants**: These include the emulsifiers Span-80 (sorbitan monooleate) and dioctyl sodium sulfosuccinate (DOSS), used in some foods. DOSS is also used as a stool softener. Industrial uses for DOSS and Span-80 include as dispersants of petroleum oil spills in rivers, lakes, and oceans.

- **Triphenyltin (TPTH)**: A fungicide and miticide used on crops. Also used on fishing nets, including in the containment industrial fishing industry where millions of fish can be kept in coastal water fish farms.

  According to the U.S. Environmental Protection Agency, TPTH is classified as a probable human carcinogen in "all routes of exposure (oral, dermal, and inhalation)." In tests done on rats, TPTH induced pituitary and testicular tumors. In mice, it induced liver tumors. Animal tests also identified the chemical as causing "developmental effects." The chemical also ends up as water pollution.

  TPTH is used on potatoes, sugar beets, and pecans. The EPA information about the chemical's use on produce say farm workers exposed to the chemical have cancer risk estimates that are "unacceptable." The chemical is sprayed on crops, including by small airplane.

Farmers aren't even supposed to feed crops treated with the chemical to farmed animals. As the EPA states: "There is an enforceable feeding restriction on TPTH labels against feeding sugar beet tops to livestock."

Perhaps nobody should be exposed to this terrible chemical.

Research other pesticides, miticides, fungicides, and farming chemicals. You will learn why there are more reasons to support organic family produce farmers. And, where possible, to grow your own food – and nurture wild edibles.

Obesogens alter gut microbiome, and increase disease risk

As mentioned, obesogens alter the gut microbiome. This can play a role in leaky gut syndrome, inflammation, and various types of diseases, including of the cardiovascular system, and the kidneys, and a compromised autoimmune system.

Obesogens increase the risk of experiencing glucose intolerance, insulin resistance, and type 2 diabetes, and also organ cancers, including of the prostate and breasts. And, weight gain, including hard-to-lose weight.

"A study analyzing National Health and Nutrition Examination Survey (NHANES) data compared BMI (body mass index) between U.S. adults in 1988 and 2006, and found a 2.3-gm/m increase in adult BMI in 2006 compared with 1988, even as the same amount of caloric intake and energy expenditure. Moreover, the quality of carbohydrate calories consumed (high vs low glycemic load) appears to be more important than the total quantity of calories consumed. Genetics is widely believed to be associated with obesity; however, known gene variants can explain only 2.7% of the individual variation in BMI. Therefore, the 2 most commonly given explanations – genetics and energy balance – cannot fully explain the substantial increase in obesity incidence observed worldwide.

Multiple environmental factors can affect obesity susceptibility. These include the gut microbiome composition, stress, and disrupted circadian rhythms, to name a few. Environmental stressors experienced during fetal development have significant impacts on obesity susceptibility later in life."
– Environmental Obesogens and Their Impact on Susceptibility to Obesity: New Mechanisms and Chemicals, by Riann Jenay Eguquiza, and Bruce Bumberg; *Endocrinology* Journal; March 2020

Reducing obesogen exposure

A plant-based, organic diet free of processed foods reduces obesogen exposure. As does avoiding canned food, not using non-stick cookware, using wood instead of plastic cutting boards, using non-toxic cleansers, and taking other measures to reduce your exposure to hormone disrupting and problematic chemicals.

The more your diet consists of organically-grown foods, and the less it consists of foods grown using chemicals, the lower your exposure to obesogens.

Eliminating meat, milk, and eggs from your diet also reduces obesogens.

Problematic substances in animal protein

While eating animal protein can include problematic substances, including obesogens, highly heating animal protein can create AGEs, the chemicals harmful to body tissues, and that increase risks of cancer, and cardiovascular, liver, and kidney diseases, diseases of dementia, and autoimmune disorders.

Cooking animal products creates some of the same toxins that exist in cigarette smoke and engine exhaust.

Rely on foods as close to their natural state as possible. When you do so, your body and health are more likely to conform to true health.

Non-foods

I was once with a girlfriend who looked at a food buffet and said, "non-foods."

She was right. The buffet spread consisted of what people shouldn't be eating.

It's interesting what modern people will put in their mouths, chew, and swallow.

What modern people eat often contains the substances it takes to experience common degenerative, chronic, and otherwise debilitating diseases.

Considering what many people eat, it should be no surprise that pharmacies, medical centers, and dialysis clinics are so common in every city and town.

People are experiencing illnesses in tune with what they are ingesting: Often this means salty, sugary, oily, processed, chemically-saturated, ultra-processed garbage out of tune with the chemistry and energies of nature.

Bad diet and lack of exercise are so common in modern society many children never experience any higher level of fitness. Instead, they are more likely to be overweight. Before many people reach young adulthood, maladies like diabetes, and cardiovascular and kidney disease are already in play. The problem is the food, and the lack of exercise, and the nutritional ignorance of those they could learn from, and school lunch programs, and the misinformation about nutrition spread in advertising. And the easy access to fast foods and junk snack shops.

If a food is advertised, it is probably very specifically not what you should put in your mouth – if you want to experience the best of health.

Toxic foods result in problems within you, and in wildlife

Much of what is sold in grocery stores shouldn't be considered food. Much of it takes an enormous amount of resources to produce, package, and distribute – then leaves behind a variety of pollutants, from plastics and chemically coated materials, to toxic ingredients saturating nature and wildlife.

When the amount of resources used to produce food and packaging – and to ship and market all of that stuff – is taken into consideration, it is easy to understand why overconsumption can be considered disrespectful to the environment, wildlife, and the Earth we all depend on.

Once into the habit of overeating, not only are people wasting their money, time, and health, they also are wasting water, fuel, and other resources used to produce, package, ship, market, and prepare the food.

Both overeating and obesity increase the risks of experiencing a wide variety of health issues, including cancer, and cardiovascular and kidney disease, and types of autoimmune disorders.

AB418: California State Assembly Bill 418

As I was writing this page there were news stories about a bill being called "controversial." Assembly Bill 418: AB418 was introduced into the California State Assembly to ban certain toxic ingredients from foods being sold – or manufactured – in the state of California. The ingredients are known to cause a variety of health problems, including kidney, liver, and cardiovascular disease, nerve disorders, behavioral and mental health issues, miscarriages, autoimmune dysfunction, and cancer.

Some people were angry about the possibility of the bill becoming law. As if it is a bad thing to protect consumer health. The industries making money from the products worked against the AB418.

The chemicals AB418 seeks to prohibit include bromated vegetable oil, potassium bromate, propylparabens, red dye No. 3, and titanium oxide.

The European Union banned the same chemicals.

- **Bromated vegetable oil**: Used as an ingredient in canned and bottled beverages, including to prevent citrus flavoring from separating and floating to the surface.

- **Potassium bromate**: Used in baked foods to strengthen dough and make it rise higher. See the section in this book about potassium bromate. Learn which foods contain this additive, and how you can avoid it.

- **Propylparabens**: Used as an antimicrobial food preservative.

- **Red dye No. 3**: Shown to disrupt the behavior of children, interfere with attention spans, and with brain function.
Why would anyone allow their child to consume foods containing the chemical?
    On food labels, it is often listed as "FD&C Red #3." In addition to candy, it's an ingredient in many processed foods. Ironically, it is also in some pharmaceutical drugs.

- **Titanium oxide**: A white color and smooth texturizer used in candy and processed foods.

Trade groups working against your health

What is there to be angry about by banning such harmful chemicals?

The National Confectioners Association – a trade group based in Washington D.C. – expressed opposition to AB418. They pointed out that the chemicals have been approved as safe for use by the U.S. Food and Drug Administration.

The Confectioners Association statement said "Ingredients that would be banned under the proposal have all been approved by the U.S. Food and Drug Administration. Food safety is the number one priority for U.S. confectionery companies, and we do not use any ingredients in our products that do not comply with the FDA's strictest safety standards."

The National Confectioners Association is a trade group working to protect the financial interests of businesses, and is funded by them. It's not there to protect the health of humans, the environment (where all of those chemicals end up – in the water, soil, and air), or wildlife.

The FDA is hardly flawless in their decisions. The FDA allows all sorts of artificial chemical colorants, preservatives, texturizers, flavorings, scents, and other synthetic chemical additives in food, beverages, and drugs. Chemicals known to play a role in adverse health conditions, including brain and nerve dysfunction, liver and cardiovascular and kidney problems, hormonal imbalance, thyroid issues, learning disabilities, skin issues, allergies, cancers, birth defects, and autoimmune disorders.

Considering that many of the chemicals are used in candy, and children eat more candy than adults, what the National Confectioners Association is fighting against is the health of children – including the long-term impact of consuming chemicals known to cause human disease, defects, and dysfunction.

Supporters of AB418 included The Environmental Working Group and the National Institute of Environmental Health Sciences.

The Environmental Working Group – which works to protect humans and the environment – issued a statement in relation to AB418, stating: "We know they are harmful and that children are likely eating more of these chemicals than adults. It makes no sense that the same products food manufacturers sell in California are sold in the European Union, but without these toxic chemicals."

What is it that the U.S. confectioner's trade group is protesting, when it is easy to understand the chemicals aren't needed? The trade group is funded by those who make money by selling the chemicals, and foods containing them.

Note: AB418 passed in 2023, and is to go into effect in 2027.

As California is the fifth-largest economy in the world, what California rules on often impacts the global market. Companies want to make what they can sell in California. If things are banned in California, they are less likely to be sold in other regions of the world.

I mention this because most people are unaware of the chemicals in processed foods, and what the chemicals can do to health, to wildlife, and to the environment.

It becomes part of you, us, and wildlife

What you eat ends up in your tissues, in the environment, and in wildlife.

Everything from fish and other life forms in the rivers, lakes, and oceans, to the mammals, reptiles, and birds throughout the wild are being found with residues of pharmaceutical drugs and food chemicals in their tissues. Just as those chemicals cause adverse health issues in humans, they also impact the health of wildlife.

Cell health: sirtuins, telomeres, and the mitochondria

A balanced diet with adequate calories plays a role in cell lifespan. An explanation of sirtuins and telomeres provides an understanding of this.

When the mitochondria structure inside every one of your cells is provided with nutrients, it releases the SIRT3 (sirtuin homologue 3) and SIRT4 (sirtuin homologue 4) enzymes that strengthen the cell energy.

Biologically younger

On a clean, highly nutritious diet, and a healthy, active lifestyle your cells live longer and are more healthful. This is one reason why people who follow a healthful, clean, fresh foods diet, and who remain physically active appear younger than those who do not. They are literally biologically younger than people of the same age who eat low-quality foods, who consume too many calories, and who don't get adequate exercise.

Mitochondria, cell death, and calorie restriction

David Sinclair, an assistant professor of pathology at Harvard Medical School, was involved in a study revealing the presence of the SIRT3 and SIRT4 enzymes and how they protect cells by preventing the mitochondria from releasing proteins leading to cell death.

Reasonable calorie restriction rather than gluttonous calorie overload is one key to better health.

(I am NOT advocating the false and dangerous concept of breatharianism, or the total elimination of food.)

Mitochondria nutrients

The mitochondria are protected by the antioxidants in edible plant matter, and by exercise, by a regular sleep pattern, and by avoiding smoking, addictive drugs, and junk food.

Regular exercise is especially helpful for maintaining mitochondrial health, and triggers mitochondrial biogenesis – which is the formation of mitochondria. Part of the muscle-strengthening happening when someone exercises is exactly the formation of more mitochondria material in the muscles.

Endurance athletes have larger and more mitochondria in their muscle cells, which increases their energy production – because mitochondria convert food energy into cell energy.

Combined with stronger muscles, including the heart, athletes are able to generate more energy, and use it more quickly, allowing them to run and otherwise move faster, and for a longer period of time than those who do not exercise.

"Skeletal muscles require the proper production and distribution of energy to sustain their work. To ensure this requirement is met, mitochondria form large networks within skeletal muscle cells, and during exercise, they can enhance their function.

The modulation of mitochondrial activity by exercise is not only fundamental for physical performance, but also a key point for whole-organism well-being.

Exercise is a physical activity that works the body at greater intensity than usual movements. To work at higher intensity, the body, particularly the skeletal muscles and the cardiovascular system, requires an extra supply of energy. Mitochondria are the main energy suppliers that coordinate AT production, reactive oxygen species (ROS) production, and calcium signaling, which are fundamental processes for sustaining body activity during exercise.

Endurance exercise training can increase the mitochondrial content per gram of tissue as well as the mitochondrial composition."
– Stay Fit, Stay Young: Mitochondria in Movement: The Role of Exercise in the New Mitochondrial Paradigm; *Oxidative Medicine and Cellular Longevity* journal; Jan. 2021

These are all reasons why this clean, low fat, plant-based diet is also helpful for athletic performance. As is daily cardio exercise.

Sirtuins and caloric intake

Sinclair's lab released a number of studies based on the impact of caloric intake on cell health, and the study of sirtuins, which manage cell protein maintenance of intercellular structures.

Sinclair's team concluded that low caloric intake rather than high caloric intake activates a gene that triggers the production of the NAMPT (nicotinamide phosphori-bosyltransferase) enzyme that signals for the production of the NAD (nicotinamide adenine dinucleotide) molecule, which helps to maintain cellular metabolism. The increase in the NAD triggers the SIRT3 and SIRT4 genes to release their enzymes.

Telomeres

The 2009 Nobel Prize in Physiology or Medicine was awarded to three American scientists, Elizabeth Blackburn, Carol Greider, and Jack Szostak for their landmark work discovering key aspects of how telomeres and telomerase enzymes work in aging, in protecting chromosomes, and in disease mechanisms, including the development of cancer.

Telomeres are repetitive DNA buffer caps on the ends of chromosomes where the DNA molecules carrying genes are packed. The telomeres protect the chromosomes from degradation, which plays a role in aging and disease prevention. Telomeres also prevent the chromosomes within cells from fusing.

The scientists also identified the enzyme that makes telomere DNA, naming it telomerase. When the cells divide, the telomeres are consumed, but are replenished by the telomerase enzyme, helping to complete the formation of the cell.

Cell replication and life

Understanding the way telomeres function helps in the understanding of cell life, and the length of human life.

Each time cells replicate the telomere becomes shorter. Cells of a newborn will replicate nearly 100 times, while cells of an elderly person may replicate only about 25 times.

Cancer cells have the ability to maintain their telomerase enzyme activity, which allows the cancer cells to preserve the telomere length on the ends of their chromosomes, and this allows for cancer cells to keep replicating many more times than a normal, healthy cell.

People who follow a healthful lifestyle, including a nutritious, plant-based diet free from damaged oils, and have regular patterns of exercise and sleep, and who avoid addictive substances have been found to maintain longer telomeres than those who are lacking in health through an unhealthful diet, lack of exercise, and addictions.

Microscopic youth

The length of the telomeres helps to determine how many times a cell can replicate. This is why it is said those who follow a healthful lifestyle have younger cells – which means their cells appear to be younger on a microscopic level, and can replicate more times than those of people who do not lead a healthful lifestyle.

In other words, those who take care of themselves are biologically younger – when their cells are compared to those of people of the same age who lead an unhealthful lifestyle.

Molecular clock

"The gradual shrinking of telomeres negatively affects the replicative capacity of human adult stem cells, the cells that restore damaged tissues and/or replenish aging organs in our bodies. The activity of telomerase in adult stem cells merely slows down the countdown of the molecular clock, and does not completely immortalize these cells. Therefore, adult stem cells become exhausted in aged individuals due to telomere length shortening that results in increased healing times and organ tissue degradation from inadequate cell populations."
– Hidden secret of immortality enzyme telomerase; ScienceDaily.com

Telomere damage

Situations found to reduce telomere length include lack of exercise and otherwise inadequate stress relief; substance abuse; a diet high in clarified sugars, a diet rich in highly heated fats (such as in griddled, broiled, seared, grilled, fried, and oil sautéed foods), and other less than healthful foods; a diet rich in acrylamides and glycotoxins, and other chemicals formed when certain foods are cooked to high temperatures; an acidic diet; a diet lacking in the antioxidants contained in fresh fruits and vegetables; low levels of vitamin D; insulin intolerance; and obesity.

Raising telomerase enzyme levels

In 2008 Dr. Dean Ornish of the Preventative Medicine Research Institute in Sausalito, California, cooperated with doctors at U.C. San Francisco, to conduct a study involving 30 men with low-risk prostate cancer. By placing them on a regular exercise program combined with a diet low in fat and refined sugars, but rich in fruits, vegetables, and whole vegan foods, he was able to raise the telomerase enzyme levels in their blood by 29 percent.

Twins and telomeres: anti-aging effect of exercise

A study conducted by researchers at Kings College London with colleagues from New Jersey Medical School and published in the February 2008 edition of the *Archives of Internal Medicine* concluded that exercise may have more to do with longevity than do genes. The study included more than 2,400 volunteers who were twins between the ages of 18 and 81. It found twins who were smokers, were overweight, and especially those who engaged in the least amount of exercise had telomeres shorter than those of their twin who lived a more healthful lifestyle. The telomeres were especially more prominent in those who remained physically active. When identical twins were studied, it showed the identical twin who was more active had significantly more prominent telomere length on the chromosomes in their white blood cells. The researchers conclude: "Adults who partake in regular physical activity are biologically younger than sedentary individuals." Dr. Tim Spector of Kings College said, "A sedentary lifestyle appears to have an effect on telomere dynamics – thus providing a powerful message that could be used by clinicians to promote the potentially anti-aging effect of regular exercise."

You can maintain healthful telomerase enzyme levels and longer telomere caps by engaging in daily exercise, following a nutritious plant-based diet free from junk ingredients, maintaining a regular sleep schedule and a healthful weight, and by not smoking, or using alcohol.

Prevention

It is clear that taking in a healthful amount of calories from a clean diet is key to maintaining healthful weight and energy, and preventing such health situations as cancer, organ dysfunction, and heart and kidney disease, nerve issues, and autoimmune disorders, including diabetes, arthritis, lupus, and asthma.

Avoid purchasing foods that trigger overeating.

Head to the produce section for fruits and vegetables – and avoid the snack and processed foods sections.

Learn to make foods from scratch in healthy serving sizes, as that is less expensive, and healthier.

Learn to grow sprouts, and include sprouts as an inexpensive, richly nutritious, regular part of your daily diet. Broccoli sprouts are particularly beneficial.

Read the parts of this book about the gut biome, and follow a diet protective of your intestinal bacteria.

Decrease the amount of advanced glycation end products (AGEs) in your diet by avoiding processed foods.

Depend more on fruits, vegetables, sprouts, nuts, seeds, beans, and seaweeds, and use ways of cooking (steaming, stewing, and boiling, instead of frying, grilling, searing, broiling, microwaving, etc.) that are less likely to create the problematic heat-generated chemicals.

"Diabetes, hypertension, and obesity are major contributors to the global burden of chronic kidney disease. A recent umbrella review confirms that vegetarian diets in the general population correlate with a reduced risk of diabetes, dyslipidemia, and ischemic cardiac disease. Switching from an omnivorous diet to a plant-based diet has also proven able, as evidenced by a recent meta-analysis, to significantly reduce blood pressure, more so in vegan diets than in lacto-ovo-vegetarian diets [dairy and eggs]. Plant-based diets also have beneficial effects on body weight, as evidenced by observational studies, which show that the body mass index, in a given population, is generally higher among omnivores and gradually decreases in parallel with the reduction in the consumption of animal products and in those who follow a plant-based diet, reaching the lowest values among those who follow a vegan diet. Similarly, numerous interventional studies have demonstrated the efficacy of the plant-based diet, which is stronger in vegan diets, in reducing body weight through various possible mechanisms, including a reduced caloric intake (linked to the increased intake of foods with low caloric density and high fiber content), an improvement in the functioning of the intestinal microbiota, and increased insulin sensitivity. In another umbrella review, the vegan diet was found to be effective in reducing body weight. The incidence of diabetes mellitus as well as metabolic

133

syndrome is also halved in those who follow a vegetarian diet, compared to those who follow an omnivorous diet. Furthermore, in interventional studies, for diabetics, switching to a vegan diet compared to a conventional American diet resulted in improved glycemic control, weight loss, a reduced need for diabetes medications, and improved lipid profile."

– The Role of Plant-Based Diets in Preventing and Mitigating Chronic Kidney Disease; *Journal of Clinical Medicine*; Sept. 2023

Raw vegan and raw vegan fusion

Because of the health issues related to heat-generated substances in cooked foods, some people experiencing health problems choose to follow a raw vegan diet as part of their healing – perhaps for a season, or for years. This might include following the living foods dietary guidelines taught at the Ann Wigmore Natural Health Institute in Puerto Rico.

The food choices advised at Wigmore's retreat certainly eliminate many toxins, and infuse the body with true, clean botanical nutrients.

Others will go for raw vegan fusion, which is a diet of raw vegan foods, and also including some boiled, stewed, or steamed foods – but less reliant on (or containing no) highly heated foods. Bottled oils are also likely out of the picture.

Vibrant health

A clean, plant-based diet that also does not include fried and oil sauteed foods is rich in antioxidants, including polyphenols (including flavonoids like quercetin), and other mitochondria nutrients is what you want for experiencing vibrant health.

"Polyphenols are naturally occurring compounds with similar structures (several hydroxyl groups on aromatic rings) and are mainly found in fruits and vegetables. Polyphenols are known to regulate free radical scavenging, cellular signaling and transduction, gene expression, and cellular communication. Two of the best-studied polyphenols are resveratrol, which is found in red wine, and quercetin, which is mainly found in apples and onions. Both quercetin and resveratrol have been extensively studied by exercise physiologists, as they are known to promote mitochondrial biogenesis."

– Stay Fit, Stay Young: Mitochondria in Movement: The Role of Exercise in the New Mitochondrial Paradigm; *Oxidative Medicine and Cellular Longevity* journal; Jan. 2021

The diet advocated in this book combined with daily exercise absolutely helps to protect against metabolic syndrome, including by reducing risks of cardiovascular disease, diabetes, intestinal disorders, kidney disease, and obesity.

I follow a plant-based, vegan diet that is free of all meat (including beef, pork, chicken, turkey, fish, amphibians, reptiles, and crustaceans), dairy (milk, butter, cream, cheese, yogurt, kefir, ice cream, and foods containing milk extracts, including casein and whey protein), and eggs (including mayonnaise, and any food containing eggs). I do have some steamed, boiled, or stewed foods, all strictly vegan.

Dietary rejuvenation

"Dietary contributors to disease are easily swept aside, as our culture assumes it is normal to be chronically medicated to regulate cholesterol, blood pressure, and blood sugar."
– Neal Barnard

A plant-based/vegan diet free of fried and sauteed oils, sugar and oil extracts, and processed and synthetic substances promotes the detoxification of the body by unclogging the system through unadulterated, whole foods. By providing high-quality nutrients, it rejuvenates the cellular structures – including everything from the cell membrane to the mitochondria, from the bones to the brain, and from head to toe. It helps in the refinement of the body, especially when combined with daily exercise.

A clean diet helps a person to flourish in health, and reverse damage caused by unhealthful living, including from toxic and dulling foods, laziness, addictions, and other life matters.

The pitch of your being

"At the root of all power and motion, there is music and rhythm, the play of patterned frequencies against the matrix of time. We know that every particle in the physical universe takes its characteristics from the pitch and pattern and overtones of its particular frequencies, it is singing. Before we make music, music makes us."
– Joachim-Ernst Berendt

A clean diet combined with daily exercise and intentional, goal-oriented living utilizing talents, skills, and intellect rearranges the pitch of your being. It clears the garbage from your system, and improves your nerve system and ability for your brain to function.

By allowing for cellular structures to release waste matter and residues, a highly nutritious diet improves your organs, nerves, blood flow, the communication between cells, and the function of your entire system, all the way to your molecular structures.

Use this health to create a life right for you.

While you may have been living under a slothful and struggling energy level as the result of consuming deadening foods saturated with what your body absolutely does not need, a clean diet energizes you in ways you may have never felt. You might feel as if your energy frequencies are finally intact.

A clean diet combined with daily exercise increases the amount of the telomerase enzyme in your system, allowing the telomeres on your chromosomes to remain structurally longer – as they do in healthier people.

Based on cell structure, cell aging, and cell function, people who follow a clean diet are biologically younger.

Wildlife diet

Wild animals have been subsisting on uncooked plant matter forever. Humans are the only creatures on the planet that cook food, adding chemicals to their foods, and extracting oils and clarifying sugars, and adding those to their foods.

Try following a diet that is more raw, and less cooked, clear of unnatural ingredients, and is free of grilled, broiled, seared, charred foods, microwaved, and fried or oil sautéed foods, and foods cooked to crispy brown. This way you will greatly reduce the AGEs in your system. You will experience less inflammation, and will have a healthier gut biome, and a stronger immune system, and likely a higher level of energy with more clarity of thought.

Superfoods

Superfoods could include seaweed powders, medicinal or apoptogenic mushrooms, and things like aloe vera, tropical berries, rare fruits, and high desert foods, including maca root powder from the Andes.

Superfoods could also be what people think of as weeds, but are edible plants rich in a variety of antioxidants, anti-inflammatories, vitamins, minerals, amino acids, and other nutrients.

Among the foods some classify as superfoods are camu camu, lucuma, acai fruit, and maqui berry powders. There is also moringa leaf powder, and matcha.

Everything from goji berries to black pepper, ginger, ginseng, mesquite powder, turmeric, nori, dulse, fenugreek, and various types of berries and herbs are touted as superfoods. I use many of these ingredients, but call them "food."

The term "superfood" seems a bit cartoonish. It's something used by questionable "health food gurus," who may only be nothing more than salespeople cleverly presenting themselves as some sort of inspirational health savior types.

Salicylates

Among of the benefits of growing your foods, and also getting them from local organic family farmers is you naturally improve your nutrition with fresh foods, and avoid the chemicals used to grow corporate foods, while also reducing the defensive plant chemistry of unripe produce.

There are plant chemicals called salicylates. They protect plants from insects, birds, and other wildlife, until the plant chemistry is ready for the wildlife to partake of the plant, or to take over the plant. Salicylates also work to protect the plants from bacteria and fungi. The chemicals naturally become less present in ripe fruits and vegetables.

When you continually eat unripe fruits and vegetables salicylates can build up in your tissues. They have been linked to emotional issues, such as depression, fatigue, hyperactivity, and lack of attention and concentration. Physical reactions indicating salicylate sensitivity can include itchy and puffy eyes, nausea, stomach upset, rashes, sinus issues, and swelling in the feet and/or hands.

Salicylism, which is an overexposure to salicylates, is similar to aspirin poisoning. Aspirin is a salicylate-based drug, and can cause a pharmacological reaction in people sensitive to salicylates.

While it is unlikely you will avoid all salicylates – and there are some naturally present in some of the foods you eat, and humans can naturally handle some salicylate exposure – people with histories of headaches and asthma may also want to steer clear of foods and products rich in salicylates.

Because salicylates may also be used in preservatives, perfumes, and some medications, those with sensitivity to salicylates would benefit by understanding which products might contain them.

While you will be consuming some salicylates when you eat fruits and vegetables, there is an amount the system can tolerate, but continually consuming unripe fruits and vegetables may be problematic for people who are more sensitive to salicylates.

Salicylates in mass marketed and processed foods

Eating whole fruits and vegetables, even unripe ones, is not going to expose a person to the amounts of salicylates contained in processed and packaged foods made from unripe fruits and vegetables, such as jams and jellies made using unripe fruit, orange juice made using unripe oranges, or tomato sauces, salsa, or catsup made using unripe tomatoes. The salicylates would be much more present in the pureed, boiled down, dehydrated, or otherwise concentrated foods made of unripe produce. There would be many more tomatoes in a cup of tomato sauce or diced, dried tomatoes when compared to a cup of chopped, fresh tomatoes.

Leukotrienes the inflammatory mediators

A plant-based diet rich in raw fruits and vegetables reduces inflammatory mediators called leukotrienes, and reduces sensitivity to salicylates, and also reduces inflammatory diseases and autoimmune disorders (including arthritis, diabetes, asthma, lupus, and others).

"In addition to asthma, leukotrienes have shown to play a role in the development of cardiovascular disease. Researchers have noted that atherosclerotic vascular lesions express the entire biochemical machinery necessary for leukotriene production, including 5-lipooxygenase, FLAP, and other distal enzymes important for leukotriene synthesis. Moreover, levels of 5-lipooxygenase within atherosclerotic vessels correlates with disease severity.

Leukotrienes have a connection to various cancers. Chronic inflammation leads to an increased risk of certain cancers. For example, the chronic inflammation provoked buy inflammatory bowel disease (IBD) appears to promote the transformation to colorectal adenocarcinoma"
– Physiology, Leukotrienes; *StatPearls* journal; Aug. 2023

What decreases the likelihood of experiencing cardiovascular disease, autoimmune disorders, and inflammation? A clean, plant-based diet.

Those are all reasons to go for more locally and organically grown foods free of synthetic chemicals, and to make foods from scratch. And, where possible, to grow your own, even if it means planting and nurturing wild edibles, and planting fruiting trees and bushes on nearby wild land (which would also benefit native wildlife).

Ripening agents

Fruits and vegetables shipped from far away, or otherwise that may have been picked while they were not yet ripe, often have ripening agents applied to them, such as bethylene, ethylene, ethane, ethephon, and calcium carbide. This is done when arriving in the destination country or region to trigger the ripening process. Because the residues of ripening agents may not be the healthiest things to ingest, it could be beneficial to use vinegar and water to rinse, soak, or otherwise wash fruits and vegetables from distant countries.

Calcium carbide releases acetylene gas, which triggers the ripening of fruit.

Acetylene has been found to reduce oxygen transfer to the brain, but is found in such small amounts when used as a ripening agent that it has been determined a non-issue.

The reason calcium carbide has been banned as a ripening agent in some countries is because it can contain trace amounts of arsenic and phosphorus, which can end up as residues on produce.

One reason why truly fresh, locally grown and ripe fruits and vegetables may taste better than those shipped from far away is because of the artificial ripening processes the shipped fruits and vegetables may have gone through.

Anyone who has had a vegetable garden or fruit trees likely knows how it is that fresh fruits and veggies taste better than store-bought. All of the days, or weeks, or months of shipping and the manipulation the store-bought produce went through is part of the flavor issue.

Fruits and vegetables that may be treated with ripening agents include apples, beets, bell peppers, blackberries, blueberries, cherries, citrus, cranberries, currants, figs, mangoes, papayas, pears, and tomatoes. Coffee also is often treated with ripening agents, and this can play into why it irritates those with IBD.

"Calcium Carbide can be a toxic substance, both for consumers and workers involved in fruit production. Calcium Carbide irritates the oral and nasal mucosae, in addition to causing gastrointestinal discomfort. Acetylene gas is soluble in water, and can buildup in fruits and affect the neurological system. The impurities found in Calcium Carbide, such as traces of arsenic and phosphorus, can lead to acute irritation of the mouth and nose, vomiting, skin ulcers, and even kidney damage."
– Substances used in the ripening of fruits can cause kidney damage and water and electrolytic disorders; *Brazilian Journal of Nephrology*; Nov. 2023

"Acetylene gas can accumulate in fruits when large amounts are used to ripen it. It may be possible to have negative health effects from eating massive quantities of fruits that have stored acetylene gas. This could include nervous system problems like dizziness, fatigue, and confusion.

But if you live in the U.S., you may not have to worry about eating fruit ripened with calcium carbide. Ethylene is often used when fruits are artificially ripened in the U.S. Many countries have banned the use of calcium carbide in fruit ripening. But some fruit producers still use it illegally to keep costs down."
– Calcium Carbide for Fruit Ripening; GoodRx; March 2024

"Studies have found that chemically ripened mangoes contain higher levels of toxins compared to naturally ripened ones, which can be dangerous when eaten regularly, or consumed in large amounts by people with weak immune systems, or other existing medical conditions.

It has also been shown that workers involved in growing and handling these fruits may suffer from long-term exposure if exposed concentrations of certain toxic substances exceed acceptable levels for safety standards set forth by various organizations like OSHA (Occupational Safety and Health Administration).

Calcium carbide and ethrel are toxic to both humans, birds, and other animals. They can cause a range of adverse health effects, including skin irritation, respiratory issues, dizziness, nausea, and headaches. Long-term exposure may also lead to organ damage or cancer in some cases."

– Study of food toxicology of toxins artificially introduced into the food or fruits; *Toxicology Research* journal; July 2023

Chemicals that have been used to ripen fruits have been found to be toxic to wildlife, including through breathing the vapors, or eating foods tainted with the chemicals. Long-term exposure can lead do damage to the bones and blood, kidneys, liver, and other tissues. Exposure can cause breathing difficulties, cognitive decline, convulsions, diarrhea, dizziness, hypoxia, vomiting, seizures, ulcers, and even death. These are reasons why various countries have banned or limited the use of these chemicals.

This is not to say you should avoid all fruits and vegetables from outside of your region – especially if those are the only ones available to you. It is important to have the nutrients from fruits and vegetables in your diet. But, it is more beneficial to eat the actual fruits and vegetables – rather than to consume processed foods containing fruits and vegetables, such as canned and bottled products – or jellies, jams, and juices.

If you can't get fruits and vegetables whole and unheated, one choice is frozen foods. Another choice is to use dehydrated organic fruits and vegetables, or powders like Infinity Greens. Another choice is to use foods sold in glass jars, with canned foods being the last choice.

Inflammation

There are many reasons why certain foods could lead to inflammation, and often because the foods have been highly heated, contain extracts or clarified substances, or synthetic chemicals.

"Acute inflammation is your body's natural response to illness, injury, or infection, and usually resolves on its own.

But there's another kind of inflammation – the kind that affects the whole body – which is called systemic. Systemic inflammation can become chronic; it can persist for months, or even years.

Chronic, systemic inflammation is a factor in diseases such as obesity, metabolic syndrome, pre-diabetes, type 2 diabetes, heart disease, inflammatory bowel disease, including Crohn's disease, and ulcerative colitis, some forms of cancer, arthritis, and Alzheimer's disease.

What foods cause inflammation? Unfortunately, a lot of them. In particular, experts recommend avoiding these inflammatory foods:
- Red meat, such as steak and hamburgers
- Processed meat, such as bologna, bacon, sausage, and lunchmeat
- Commercial baked goods, such as snack cakes, pies, cookies, and brownies

- Bread and pasta made with white flower
- Deep fried items, such as French fries, fried chicken, chips, and donuts
- Foods high in added sugar, such as candy, jelly, and syrup
- Sugar-sweetened beverages, such as soda, bottled or canned tea drinks, and sports drinks
- Trans fats, found in margarine, microwave popcorn, refrigerated biscuits, and dough, and nondairy coffee creamers
  – Anti-inflammatory Diet: What is inflammation?; Johns Hopkins Medicine

Along with the list above, processed foods, foods cooked at high temperatures, those containing clarified sugars and extracted oils, and anything grilled, broiled, fried, seared, oil sautéed, charred, torched, or griddled, and also refined carbohydrates, "instant" foods, and bottled sauces and dressings (containing questionable ingredients), are what can be considered inflammatory foods.

Fruits, vegetables, sprouts, and raw nuts and seeds, and seaweeds, and beans are rich in anti-inflammatories and anti-oxidants. Berries are particularly rich in them.

A key to reducing inflammation

Generally, the diet advocated in this book, including the section about soaking, germinating, sprouting, and otherwise activating or enlivening foods, helps to reduce inflammation. The advice about eating fruits and vegetables of a variety of colors, and staying away from processed foods, is also about preventing and reducing inflammation.

Mediterranean diet

People seeking to reduce inflammation often turn to the "Mediterranean diet," or whatever their view of it is.

Some pretty unhealthy foods can be considered to be part of the "Mediterranean diet."

Simply because some food product is promoted as within the "Mediterranean diet" doesn't mean it is something that is going to reduce inflammation, improve cardiovascular health, kidney health, or any other area of health. It depends on the ingredients, how they were grown, and how they were prepared.

There are many foods people consider to be healthy, but either aren't, or simply are not healthy. There may be ingredients in the foods that can be health negating, including damaged and rancid oils, clarified substances, salts, and synthetic chemicals. There are also the forms of cooking foods that increase inflammatory substances (AGEs). There are foods that are more helpful for the gut biome, and those that damage both the gut biome and the intestinal lining.

If someone is following the "Mediterranean diet," It is best to make most of it raw vegetables (including plenty of raw garlic), and raw fruit, and stay away from ingredients that would increase inflammation, and that would damage the gut microorganisms.

Olive oil, inflammation, and C-reactive protein

"In the 19th century, it was unusual to eat processed food that was preserved in a box, a bag, or a can. A common preservative in this packaging method was processed oil.

At the same time, these oils were increasingly used for cooking at home. As the restaurant industry flourished, offering more availability and variety, the public developed a habit of eating out several times a week, exposing themselves to restaurant meals that were frequently prepared with oil. A cardiovascular disease epidemic onset seemed to coincide with the widespread exposure to oils. There is now science both in animal and human studies that indicate how oils promote vascular injury."

— Is Oil Healthy?, by Caldwell B. Esselstyn, MD; *International Journal of Disease Reversal and Prevention*; 2019

Some think if you include a lot of olive oil in the diet that is some sort of health elixir.

Olive oil is about 15% saturated fat, a substance identified as contributing to cardiovascular disease. Heating the oil to high temperatures also degrades it, making it stickier, and more unhealthy, and also contributing to cardiovascular plaque.

There are some pretty low-quality olive oils. Some oils are sold as olive oil when they consist of a cheaper oil, or are only partially olive oil.

Including oil in the diet also increase the liver's production of C-reactive protein, which is an indication of inflammation. This also increases the risk of cardiovascular disease, heart attacks, and strokes. What increases inflammation and cardiovascular disease also increases the risks of kidney disease, autoimmune disorders, and cancer.

People with certain conditions test higher for C-reactive protein. The conditions include bacterial infection, and certain autoimmune disorders, including asthma, Crohn's disease, inflammatory bowel disease, lupus, pericarditis (inflamed lining of the heart), rheumatoid arthritis, and ulcerative colitis. Other conditions that may also play a role in high levels of C-reactive protein are dehydration, hepatitis, HIV/AIDS, kidney disease, and certain types of cancer.

It's best to avoid bottled oils, including avoiding olive oil. You get enough oil from every cell of every fruit, vegetables, sprout, nut, seed, bean, and legume, and if you also eat sea vegetables.

"This latest study adds to growing evidence that olive oil – which is pure liquid fat, with most other nutrients, including fiber, stripped away – is not a health food.

Prominent whole-food, plant-based physicians such as Caldwell Esselstyn, M.C., have long recommended consuming low-fat whole foods, plant-based diets with little to no added oils for optimal heart health. In 2019, Esselstyn authored an editorial in the *International Journal of Disease Reversal and Prevention* highlighting scientific evidence linking oil consumption with damage to the arteries."

— Studying the effects of olive oil in plant-based diets, by Courtney Davison; ForksOverKnives.com; Jul. 2024

"Both plant-based diet patterns [with olive oil, or without] improved cardiometabolic risk profiles compared with baseline diets, with more pronounced decreases in LDL-cholesterol after the low extra virgin olive oil. Addition of extra virgin olive oil after following a low intake [olive oil] pattern may impede further lipid reduction."

– Recipe for Heart Health: A Randomized Crossover Trial on Cardiometabolic Effects of Extra Virgin Olive Oil Within a Whole-Food Plant-Based Vegan Diet; *Journal of the American Heart Association*; July 2024

Feta: a rich source of cholesterol, saturated fat, and the proinflammatory Neu5GC molecule

Some think that because feta cheese is in the Mediterranean diet, it means you can eat lots of feta cheese, loading it into salads and other dishes. Feta also contains saturated fat, and cholesterol, and the Neu5Gc molecule that can make cancer more aggressive.

There are vegan versions of feta cheese free of the problematic substances. It also is easy to make a vegan version of fetta. One recipe for vegan feta is on the PlantBasedKidneys site.

"Researchers from Israel, France, Italy, and the United States have found a direct molecular link between meat and dairy diets and the development of antibodies in the blood that increase the risk of cancer.

This connection may explain the high incidence of cancer in people who consume large amounts of dairy products and red meat, similar to the link between high cholesterol and heart disease.

Roquefort and sheep feta cheese as well as sheep yogurt have high amounts of Neu5Gc sugar [molecule] per gram, followed by sausage and steak."

– Dairy and red meat increase risk of colorectal cancer: High consumption of certain cheeses, sheep yogurt, sausage, and steak found to cause antibodies that contribute to cancer; Israel21c.org; Oct. 2020

Gut health to reduce inflammation

The foods you eat can either keep the gut healthy, or degrade it.

What you eat either prevents or promotes the possibility of experiencing leaky gut syndrome.

Your food choices either promote or reduce the risk of experiencing inflammation, and autoimmune disorders, and cardiovascular, liver, thyroid, and kidney disease, and various types of cancer.

Building and encouraging a healthy gut microbiome can include enlivening foods, including by soaking nuts, seeds, beans, and some grains, and in fermenting others.

Nurturing the gut biome includes getting rid of what isn't good, but having what is rich in vitamins, minerals, enzymes, and antioxidants, polyphenols, and inulin. It includes eating deeply-colored fruits and vegetables. It involves getting the essential fatty acids naturally present in edible plants. It is about ingesting the natural nutritional and health-promoting components of fruits, vegetables, sprouts, and other edible plants.

Encouraging a healthy gut biome includes providing what the gut needs: the fiber from edible plants that then work as prebiotics. It also is helpful to eat fermented foods containing probiotics, like sauerkraut, kimchi, and fermented coconut yogurt, and fermented nut cheeses.

"Probiotics are defined as 'live microorganisms which when administered in adequate amount confer a health benefit on the host' and represent a very direct means of modulating the composition of the gut microbiota by adding exogenous microorganisms. The most common probiotics are lactobacilli and bifidobacteria."
– The way to a man's heart is through his gut microbiota – dietary pro- and prebiotics for the management of cardiovascular risk, by Karen M. Tuohy, Francesca Fava, and Roberto Viola; *Proceedings of the Nutrition Society* journal; Feb. 2014

Some people will tell you the way to get probiotics is by eating yogurt. You can get probiotics in a number of ways, and not by eating the teat excretions of cows that contain health-depleting substances. There are plenty of vegan sources of probiotics, including fermented foods, but also vegan probiotic supplements.

Leaky gut, a healthy gut biome, and autoimmune disorders

Having healthy gut microbes helps to prevent leaky gut syndrome. Leaky gut allows undigested proteins into the blood system, which can damage the kidneys, and lead to – or worsen – autoimmune disorders, including arthritis, lupus, asthma, diabetes, and others.

The foreign proteins that make it through a damaged gut lining can land in soft tissues, including the joints, spine, and cartilage, but also the eyes, and other tissues. Inflammation ensues. This process can trigger the body to form antibodies to attack the foreign proteins. It also can attack similar proteins the body makes. The situation turns into a mess, and is labeled "an autoimmune disorder."

Gut bacteria and dysbiosis

Unhealthy bacteria in your gut from eating a bad diet can also cause leaky gut syndrome, and the variety of associated health problems.

The imbalance of microbial species in the microbiome of the gut is a situation called dysbiosis. The immune system then gets out of balance, and illnesses can settle in.

Celiac disease

Celiac disease is a situation also involving leaky gut, which is related to gluten from wheat, barley, and rye. People with Celiac would also be wise to avoid dairy products, and fried and oil sautéed foods.

If you have leaky gut issues, and you are also eating meat, dairy, and eggs, the undigested proteins from those can get into your bloodstream. This can magnify autoimmune responses, inflammation, and damage to your joints, organs, and other tissues.

The above is unlikely to happen with plant proteins. It's the animal proteins from meat, dairy, and eggs that are the problem. But also, the gut can be damaged by rancid oils, substance abuse, and certain medications, synthetic food additives, industrial residues, and the residues of farming chemicals.

As mentioned earlier, the antibodies your body makes to attack the foreign animal proteins are also likely attacking similar proteins your body makes. The situation is of "dis ease."

Gluten-free menu items might contain gluten

If you are avoiding gluten because you have celiac, have a history of depression and/or anxiety, or for some other situation, know that many products labeled "gluten-free" may contain gluten. Many restaurants also list items on the menu as gluten-free, when the items do contain gluten.

"Even tiny amounts of gluten in foods are troublesome for people with celiac disease, and restaurants may be the hardest places to avoid the protein, finds a new study. More than half of gluten-free pizza and pasta dishes in restaurants tested positive for the presence of gluten; about one-third of supposedly gluten-free foods had detectable gluten. Gluten-free pasta samples were positive in 51 percent of tests; gluten-free pizza contained gluten for 53 percent.

Gluten was detected in 27 percent of breakfasts, 29 percent of lunches, and 34 percent of dinners."

– Study measures gluten in gluten-free labeled restaurant food; Columbia University's Mallman School of Public Health; April 2019

Autoimmune diseases

Those with autoimmune diseases often also have kidney issues.

Addison disease, celiac disease, chronic inflammatory demyelinating polyneuropathy, diabetes, fibromyalgia, giant cell myocarditis, Guillain-Barre syndrome, Hashimoto thyroiditis, lupus, multiple sclerosis, myasthenia gravis, myositis, polymyalgia rheumatica, psoriasis, psoriatic arthritis, rheumatoid arthritis, scleroderma, Sjogren's syndrome, and vasculitis are some autoimmune diseases. Some, including lupus and diabetes, are more likely to impact the kidneys than others.

As mentioned elsewhere, the diet in this book is likely to greatly help prevent pre-diabetes (often first diagnosed as insulin resistance), lower the risk of experiencing type 2 diabetes, and reduce the problems related to type 1 diabetes. It will also reduce the risk of experiencing – and the intensity of – some types of arthritis, and celiac disease, lupus, and some other autoimmune diseases.

Exercise is key to help prevent and reduce the risks of experiencing autoimmune disorders

A healthful diet is one major key to reduce the risk of autoimmune and other diseases. Another key is regular daily exercise – preferably in the morning, with movement throughout the day, and with a less intense evening session.

"Physical exercise has been shown to induce beneficial metabolic changes in and of itself. Many researchers have shown that exercise is more helpful than pharmaceuticals in the secondary prevention of cerebral vascular disease, and is as efficient as drugs in preventing the development of diabetes, not to mention that exercise is very inexpensive compared with medications. It has been solidly demonstrated that aerobic exercise improves insulin resistance in children, adolescents, and adults. Long interventions (>6 months) show major health benefits, including improved glucose control and decreased serum lipids, with favorable anthropometric changes. Exercise has also been shown to diminish concentrations of circulating AGEs [advanced glycogen end products that cause inflammation, and play a role in everything from cardiovascular and kidney disease, to autoimmune disorders, cancer, and other chronic and degenerative conditions.]."

– Dietary Advanced Glycation End Products and Their Role in Health and Disease; *Advances in Nutrition* journal; July 2015

Lupus and Sjogren's syndrome

I have friends with lupus and Sjogren's syndrome, and who follow a vegan diet to help manage their situations.

"In a recent case report published by the journal *Frontiers in Nutrition*, researchers discuss three case studies wherein women (ages 40, 54, and 45 years) suffering from Sjogren's syndrome (SS), and systemic lupus erythematosus (SLE), reported remission of their symptoms following switching their diets to customized plant-based nutritional regimes."

– Plant-based diets trigger remission in Sjogren's syndrome and lupus cases, by Jugo Francisco de Souza; *News: Medical Life Sciences*; Feb, 24

"Systemic lupus erythematosus patients who changed their eating patterns to incorporate more plant-based foods while limiting processed foods and animal products reported improvements in their disease symptoms.

The majority (>80%) of respondents that undertook new eating patterns with increased vegetable intake and/or decreased intake of processed foods, sugar, gluten, dairy, and carbohydrates reported benefitting from their dietary change. Symptom severity ratings after these dietary changes were significantly lower than before (21.3% decrease, $p<0.0001$). The greatest decreases in symptom severity were provided by low/no dairy (27.1% decrease), low/no processed foods (26.6% decrease) and vegan (26% decrease) eating patterns ($p<0.0001$). Weight loss, fatigue, joint/muscle pain and mood were the most cited symptoms that improved with dietary change."

– Plant-based dietary changes may improve symptoms in patients with systemic lupus erythematosus; *Lupus* journal; Jan. 2022

"With lupus, the researchers didn't mess around. Each day, the study subjects were to eat a pound of leavy greens and cruciferous vegetables like kale, fruits like berries, and lots of chia or flax, and drink a gallon of water. We're talking about a green smoothie diet to extinguish lupus flares. (Not, though, that if your kidneys are already compromised, this should be done under physician supervision so they can monitor your electrolytes like potassium and make sure you don't get overloaded with fluid.) Bottom line? With such remarkable improvements due to dietary changes alone, the hope is that researchers will take up the mantle and formally put it to the test.

Reversals of autoimmune inflammatory skin diseases can be particularly striking visually. A woman with a 35-year history of psoriasis that had been unsuccessfully managed for 19 years with drugs suffered from other autoimmune conditions, including Sjogren's syndrome. She was put on an extraordinarily healthy diet packed with greens and other vegetables, fruits, nuts, seeds, avocados, and some whole grains, and boom! Within one year, she went from 40 percent of her entire body surface area inflamed and effected down to 0 percent, completely clear, and as a bonus, her Sjogren's symptoms resolved, too, while helping to normalize her weight and cholesterol."

– Eating an Anti-Inflammatory Diet for Lupus, by Michael Greger M.D.; NutritionFacts.org; DrGreger.org; Oct. 2024

"Systemic lupus erythematosus (SLE) is a chronic multisystem autoimmune rheumatic disease in which disease flares are interspersed with episodes of remission. In contrast to organ-specific autoimmune diseases SLE comprises a constellation of signs and symptoms that can affect multiple organ systems.

A plant-based diet may have a beneficial effect on SLE patients, due not only to the direct action of nutrients on the immune system and inflammation, but also to an indirect effect on insulin resistance, obesity, and associated comorbidities.

Accelerated atherosclerosis is a significant comorbidity and the leading cause of death for patients with SLE. Patients are also more likely to experience metabolic syndrome leading to type II diabetes, obesity, and chronic kidney disease. A plant-based diet is a safe and efficacious prophylaxis and treatment for all these comorbidities.

Three small interventional studies with a plant-based diet showed a beneficial effect on patients' symptoms and therefore quality of life. A plant-based diet has the advantages of having no adverse reactions or contraindications, and can be an effective adjunct to standard treatments."

– Lupus – Prevention and Treatment with a Plant-Based Diet, by Steward Rose and Amanda Strombom; *Orthopedics and Rheumatology Journal*; Feb. 16, 2023

Intestinal tract and mood chemicals

The intestinal tract is where many mood chemicals are formed. It is why you often feel your emotions in your belly. There is a direct correlation between the chemistry of your intestinal tract, and the molecules of emotion within your brain, nerves, heart, lungs, and other organs and tissues. It all works in sync with what your intestines are doing. This also has to do with what you eat to nurture the balance of gut flora.

Because so many beneficial molecules – including those relating to and regulating emotions – are formed in the intestinal tract, following a low-fat, plant-based diet with an abundance of raw vegetables and whole, unprocessed foods free of synthetic chemicals also will likely improve mood and sleep while decreasing stress, anxiety, frustration, and irritability.

The intestinal lining can heal rather quickly. People switching to a clean diet often find they feel much better within weeks.

Leaky gut syndrome and the gut microbiota

Leaky gut is often part of, associated with, or plays a role in causing celiac, Chron's disease, ulcerative colitis, reflux, heartburn, and other intestinal problems, and gluten intolerance, candida, skin conditions, arthritis, and other issues.

A clean, low-fat, plant-based diet promotes a healthy population of gut microbiota, and helps to prevent inflammation of the intestinal tract as well as of tissues throughout the body.

The gut biome also plays a role in brain function, in a multi-network process called the gut-brain axis. This involves the autonomic nervous system, the enteric neural system, the central nervous system, and the immune and endocrine systems.

The health of the gut biome has such an impact on the brain that it can play a role in altering the function of the amygdala, hippocampus, and other areas of the brain. In this way, the gut microbiota influences behavior. It reveals how no system in the body acts alone.

The connection between the gut microbiota and the function of the nerve system should be of no surprise, considering that the emotional chemicals largely originate in the digestive tract.

A healthy gut microbiota includes a variety of archaea (another variety of single-celled organisms), bacteria, fungi, protozoans, viruses, and yeasts. Among these are Actinobacteria (Actinomycetota), Bacteroidetes (Bacteroidota), Firmicutes (Bacillota), Lactobacillae (Lactobacillus), streptococci, and Enterobacteria (Enterobacteriaceae). These all exist in symbiosis. That is, in a healthy gut.

When the gut microorganisms are out of balance, it is called dysbiosis – which can lead to a variety of health problems.

Most often, dysbiosis is caused by an unhealthful diet. Dysbiosis can also be the result of environmental toxins, a response to certain drugs and addictive substances, and by things like food poisoning and contagious illnesses.

It is estimated there are at least tens of trillions of microorganisms in your alimentary tract – from your mouth to your stomach and throughout the intestines. These organisms assist in digestion, including breaking down and fermenting what you eat, extracting nutrients from what you eat, and metabolizing (making) certain nutrients from those substances.

The organisms form certain enzymes play roles in metabolizing polysaccharides and proteins. To do this, organisms also use what you ingest so they can exist, and this is part of the symbiosis.

The gut microorganisms also break down what would be harmful substances.

The gut microbiome is a trillion times more complex than what this book has room to describe.

Some of the vital nutrients the gut microbiota metabolize (create) include branched-chain amino acids, lipopolysaccharides, secondary bile acids, short-chain fatty acids, trimethylamine, and indoles and derivatives of them.

Indoles and the gut barrier structure

Indoles are anti-inflammatory, work to neutralize free radicals, prevent oxidative stress, and are key to maintaining the permeability and mucus barrier of the intestines. They help beneficial bacteria to survive, and inhibit the growth of problematic bacteria. They also play a role in the function of the endothelial cells lining the intestines, and the cardiovascular and lymph systems.

147

"The function of the intestinal barrier is strongly linked to intestinal health and plays a critical role in animal health. The gut barrier isolates the host from the microorganisms in the intestinal cavity, and limits the movement of microorganisms and molecules from the intestinal lumen. The intestinal mucosal barrier consists of four main component: immune barrier, biological barrier, mechanical barrier, and mucus barrier. In the intestine, lymphoid tissues and immune cells make up the immunological barrier. The biological barrier is made of intestinal flora. The mechanical barrier consists of tight junctions and underlying gut epithelium. Chemicals such as lysozyme and digestive enzymes secreted by the intestines form the mucus barrier. An intact mucosal barrier system prevents microorganisms and products from migrating into the blood. Once the gut barrier is damaged and intestinal permeability increases, bacteria and their products, such as endotoxins, will translocate and activate the mononuclear macrophage system, promoting the production of a large number of inflammatory elements, such as interleukin-6 and tumor necrosis factor-a leads to a chronic microinflammatory state. Indoles are crucial in controlling intestinal barrier efficacy, including modulation of inflammatory and immunological responses, reduction of epithelial permeability, mucus production, and tight junction formation."

– Dual Role of Indoles Derived From Intestinal Microbiota on Human Health; *Frontiers of Immunology* journal; June 2022

Biochemical factory within your digestive tract plays into all areas of health

You have a biochemical factory operating within your digestive tract every day, and night. It plays into everything from the health of the intestinal lining to the function of everything from your brain and nerves to your bones and blood, heart, spleen, pancreas, liver, adrenal glands, kidneys, and all parts of you.

Your stress levels, sleep, mood, immunity, metabolism, and energy and hormone levels are impacted by the health of your gut microbiota.

A healthy gut microbiota stabilizes the systems, and protects your brain, nerves, and general health, and helps to prevent development of autoimmune and nerve disorders, and cancer.

Certain microbiota are more present in different parts of the gastrointestinal tract. The colon is more likely to have the Bacteriodetes Bacteroidaceae, Prevotellaceae, and Rikenellaceae, and the small intestine hosts a different variety of bacteria. Part of this is because of the differences in acidity, movement, and temperature in the various parts of the intestines. Also, certain bacteria in the lower intestines feed on what is produced by bacteria in the upper intestines.

The gut microbiota changes throughout life. It is a different composition in infants compared to toddlers – who then have a microbiota similar to adults. The composition of the microbiota changes in late adulthood. It is all influenced by diet, other substances, sleep, exercise, and other matters.

Infants get their initial microbiota from the vaginal tract (maternal microbiota). Babies born by cesarean are found to get a different combination of microorganisms from the skin of the mother, and might have a different variety of health concerns.

People who eat an unhealthy diet have a different composition of gut microbiota than those who eat a healthy diet. Those who follow a low fat, plant-based diet are likely to have a more diverse gut microbiota than those who eat a diet heavy in animal protein, oil, and processed foods. The same goes for the varieties of microorganisms found in the lungs, and on the skin.

"Depending on the localized regions, microbiota can be classified into gut, oral, respiratory, and skin microbiota. The microbial communities are in symbiosis with the host, contributing to homeostasis and regulating immune function. However, microbiota dysbiosis can lead to dysregulation of bodily functions and diseases including cardiovascular diseases, cancers, respiratory diseases, etc.

Generally, the gut microbiota is composed of 6 phyla including Firmicutes, Bacteroidetes Actinobacteria, Proteobacteria, Fusobacteria, and Verrucomicorbia, among which Firmicutes and Bacteroidetes are the major types."
– Microbiota in health and disease; *Signal Transduction and Targeted Therapy* journal; April 2022

Short-chain fatty acids produced by fiber fermentation in the gut

Following a plant-based diet forms vitally important short-chain fatty acids (SCFAs) in the gut.

SCFAs help protect against kidney inflammation and fibrosis, and colon cancer, and many other issues.

"Increased concentrations of SCFAs in feces and blood circulation are associated with decreased levels of inflammatory cytokines and chemokines in the kidney via GPR43 or GPR109A. SFCAs, especially propionate, attenuate the expression of monocyte chemotactic protein-1 stimulated by TNF-a by inhibiting the phosphorylation of p38 and JNK in human renal cortical epithelial cells, thereby inhibiting renal inflammation and fibrosis. Clinical studies have shown that butyrate levels in healthy volunteers are three times higher than those in chronic kidney disease patients. Administration of butyrate to rats with nephropathy improves renal fibrosis, reduces trimethylamine, and trimethylamine N-oxide in the serum and feces, and improves CKD progression in rats. Diabetic mice given a high-fiber diet showed improved intestinal microecology, increased intestinal and systemic SCFAs, and inhibited kidney injury caused by GPR43 and GPR109a. These findings indicate that an imbalance in the intestinal microbiota of patients with CKD affects their SCFA metabolites, and the reduction of propionate and butyrate enhances the progression of CKD. Therefore, supplementing SCFAs directly or modulating the gut microbiota that favors the production of SCFAs through dietary fiber or nutritional therapy may have a positive impact on the management of chronic renal failure."
– Short-chain fatty acids in disease; *Cell Communication and Signaling* journal; Aug. 2023

With a healthy microbiome, and the presence of SCFAs resulting from the fermentation of fiber in the gut, inflammation levels are kept in check, and the immune system is strengthened, reducing the risk of a variety of chronic and degenerative disorders, balancing appetite, and improving nutritional absorption, mood, and brain function.

The health of everything from your digestive, immune, cardiovascular, lymph, and nerve systems, and the kidneys, liver, spleen, pancreas, and other organs are dependent on short-chain fatty acids, and other components of the intestinal microbiome.

"Short-chain fatty acids affect intestinal motility, barrier function, and host metabolism. Furthermore, SCFAs play important regulatory roles in local, intermediate, and peripheral metabolisms. Acetate, propionate, and butyrate are the major SCFAs, they are involved I the regulation of immunity, apoptosis, inflammation, and lipid metabolism.

The human intestine contains a complex and diverse symbiotic microbial system that is mainly composed of bacteria, fungi, viruses, archaea, and protozoans. Microbiota-derived metabolites are crucial mediators of host-microbial interactions. Recent studies have shown that the main metabolites of intestinal microbiota include short-chain fatty acids, secondary bile acids, trimethylamine, lipopolysaccharides, imidazopropionic acid, branched-chain amino acids, and indole and its derivatives, which affect metabolism, immunity, and tumor development. SCFAs are mainly produced by the intestinal microbiota and indigestible carbohydrates and host secretions via anaerobic fermentation, and are one of the most important metabolite categories involved in the regulation of several biological functions.

SCFAs regulate the structure of intestinal microbiota, enhance the function of the intestinal epithelial barrier, and are beneficial in delaying disease progression through a variety of ways, such as those in type 2 diabetes, obesity, chronic kidney disease, hypertension, inflammatory bowel disease, and colorectal cancer."
– Short-chain fatty acids in disease; *Cell Communication and Signaling* journal; Aug. 2023

Acetate, butyrate, and propionate are all short-chain fatty acids derived from microbial fermentation of fiber in the gut. They can't form without fiber.

"Among 488 microbial signatures of an omnivore gut microbiome, we found species such as A. putredinis, B. wadsworthia and R. torques, that were generally linked to meat (especially red versus white meat) consumption. These species have been previously implicated in inflammatory diseases such as inflammatory bowel disease, colorectal cancer, and an overall decrease in SCFAs, and were more likely to be associated with negative cardiometabolic health outcomes. In contrast, signature microbes of a vegan gut microbiome, such as Lachnospiraceae, Butyricicoccupus sp. And R. hominis, were linked to the consumption of fruits and vegetables, for example, due to their specialized role in fiber degradation, and are commonly described as producers of SCFAs. These observations were also reflected by more signature vegan microbes associated with favorable cardiometabolic health than signature omnivore microbes, and were paralleled by pathway-level microbiome characterization."
– Gut microbiome signatures of vegan, vegetarian, and omnivore diets and associated health outcomes across 21,561 individuals; *Nature Microbiology* journal; Jan. 2025

To form the SCFAs, you need to eat plants. Plants contain fiber. Meat, dairy, and eggs do not contain fiber. Nor does bone broth, and other animal-derived ingredients like casein, whey, gelatin, or lard.

A low-fat, plant-based diet rich in raw foods, and which may include steamed and boiled foods, is beneficial for building a healthful gut biome. This helps to reduce the risks of gluten intolerance, celiac, leaking gut, irritable bowel issues*, and arthritis, and other rheumatoid and digestive issues. It reduces the risk of experiencing cancers throughout the body, and especially colorectal cancer. (*Certain inflammatory bowel issues require a particular diet, as can be advised by a gastroenterologist and/or dietician.)

A clean, low-fat, plant-based diet can be helpful for those with autoimmune disorders as they avoid gluten grains, corn, soy, bleached foods, clarified and processed sugars, and a diet also free from MSG, and synthetic chemical food additives (colorings, flavorings, scents, preservatives, and texturizing agents).

Butyrate, propionate, and intestinal, renal, and cardiovascular health

"Butyrate is a short-chain fatty acid made by good bacteria in the gut as a byproduct of fiber digestion. Butyrate signals the immune system that the gut bacteria are in the desirable range. When the butyrate level becomes low due to inadequate fiber intake, the body produces an inflammatory reaction.

Butyrate has been shown to have numerous positive effects: Suppressing or preventing cancer. Suppressing hunger. Inhibiting growth of bad bacteria. Increasing mineral absorption. Decreasing incidence of obesity. Assisting in activating programmed cell death.

A plant-based diet, one rich in fiber and resistant starch, produces and feeds good gut bacteria."
– Butyrate; NutritionFacts.org

Butyrate has been the focus of those wanting to improve their gut health. As explained, it is a short-chain fatty acid metabolized in the gut by the fermentation of fiber. As in, from plants. Butyrate play a role in maintaining the homeostasis (balance) of the intestines, specifically protecting the lining of the intestines, and preventing leaky gut. It helps to prevent inflammation, autoimmune disorders, renal fibrosis, and the growth of cancer.

Butyrate is used as energy by colonocytes, which are the epithelial cells lining the colon. This is one reason why, without an adequate amount of fiber in the diet, colon health degrades. The colonocyte cells are involved with digestion, nutrient and water absorption, electrolyte balance, and are rich in mitochondria, which transfer food energy into cell energy. This also helps to reveal why keeping a healthful gut microbiome is vitally important for health.

"Butyrate is formed in the gut during bacterial fermentation of dietary fiber, and is attributed to numerous beneficial effects on the host metabolism.

The gut microbiota is now recognized as a 'new organ,' and its role in health and disease has become widely acknowledge. Emerging evidence supports the hypothesis that gut microbiota dysbiosis is closely related to the development of non-communicable diseases, including cardiovascular disease, colorectal cancer, obesity, or type 2 diabetes. Host-microbiome interactions are heterogenous and multifaceted, some of them being mediated by microbial fermentation products.

Short-chain fatty acids, acetate, butyrate, and propionate, are primary products of microbial fermentation of dietary fiber in the colon."
– Determination of Butyrate Synthesis Capacity in Gut Microbiota; *Biomolecules* journal; Sept. 2021

"Butyrate has multiple physiological activities, including providing energy to colonocytes and improving the intestinal barrier via the upregulation of tight junctions. Butyrate lowers systemic inflammation by preventing lipopolysaccharide (LPS) from crossing the intestinal wall and entering the bloodstream. The intervention studies included in the review have reported an increase in the butyrate-producing bacteria, such as Ruminococcaceae, Lachnospiraceae, Coprococcus, Roseburia, Blautia, Alistipes, and Faecalibacterium prausnitzii. Substantial evidence shows that acetate, propionate, and butyrate have preventive effect against various diseases, including type 2 diabetes, inflammatory bowel disease, and immunological diseases. SCFAs, for instance, have been demonstrated to boost immunity in the host. They are also crucial for neuron function and maturation and for maintaining the blood-brain barrier function. SFCAs also promote metabolism and play a significant role in preventing or treating obesity. The considerable body weight reduction observed in vegan and vegetarian intervention diets strongly supports the claim."

– Effect of Plant-Based Diets on Gut Microbiota: A Systematic Review of Interventional Studies; *Nutrients* journal; Mar. 2023

"Butyrate inhibits the occurrence and development of colon cancer by regulating the expression of tumor suppressor genes and promoting apoptosis. As an energy metabolite, butyrate promotes the proliferation of normal colon cells."

– Short-chain fatty acids in disease; *Cell Communication and Signaling* journal; Aug. 2023

"One approach to improving the quality of life and lifespan of chronic kidney disease patients is to focus on dietary managements. For these patients, some dietary recommendations are clear, such as reducing protein intake. However, increasing dietary fiber intake has less adherence despite evidence of its multiple salutogenic [supporting human well-being] effects. Short-chain fatty acids are the main final metabolic products of carbohydrate and protein fermentation by the gut microbiota. Acetate, propionate, and butyrate are the most abundant short-chain fatty acids, with the latter being the main energy source of colonocytes. Short-chain fatty acids enter the systemic circulation through colonocytes by active transporters or passive diffusion.

Through their ability to reach the peripheral circulation, propionate and butyrate can exert several physiological functions in multiple organs, and interfere in a variety of pathological disorders. Short-chain fatty acids are key to maintaining the integrity of the intestinal barrier, and can modulate immune system activation, reduce systemic inflammation, and counteract the production of uraemic toxins produced by proteolytic bacteria, among other activities."

– Propionate and butyrate counteract renal damage and progression to chronic kidney disease; *Nephrology Dialysis Transplantation* journal; Jan. 2025

Those with chronic kidney disease typically test lower for short-chain fatty acid activity.

The metabolization of short-chain fatty acids can be increased by following a plant-based diet, and eliminating animal protein and extracted oils, as this will increase the fiber in the diet, and increase the variety of microorganisms in the gut biome.

The more animal protein and oily foods you eat, the lower the variety of microorganisms in the gastrointestinal tract, and the lower your intestinal production of short-chain fatty acids. Animal protein also increases the unhealthful organisms in the gut, resulting in TMAO (Trimethylamine N-oxide), which is linked to neurological decline, and both cardiovascular and kidney inflammation, and to strokes and heart attacks, and kidney failure.

What you don't want to follow is a diet that increases the amount of TMAO in your system. It is produced by the liver, and is oxidized from trimethylamine (TMA), metabolized in the gut by eating certain foods, mostly animal protein.

Foods that increase the liver's production of TMAO are red meat, pork, poultry, eggs, fish, and dairy.

"TMAO is mainly formed from nutritional substances from the metabolism of phosphatidylcholine/choline, carnitine, betaine, dimethylglycine, and ergothioneine by intestinal microflora in the colon. Its level is determined by many factors, such as age, gender, diet, intestinal microflora composition, kidney function, and also liver flavin monooxygenase activity. Many studies report a positive relationship between the level of TMAO concentration and the development of various diseases, such as cardiovascular diseases, and cardiorenal disorders, including atherosclerosis, hypertension, ischemic stroke, atrial fibrillation, heart failure, acute myocardial infarction, and chronic kidney disease, and also diabetes mellitus, metabolic syndrome, cancers (stomach, colon), as well as neurological disorders."
– Trimethylamine N-oxide (TMAO) in human health; *Experimental and Clinical Sciences Journal*; Feb. 2021

Eliminate animal protein from your diet, and you automatically decrease the amount of TMAO in your system.

In other words: to help prevent kidney and cardiovascular disease, neural degradation, and autoimmune disorders: Eat plants. Not animals, eggs, or dairy. And not damaged and rancid oils.

As suggested elsewhere, look at the recipes on the ForksOverKnives site, or in the Forks Over Knives recipe books, which are all plant-based, and oil-free. There is also the PlantBasedKidneys site, which has a variety of recipes, some containing avocado oil (which I omit).

Lowering risk: eliminating bottled oils

In his book *Prevent and Reverse Heart Disease*; Dr. Caldwell Esselstyn discourages the use of bottled oils (including olive oil, coconut oil, corn oil, seed oils, and other oils). So does Dr. John McDougall, author of *The Starch Solution*. Their advice is excellent not only for those who want to avoid heart disease while also lowering their risk of cancer and weight gain, but also for those with gluten, celiac, leaky gut, and other digestive issues, and/or who have kidney issues.

Soy and sugars and celiac

Soy and processed sugars can also be problematic for those with celiac. Esselstyn's diet includes soy.

Both the diet encouraged in this book and suggested by Esselstyn discourage the use of processed sugars (white [beet, cane] sugar, corn syrup, agave, rice syrup, etc.). Esselstyn's book provides recipes containing small amounts of sugar as an option. Both diets may or may not include maple syrup, depending on personal preference. (Consider using date sugar, lucuma fruit powder, monk fruit powder, or stevia instead.)

Desiring something sweet? Eat a piece of organically-grown fruit, and/or berries. Where possible, grow some.

Leaky gut and the intestinal barrier

Leaky gut is a condition in which larger molecules not being effectively broken down in the natural digestive processes within the mouth, stomach, and intestines pass through a damaged intestinal barrier – the intestinal mucosa. Typically, the barrier had been damaged by bad foods, heated and/or rancid oils, AGEs, synthetic food chemicals, and animal protein. The intestinal lining also can be damaged by infectious agents (bacterial, protozoan, viral), pharmaceutical drugs (steroids, NSAIDS [nonsteroidal anti-inflammatory medications], cytotoxic drugs, and hormones [including birth control pills]), chemotherapy, radiation, and toxins. A depletion of the beneficial intestinal bacteria ("friendly flora") – such as from taking antibiotics, colloidal silver, antacid products, and from alcohol abuse, consuming processed sugars, and unhealthful diet – can also play a role in leaky gut.

The larger molecules getting through the damaged intestinal barrier then enter into the bloodstream and act as antigens, which are foreign proteins, bacteria, and other substances that trigger immune system responses. These antigens can play a role in autoimmune disorders, including certain types of arthritis and rheumatic diseases as the immune system develops autoantibodies that then attack the antigens. This is especially so as the antigens land in the soft tissues of the joints – everything from the jaw, neck, spine, shoulders, hips, elbows, knees, ankles, feet, wrists, and hands.

As you follow a clean diet, you may find many of your health challenges greatly reduced, or eliminated. Part of this will because you healed your intestinal tract, and improved your gut microbiome, level of nutrition, blood system, and kidney, liver, heart, neural, and brain function.

The liver and leaky gut

While the liver can deal with some of the antigens, under the condition of leaky gut the amount of antigens entering the bloodstream can overwhelm the liver, keeping the antigens in the bloodstream. They may then settle in the various tissues of the body, including connective tissues and muscles, and other soft tissues, where they can trigger inflammation. The inflammation is the body displaying activities of attacking its own tissues, and is labeled as an "autoimmune disorder."

Musculoskeletal complications and inflammatory bowel disease

"Musculoskeletal complications are frequent and well-recognized manifestations in IBD (inflammatory bowel disease), and affect up to 33 percent of patients with IBD. The strong link between the bowel and the osteo-articular system is suggested by many clinical and experimental observations."

– Rheumatic Manifestations of Inflammatory Bowel Disease; *World Journal of Gastroenterology*, Nov. 2009

As mentioned elsewhere, a gastroenterologist can help determine what sort of bowel issues you may have, and offer solutions, including a restricted diet.

Harming your gut biome

What can harm your gut biome, for various reasons, are processed foods containing synthetic chemicals, including artificial sweeteners, colorings, flavors, scents, and texturing agents, and foods cooked at high temperatures, including roasted, seared, grilled, broiled, toasted, rotisserieed, fried, oil sautéed, and microwaved foods.

What also can harm your gut microbiota are industrial chemicals, including those found in some processed foods, and certain types of food packaging, in foods grown using chemicals, and in fish, beef, pork, chicken, turkey, and other meats, and in dairy, and eggs, and in some cosmetics, soaps, cleansers, and in most plastics.

"Endocrine disruptive chemicals (EDCs) have been implicated in disease states such as insulin resistance, glucose intolerance, type 2 diabetes, and obesity, breast and prostate cancer, as well as reproductive development disorders. In addition to their direct effects on physiology, exposure to EDCs, such as BPA, disturbs gut microbial composition. This may lead to changes in host lipid metabolism, among other effects. It was proposed that environmental obesogens could cause gut dysbiosis which might lead to inflammation and insulin resistance. The gut employs a multilayers mucus structure to maintain distanced between the gut epithelial cells and the gut microbiota as a protective mechanism. EDCs could increase the permeability of the small intestine, increasing the likelihood that bacterial pathogens will enter the body's circulation and target other organs. Food additives, such as artificial sweeteners, and contaminants such as pesticide residues can interfere with the gut microbiota and gut barrier function which could lead to intestinal, metabolic, and autoimmune disorders. Notably, obesity and type 2 diabetes were found to be associated with intestinal dysbiosis and gut barrier disruption."

– Obesogens: How they are identified and molecular mechanisms underlying their action; *Frontiers of Endocrinology* journal; Nov. 2021

Harming your gut biome includes eating a diet that increases problematic gut bacteria, while reducing the good gut bacteria that help in the digestion of food, absorption of nutrients, the creation of short-chain fatty acids, and protecting the lining of the stomach and intestines.

"Metabolic diseases include obesity, type 2 diabetes, non-alcoholic fatty liver disease, thyroid disease, hyperuricemia, hyperlipidemia, and others. The gut microbiota and short-chain fatty acids affect host metabolism, and dysbiosis is believed to be one of the main causes of common metabolic diseases in humans."

– Short-chain fatty acids in disease; *Cell Communication and Signaling* journal; Aug. 2023

Eating what reduces the good gut bacteria increases your risk of experiencing a variety of health problems, including unwanted weight gain, cardiovascular, liver, and kidney disease, and autoimmune disorders – including those that increase the risk of diseases of dementia.

Red meat degrades the gut microbiota, and Earth's biome

"Red meat was a strong driver of omnivore microbiomes, with corresponding signature microbiomes negatively correlated with host cardiometabolic health. Conversely, vegan signature microbiomes were correlated with favorable cardiometabolic markers, and were enriched in omnivores consuming more plant-based foods.

Diet is inextricably linked to human health. Globally, poor diets low in unprocessed, plant-based foods cause more deaths than any other risk factor, with cardiovascular disease, cancers, and type 2 diabetes as the leading causes of diet-related deaths. Unhealthy diets also carry a wide range of negative environmental impacts. Animal-based foods contribute comparably more than plant-based foods to global environmental change through their impact on climate, land, and freshwater use, and biodiversity. Consequently, there is increased interest in diets with higher fractions of plant-based foods that decrease both risk of disease, and negative environmental impact.

The gut microbiome plays an integral role in human health that can be modified by diet. For example, fermentation of otherwise indigestible plant polysaccharides by gut microbes contributes to a health, non-inflamed gut barrier and maintenance of gut homeostasis through the production of short-chain fatty acids and immune system crosstalk. Moreover, plants contain polyphenols, the products of plant secondary metabolism, that are known to promote beneficial bacteria that prevent inflammation, enhance the gut barrier, and hinder potential pathogens.

By contrast, a diet rich in animal foods leads to increased protein fermentation, which may result in a leaky mucosa, local and systemic inflammation, and reduced production of short-chain fatty acids. For example, the breakdown of certain animal proteins is linked to the synthesis of gut microbial trimethylamine (TMP), which is oxidized in the liver to trimethylamine N-oxide (TMAO). TMAO has been implicated in various cardiovascular diseases and is a potential contributing factor to colorectal cancer."

– Gut microbiome signatures of vegan, vegetarian, and omnivore diets are associated with health outcomes across 21,561 individuals; *Nature Microbiology*; Jan. 2025

Gut biome plays into many of our cellular processes

A healthy gut biome assists in the absorption of vitamins and minerals, and helps to metabolize short-chain fatty acids, and also polyphenols in a variety of edible plants. This plays into processes within the body, from brain, cardiovascular, muscle, liver, kidney, pancreas, spleen, and other organ functions, to mood, sleep, and energy, and autoimmune system functions.

"The greater the variety of plant-based foods we consume, the greater the diversity of beneficial microbes in our gut. This is because different plant-based foods contain different types of fiber, and each fiber can stimulate the growth of different types of health-promoting microbes. These microbes work together to improve our gut health, so the more diversity of health-associated microbes in our gut microbiome, the better our chances of gut health."

– Nicola Segata, PhD, Department of Cellular Computational, and Integrative Biology (CIBIO) at Universita di Trento, Italy

While it is good to include a variety of fruits, vegetables, sprouts, nuts, seeds, grains, legumes, and seaweeds in our diet, we don't have to include such a wide variety every single day. Too much variety all at once can be a bit much, and cause intestinal upset as each plant substance is vibrating at a different rate. You can be kinder to your system by spreading the variety of foods throughout a week – or month – to encourage a variety of gut microbes.

"The role of a plant-based diet in influencing obesity and inflammation was explored [and] demonstrated the positive effects of a vegan diet on the link between gut microbiota and metabolic syndrome. The authors included six obese, diabetic, and/or hypertensive individuals. The results showed lower blood glucose levels, body weight, triglycerides, total cholesterol, LDL-cholesterol, and hemoglobin A1c levels [blood sugar levels], following a month of vegan diet intervention. The number of Firmicutes [bacteria] was drastically reduced, and the abundance of Bacteroidetes was dramatically increased, due to the vegan diet therapy-induced changed gut microbiota. Even though the ratio of Firmicutes to Bacteroidetes changed, the host's enterotype did not change. This is because Prevotella and Bacteroides, which break down plant polysaccharides, grew in response to the vegan diet. In particular, the Enterobacteriaceae family of bacteria – known to cause chronic, low-grade inflammation – was found to be reduced in those following a vegan diet."

– Effect of Plant-Based Diets on Gut Microbiota: A Systematic Review of Interventional Studies; *Nutrients* journal; Mar. 2023

Probiotics

To improve your gut microbiota, consider taking a probiotic supplement for a month, and include raw sauerkraut in your diet as you also follow a clean, low-fat, plant-based diet free of extracted oils, processed foods, and synthetic chemicals.

"Probiotics are defined as live microorganisms that, when given in adequate quantities, provide health benefits to the host. Probiotics may be involved in the prevention and treatment of colorectal cancer through three different mechanisms. Firstly, probiotics inhibit the colonization of pathogenic bacterium through the release of antimicrobial peptides, reducing the luminal pH and competing directly with pathogens for nutrients. Secondly, through unique immunomodulatory effects to reduce inflammation or enhance anti-tumor immunity. Finally, probiotics increase mucin production and expression of tight junction proteins and promote epithelial restoration to enhance intestinal barrier function. These findings suggest that microbial interventions are beneficial in the treatment of colorectal cancer."

– Role of dietary nutrients and metabolism in colorectal cancer; *Asia Pacific Journal of Clinical Nutrition*; June 2024

(Research: organic vegan probiotic supplements, and raw sauerkraut.)

Meat nurtures gut bacteria that produce harmful substances

"Certain gut flora can take carnitine from the red meat we eat, or the choline concentrated in dairy, seafood, and eggs, and convert it into a toxic compound [TMAO] which may lead to an increase in our risk of heart attack, stroke, and death. This explains why those eating more plant based diets have lower blood concentrations of the stuff, but they also produce less of the toxin even if you feed them a steak [after a long term vegan diet]. You don't see the same conversion, suggesting an adaptive response of the gut microbiota in omnivores. They are what we feed them."
– Dr. Michael Greger, in the video Microbiome: We Are What They Eat; NutritionFacts.org; DrGreger.org

"The gut microbiome is a complex ecosystem compromising trillions of microorganisms that play a crucial role in human and animal health. Diet is a modulator of the gut microbiome, and animal products cause changes in gut microbiome composition and function.

Red meat may increase the gut microbiota's production of uremic toxins such as trimethylamine (TMA) n-oxide (TMAO), indoxyl sulfate, and p-cresyl sulfate. These uremic toxins are linked to a higher risk of cardiovascular death."
– Effect of Consumption of Animal Products on the Gut Microbiome Composition and Gut Health; *Food Science of Animal Resources Journal*; Sept. 2023

Some of the same studies concluding how harmful meat, dairy, and eggs are – including how eating them increases the risk of cancer, cardiovascular and kidney disease, and autoimmune disorders including diabetes and arthritis – also contain comments about how meat, dairy, and eggs are nutritious, including for getting amino acids to build protein. Such mixed messages can make a person wonder who paid for the studies, and why the same studies state how harmful meat, dairy, and eggs are, while also saying you should eat them. It's ironic, contradictory, perplexing, and suspicious advice.

You can get all the amino acids you need by eating plants. Plants also are a better form of nutrition for minerals, vitamins, anti-oxidants, anti-inflammatories, enzymes, and other nutrients. Plants contain the fiber needed for a variety of reasons, including for feeding our gut microbiome.

"L-carnitine with a TMA structure similar to that of choline and commonly found in meat, may also be converted to TMA by the gut microbiota, and contribute to the increased cardiovascular disease risk associated with high red meat consumption. They confirmed microbial involvement in TMA(O) formation from dietary l-carnitine using a stable isotope dilution method and broad spectrum antibiotic microbiota suppression in five healthy omnivorous subjects, and in germ-free and antibiotic-treated animals. Conversion of dietary l-carnitine to TMAO did not appear to occur in long-term vegans or vegetarians, suggesting an adoptive response of the gut microbiota in omnivores to TMA production from l-carnitine derived from red meat. Compared with vegans and vegetarians, omnivores [people who eat eggs] had elevated plasma TMAO concentrations and significantly higher relative abundance of fecal clostridia and peptostreptococci, groups of bacteria commonly associated with protein fermentation.

High-fat, high red meat, and low fiber diets are associated with reduced microbiota diversity, increased relative abundance of undesirable microorganisms, and increased production of toxic compounds, including the cardiotoxicant TMAO. These observations raise the intriguing possibility that gut microbiome interactions with whole-plant foods, probiotics, and prebiotics may be at the base of healthy eating pyramids."

– The way to a man's heart is through his gut microbiota – dietary pro- and prebiotics for the management of cardiovascular risk, by Karen M. Tuohy, Francesca Fava, and Roberto Viola; *Proceedings of the Nutrition Society* journal; Feb. 2014

Meat, dairy, and eggs do not contain any fiber, and they nurture harmful bacteria – including the bacteria that produce TMA (resulting in the liver producing TMAO), and bacteria that produce indoxyl sulfate, and p-cresyl sulfate.

Mammal meat and dairy (including from cows or goats) also contain the pro-inflammatory Neu5Gc molecule that can make cancer more aggressive.

The Agency for Research on Cancer, the World Cancer Research Fund, and the American Institute for Cancer Research have all linked red meat consumption to colorectal cancer.

Chicken

The more chicken, and red meat, and other types of meat you eat, the more you are ingesting saturated fat and cholesterol – as well as other substances – that increase risks of cancer, autoimmune disorders, cardiovascular disease, neurodegeneration, and kidney disease. Chicken has been directly linked to malignant melanoma, prostate cancer, and non-Hodgkin's lymphoma.

The nutrients humans need are in plants.

"Our study showed that white meat consumption above 300 grams per week was associated with a statistically significant increased mortality risk from all cancers and gastrointestinal tract. The risk was higher for men than for women."

– Does Poultry Consumption Increase the Risk of Mortality for Gastrointestinal Cancers? A Preliminary Competing Risk Analysis; *Nutrients* journal; April 2025

"Some people think plant-based, whole foods diet is extreme. Half a million people a year will have their chests opened up and a vein taken from their leg and sewn onto their coronary artery. Some people would call that extreme."

– Caldwell Esselstyn, MD, of ForksOverKnives.com

"Stop eating chickens, for Pete's sake. For starters, whether it's the white, whether it's the dark, each three-ounce piece of chicken has roughly 70 mg of dietary cholesterol. That's on par with red meat. Secondly, we've got saturated fat. Chicken is roughly 50% fat. Of that, 30% is coming from saturated fat. That clogs our arteries, contributes to insulin resistance, and also contributes to the production of cancer and tumor cells. Next, we've got animal protein. So, the essential amino acids that are in chicken are of a composition and proportion that actually cause the liver to bump up the production of IGF-1 – insulin-like growth factor number one that contributes to the production of, again, cancer and tumor cells. Next, we got antibiotic resistance. So, these chickens are so pumped with antibiotics that it promotes drug-resistant antibiotics in the human population that we don't want to be contributing to. And we've also got carcinogens, specifically

HCAs (heterocyclic amines) [and polycyclic aromatic hydrocarbons – which have been linked to cancer risk]. These are created when you cook any type of animal flesh, but they are highest with chicken. Then, lastly, what does chicken [and all animal protein] have zero of? It has zero fiber. There's an avalanche of reasons why we want to be consuming fiber."

– Rip Esselstyn, author of *The Engine 2 Diet* and *Plant-Strong: Discover the World's Healthiest Diet*

Farming chemicals

In recent years, doctors have encouraged me to follow an organic foods diet. I had already been doing so, as most of my diet is of organically-grown foods – including what we grow in the garden.

Synthetic chemicals used on farms have been found to increase risk of diabetes, cancers of the kidney and bladder, cardiovascular disease, stroke, obesity, birth defects, miscarriages, learning disabilities, neural degradation, and other health issues. These chemicals include pesticides, herbicides, insecticides, fungicides, and miticides.

"Two widely used herbicides, pendimethalin and atrazine, may be associated with altered kidney function among pesticide applicators [farm workers]. Our findings for these herbicides are consistent with observed associations with end-stage renal disease.

Pesticides have been reported to be associated with malignant and non-malignant kidney disease.

Beyond established risk factors for CKD (e.g., diabetes, hypertension), certain pesticides have been hypothesized to contribute to CKD development.

In the Agricultural Health Study, a large prospective cohort of licensed pesticide applicators (97% male) and their spouses (99% female) in Iowa and North Carolina, several specific pesticides have been associated with end-stage renal disease."

– Pesticide Use and Kidney Function Among Farmers in the Biomarkers of Exposure and Effect in Agriculture Study; National Institutes of Health; *Environmental Research* journal; May 2021

"Your kidneys are vital organs that filter 180 liters of blood every 24 hours. Chemicals and toxins also get filtered through our kidneys. Exposure to harmful chemical substances can cause adverse effects on the kidney, ureter, or bladder. The kidney is vulnerable because of its role in filtering the blood. Some chemicals and heavy metals cause severe injury to the kidney, while others produce chronic changes that can lead to kidney failure and cancer.

In the workplace, the most common route of exposure to occupational renal disease is by inhalation [breathing a substance into the lungs], skin absorption, and swallowing.

Some examples of occupational chemical products that can contribute to kidney damage and failure are benzene, organic solvents such as fuels, paints, and degreasing agents. Agrochemicals such as fertilizers and pesticides can also cause kidney illness. Workplace exposure to heavy metals such as cadmium and lead are also known to cause toxic injury to the kidneys."

– Workplace Chemical Hazards: Renal Disease; Chemscape.com

"There are risks associated with pesticide use. In addition to causing acute poisoning, they area also associated with increased cancer risks, among other diseases.

Our understanding of the role of occupational exposures, including pesticides, on end stage renal disease development in humans is growing.

Pesticides could be responsible for end stage renal disease progression. That is, pesticide exposure may cause accelerated worsening of already damaged renal function leading to more rapid ESRD [end-stage renal disease] development."

– Agricultural pesticide exposure and chronic kidney disease: new findings and more questions; *Occupational Environmental Medicine* journal; Sept. 2015

Many types of lawn and sporting field "landscape chemicals," and those used on farms have been identified as causing the progression of kidney, liver, and cardiovascular disease, and hormonal imbalance. These can include the herbicides alachlor, atrazine, metolachlor, paraquat, and pendimethalin, and the insecticide permethrin.

Then, there is glyphosate.

"In 2015, the World Health Organization announced that glyphosate is probably carcinogenic, i.e. cancer-causing. Concerns about glyphosate's impact on kidneys around from farm workers employed in the soybean fields suffering significant kidney damage despite not having typical risk factors such as diabetes and hypertension. More recent studies have shown significant alterations in kidney function in laboratory animals exposed to glyphosate, and the chemical has been shown to disrupt the microbiome in the intestine, causing a decline in the ratio of beneficial bacteria to harmful bacteria.

For consumers of soy and soybean products,, switching to organic soybeans is recommended to reduce one's exposure to glyphosate. Organic crops may still be grown using natural herbicides, but the use of chemical pesticides is forbidden for organic products."

– Dr. Dira Sooparth, Nephrologist; Bumrungrad International Hospital

The synthetic farming chemicals often are used on genetically modified feed crops grown to fatten farmed animals. Residues of those chemicals end up in the meat, milk, and eggs from farmed animals fed the chemically-laced feed crops. The chemicals also end up in the soil, rivers, aquifers, lakes, marshes, and oceans, and clouds, and rain, and in the tissues of animals, including you.

It has been found that everything from eggs to meat and dairy products from animals fed chemically-grown foods both have a weaker nutrient base, and also contain traces of harmful chemicals. This all can lead to human health issues, including kidney and cardiovascular disease, and cancers of the blood, brain, liver, reproductive organs, bones, bladder, kidneys, and other tissues.

GMOs: genetically modified crops

"Under the Non-GMO Project Standard, a genetically modified organism (GMO) is an organism to which biotechnology has been applied. This creates combinations of plant, animal, bacteria and virus genes that do not occur in nature, or through traditional crossbreeding methods.

In the absence of credible, independent, long-term feeding studies, the safety of GMOs is unknown.

Most packaged and processed foods contain ingredients derived from corn, soy, canola, and sugar beet – and the vast majority of those crops grown in North America are genetically modified.

The Non-GMO Project also considers livestock, apiculture [beekeeping], and aquaculture [farmed fish] products at high risk because genetically engineered ingredients are common in animal feed. This impacts animal-derived products such as eggs, milk, meat, honey, and seafood.

GMOs also sneak into food in the form of processed crop derivatives and inputs derived from other forms of genetic engineering, such as synthetic biology. Some examples include hydrolyzed vegetable protein, corn syrup, molasses, sucrose, textured vegetable protein, flavorings, vitamins, yeast products, flavors, proteins, sweeteners, microbes, enzymes, oils, and fats.

Because GMOs are novel life forms, biotechnology companies have been able to obtain patents to control the use and distribution of their genetically engineered seeds. Restrictive license agreements erode farmers' right to save seed [from year to year]. Relying on third-party corporations to provide farmers with both GMO seed and chemical inputs such as herbicide makes those farmers beholden to Big Ag, posing a serious threat to farmer sovereignty and to the national food security of any country where they are grown.

The most common genetically modified crops grown worldwide have been engineered for herbicide tolerance. In the first 20 years of the GMO experiment, the use of toxic herbicides, such as Roundup (glyphosate), increased fifteen fold. The use of these herbicides has led to a decline in native plants, which has downstream effects on biodiversity. Additionally, the overuse of herbicides has led to the emergence of pesticide-resistant 'superweeds' and 'superbugs,' which can only be killed by spraying more toxic chemicals."
– NonGMOProject.org

"Roundup and its active ingredient glyphosate are subject to controversy because animal and test-tube studies have linked them to various diseases. There is new evidence that glyphosate exposure may increase the relative risk of non-Hodgkin's lymphoma by 41%."
– Healthline.com

"The FDA has given the biotech industry carte blanche to produce and market any number of genetically engineered foods without mandatory agency oversight or safety testing, and without a scientific showing that these foods are safe to consume.

Twenty-nine leading scientists recently declared that animal test results linking genetically engineered foods to immune-suppression are valid.

IGF-1 [insulin-like growth factor-1, a hormone that is increased in dairy products from cows treated with genetically engineered recombinant Bovine Growth Hormone (rBHG) to produce more milk] could survive digestion, and make its way into the intestines and blood streams of consumers. These findings are significant because numerous studies demonstrate that IGF-1 is an important factor in the growth of breast cancer, prostate cancer, and colon cancer.

Genetic engineering can also alter the nutritional value of food. In 19912, the

FDA's Division of Food Chemistry & Technology and Food Contaminants Chemistry examined the problem of nutrient loss in GE foods. The scientists involved specifically warned the agency that the genetic engineering of foods could result in 'understandable alteration in the level of nutrients' of such foods. They further noted that these nutritional changes 'may escape breeders' attention unless genetically engineered plants are evaluated specifically for these changes.' Once again, the FDA ignored the findings by their own scientists, and never subjected the foods to mandatory government testing of any sort."
– GE Food & Your Health; Center for Food Safety; Feb. 2025

The altered DNA in genetically modified crops and farmed animals are rather new to Earth, and are becoming more common. Everything from tomatoes, papaya, corn, soy, and other food plants – and even some fish grown for human consumption, or fed to farmed animals – have been genetically modified. What the long-term impacts of these alterations might have on both plants, non-human animals of all varieties – and the human animal – are still a guess. It likely will take many decades to understand the implications of this experiment being conducted on all of humanity, wildlife, and nature.

Scientists have found that at least the chemicals used on genetically modified plants can cause problems with the nerves, brain, blood, liver, kidneys, and other tissues.

The most recent decades are the first in history that humans and other animals have been consuming genetically altered foods. It is an experiment.

The fear that GMOs might cause problems with human DNA could be reality, including relating to rates of certain types of cancer.

For better health, follow an organic, plant-based diet. By doing so, you will be reducing exposure to altered DNA, and to the synthetic chemicals used on crops, and the meat, dairy, and eggs from animals fed the GMO crops.

Find the organic produce farmers in your region. Locate the stores or co-ops selling organic produce, or start a co-op that does so. Learn to grow organic food. Learn about wild edibles.

Genetically modified organisms = GMOs

"A large percentage of our processed foods contain genetically modified organisms (GMOs). Unfortunately, the long-term health effects of GMO crops on humans remains unknown due to the lack of studies. However, studies on animals indicate that serious health effects are linked to GMOs. These include changes to major organs like the kidneys."
– Be aware of kidney-damaging foods; Piedmont.org; 2025

Another way to improve the quality of your food choices is to avoid genetically engineered produce. These are also more likely to have been grown using the farming chemicals you probably want to avoid.

Look for the term "non-GMO" on food labels.

Companies labeling their foods as non-GMO are aiming to supply food that has not been genetically modified.

The Non-GMO Project is a group working to protect our right to know what is in our food. The group administers a non-GMO certification process. You might have noticed their label featuring an image of a monarch butterfly. (Search: NonGMOProject.org.)

"The most familiar genetically modified organisms are modified with transgenic techniques, which have been available since the mid-90s. These GMOs are essentially living organisms whose genetic material has been artificially manipulated in a laboratory through genetic engineering, creating combinations of plant, animal, bacteria, and virus genes that do not occur in nature, or through traditional crossbreeding methods. Products of new genetic engineering techniques (e.g. CRISPR, TALEN, RNA interference, ODM, and gene drives) are also GMOs.

Most GMOs have been engineered to withstand the direct application of herbicide and/or to produce an insecticide. However, new techniques (such as CRISPR, RNA, ODM) are now being used to artificially develop other traits in plants, including resistance to browning in potatoes, and to create new organisms.

Genetically modified organisms are distinct from crops that have been bred using traditional cross breeding methods. GMOs are only created through the use of genetic engineering or biotechnology, not through processes that could occur in nature. Regardless of whether foreign DNA is used, any process where nucleic acid is engineered in a laboratory is genetic engineering, and the resulting products are GMOs. This also includes what is sometimes referred to as synthetic biology, or synbio.

Some crops have genetically modified versions that are widely commercially produced. These are corn, soy, cotton, canola, alfalfa, papaya, potato, sugar beet, and zucchini.

Many GMO corps are refined and turned into processed ingredients such as: corn starch, corn syrup, canola oil, sugar, molasses, soy lecithin, soy hemoglobin, citric acid, cellulose, maltodextrin, flavorings, vitamins, and anything that says 'vegetable,' but is not specific.

The Non-GMO Project is the leader in advocating for GMO transparency, conducting ongoing research and technical oversight of the changing GMO landscape.

Non-GMO means a product was produced without genetic engineering, and its ingredients are not derived from GMOs. Non-GMP Project Verified additionally means that a product is compliant with the Non-GMO Project Standard, which includes stringent provisions for testing, traceability, and segregation. Only Non-GMO Project Verified products are allowed to use the verification mark. Importantly, the mark includes the Project's URL, where consumers can look up the Standard to better understand what it means.

Because GMOs are novel life forms, biotechnology companies have been able to obtain patents with which to restrict their use. GMOs, therefore, post a serious threat to farmer sovereignty, and to the national food security of any country where they are grown, including the United States and Canada.

Over 80 percent of all GMOs grown worldwide are engineered for herbicide tolerance. As a result, use of toxic herbicides such as Roundup has increased 15 fold since GMOs were introduced. GMO crops are also responsible for the emergence of 'superweeds' and 'superbugs,' which can only be killed with ever

more toxic poisons like 2,4-D (a major ingredient in Agent Orange). GMOs are a direct extension of chemical agriculture and are developed and sold by the world's biggest chemical companies. The long-term impacts of GMOs are unknown, and once released into the environment these novel organisms cannot be recalled."
– NonGMOProject.org

The activities of the companies genetically engineering food plants are a danger to everyone, and the wildlife of plants, animals, bacteria, fungi, and other life forms.

Some of the GMO companies have included Aventis (France), BASF (Germany), Bayer CropScience (Germany), DOW Chemical (US), DuPont (US), Monsanto (US – acquired by Bayer in 2018), Novartis (Swiss), and Zeneca (Britain).

Your food choices might be supporting GMO companies

The very same companies listed above have been involved in the manufacture of dangerous farming chemicals that poison our food, water, soil, and air, and alter microorganisms, including our gut organisms. These chemicals have been linked to increased rates of everything from cancer, liver and kidney issues, asthma, diabetes, learning disabilities, depression, infertility, low-birth-weight babies, miscarriages, and other maladies. Why are we allowing this to happen? The way you spend your food money is either supporting these companies, or not.

If you eat fish, cows, pigs, chickens, or other farmed animals, or consume dairy or eggs, it is likely the farmed animals had been fed GMO crops, and have absorbed the toxic farming chemicals into their tissues, which then end up in you.

By avoiding any foods from born, hatched, or spawned creatures, you are also reducing your risk of exposure to GMO organisms and related chemicals.

Learn more about GMOs

- NonGMOProject.org
- OrganicItsWorthIt.org
- SayNoToGMOs.org
- ResponsibleTechnology.org
- OrganicConsumers.org

When possible, refrain from eating foods grown using toxic chemical fertilizers, insecticides, herbicides, pesticides, fungicides, miticides, defoliants, and other farming chemicals. However, it is important to get the adequate caloric intake, and to eat a variety of fruits, vegetables, and other plant matter to get the nutrients you need. Some people don't have access to organically grown foods, and can only eat what is available.

Pharmaceuticals, animal farming, and food poisoning

The pharmaceutical drugs used on farmed animals – including cows, pigs, lambs, goats, birds, and farmed fish – can also cause human health problems, and play a role in antibiotic-resistant food contaminants.

Food poisoning is often traced to the type of bacteria that flourish in the digestive tracts of cattle fed unnatural diets of grains. The grains are most often grown using synthetic chemicals, which end up as residue in the grains. The chemical residues are then in the farmed animals. Farmed animals are also commonly treated with a variety of pharmaceutical drugs, and the tissues of the animals have residues of the drugs.

What is it that you are eating when you eat bits of farmed animals, or dairy products, or eggs? It depends on what they were fed, what they were exposed to, how they were raised, what materials they were packaged in, and what sort of cooking was done to the animal protein.

Choose organic

By choosing organic foods, you will be reducing the use of toxic chemicals while supporting the organic foods industry, and protecting the health of the Earth, wildlife, and farm workers, and their communities.

While you may not be able to localize all of your food choices, you can likely do so with much of your foods. The more you rely on these safer foods, and the less you eat foods transported from distant lands, the more you will be improving the level of your nutrition while protecting wildlife and the ecosystems of both your region and the rest of the planet, and reducing your carbon footprint.

Hands in soil improves your brain, and immunity

The simple act of gardening improves your health in ways uncommonly known.

"Food is an intimate act. Food is not only our most intimate and powerful and profound connection with nature, with a larger order, it is also our most powerful and intimate connection with our culture."
– Dr. Will Tuttle, *The World Peace Diet*

Skin exposure to the beneficial mycobacterium vaccae in soil triggers the brain to release serotonin, improving mood, assisting the uptake of nutrients in the gut, and boosting the immune system (*Neuroscience* journal, April 2007).

The harvesting and smell of fresh fruits and vegetables triggers the release of dopamine in the brain. Dopamine is a feel-good chemical associated with feelings of bliss and euphoria. These are some reasons to participate in one of the oldest human activities: getting your feet and hands in soil to grow food.

"The glory of gardening: hands in the dirt, head in the sun, heart with nature. To nurture a garden is to feed not just the body, but the soul."
– Alfred Austin

An interesting book on the topic of localizing your food is Brian Halweil's *Eat Here: Homegrown Pleasures in a Global Supermarket*. There is also the book *Food Not Lawns*. As advised elsewhere, research: permaculture.

Wild edibles

Learn about wild edible plants, including dandelion, lambs quarters, minor's lettuce, mustard greens, and other wild greens rich in nutrients. Purslane is often on this list, but it is high in oxalates.

Each region has its own selection of wild edibles. Find yours, and learn how to incorporate them into your diet.

As your health improves

As your health improves with a cleaner diet and better intestine, gut microbiome, and other organ and tissue function, especially if you had been quite ill, and become much healthier, opportunities could arise you may never have considered. Things could happen you didn't know were a possibility, or were not in your idea of how your life could happen.

With improved health and a more healthful level of energy, you could find yourself feeling and thinking differently to the point you feel like a different person. Your perceptions may change. Foods, music, and designs of things may seem different to you. Activities in which you never had thought of participating in may draw your attention. The way you eat, dress, think, and play, and the general way in which you participate in and relate with life could all go through radical changes.

The higher frequency you tune into by eating more vibrant foods, getting daily morning exercise, and living a healthier lifestyle can ignite your passions in intense ways you never considered possible.

"The brain gives the heart its sight. The heart gives the brain its vision."
– Rob Kall

Pineal gland

When you follow a clean diet, the pineal gland located at the center of your brain, functions at a higher level, as does your heart, brain, and the area where most of your emotional chemistry is made: your stomach and intestines.

The function of the network of all tissues within you are related to what you eat, the health of your gut microbiome, the exercise and daily movement you get, your sleep pattern, the thoughts you choose to entertain, the practicing of your talents and skills, and the engagement of your intellect.

Cells of the pineal gland resemble the photoreceptor cells in the eyes. A low-quality diet leads to degeneration of the eyes. Similarly, low-quality foods interfere with the function of the pineal gland. The pineal gland's response to light and dark and how it interacts with the eyes also plays a role in its melatonin production. Melatonin plays a role in quality of sleep, and the sleep-wake cycle, and this plays into hormonal regulation, and electrolyte balance, as well as muscle strength, bone density, digestion, stress level, the amount of grey matter in the brain, brain function, emotional molecules produced by the gastrointestinal tract, the interaction with the gut biome and its production of certain nutrients, and the health of the intestinal lining. The function of the pineal gland is also associated with the seasonal mood disorders some people experience. All of the body systems and functions are connected.

René Descartes called the pineal gland *the seat of the soul*.

Some call the pineal gland *the third eye*.

While the cells of the eyes allow you to see and interact with structures, it is said the cells of the pineal gland allow you to interact with energy, inspiration, and what motivates you in your visualizations.

The pineal gland is strongly connected with your emotional life. It is not walled off behind the blood/brain barrier. It receives large amounts of blood, thus it is directly connected to the function and feelings and yearnings of the heart.

Fresh eyes and expression

"When you start using senses you neglected, your reward is to see the world with completely fresh eyes."
– Barbara Sher

A healthful diet and exercise schedule will get your body, heart, brain, pineal gland, muscles, digestive organs, sex organs, hormonal system, and other tissues to function better so the rest of your life can be expressed at an elevated level.

The expression of your health, energy, intellect, creativity, skills, and potential depends on you taking care of yourself, and practicing to improve.

What you do every day plays a role in your nerve wiring, including in the brain. This is why it is important to be involved in healthful life practices, and in doing what you want to do in tune with your intellect, talents, and skills.

Avoid deadening foods that dull your frequency

Avoid deadened or otherwise ultra-processed foods that lower your frequency and leave residues of toxins in your tissues, clogging and dulling your system, your daily experiences, and your life.

Follow a diet of high-quality foods that enliven your body, bring about the vibrant beauty of health, improve your level of consciousness, and allow you to dive into your potential.

"And the time came when the risk to remain tight in a bud was more painful than the risk it took to blossom."
– Anais Nin

Be engaged with what inspires you, and leads you into a better life experience, including through nutrition, exercise, and quality sleep, and in what is in tune with improving your skills.

But where do you get your protein?

All of my dietary protein is from eating plants, as I haven't consumed any animal protein in decades.

Because of many matters – including the mass breeding and killing of the farmed animals, what the animals are fed and put through, how the animal farming industry contributes to the spread of contagious diseases, and the way eating animal protein can increase inflammation, reduce beneficial gut organisms, increase the problematic gut organisms, and increase the risks of experiencing varieties of chronic, degenerative, and otherwise debilitating diseases – meat, eggs, dairy are not the best sources of protein.

The protein shortage myth

The body needs relatively little protein per calorie. Breast milk is less than 3% protein, and contains more carbohydrate, and fat. It is the ideal food for when you are growing faster than any time in your life: your first year of life. Yet, many people in commercialized society are eating somewhere over 35% protein, in the form of meat, dairy, and eggs.

You get enough protein from eating fruits, vegetables, sprouts, nuts, beans, legumes, grains, seeds, and seaweeds. As in: you get enough of the amino acids needed for your system to form your proteins. Many people don't understand this to the point they don't know what proteins are, or what they are made of – or how the body deals with proteins. Then, they are subjected to misunderstanding what foods to eat, and end up relying on the misinformation about what food is, and what food is not healthful.

Enough calories from a variety of plant sources = more than enough amino acids to make proteins

You will do fine on under 10% of your calories as protein. You will get more than this by eating enough calories of any combination of edible plants. You easily will get more if you are eating beans, legumes, lentils, and peas, or nuts, and even leafy greens and sprouts. You will get enough if you eat things that are under 6% protein, including broccoli, and sweet potatoes. Other plant foods are over 10% protein, including oatmeal.

"Think" they aren't getting enough protein

How many people do you know who have been diagnosed with protein deficiency? Not those who "think" they aren't getting enough protein. Not those who say or guess they aren't getting enough protein. Not the gym bunnies who concern themselves with protein to the point they are consuming all of those whey protein, casein protein, bone protein, soy protein, pea protein, and other protein powders on the market – which can damage their health, bones, gut biome, cardiovascular system, and kidneys. Many of those protein products have been tested positive for things like heavy metals and industrial chemicals. More on this topic in the following pages.

"Both plant and animal food can fulfill your protein needs. Once animals foods were considered superior for protein as they contain all the essential amino acids.

Dieticians now say it is not necessary to consume all the essential amino acids at one time. Instead, they can be spread over the course of a day, making it much easier for people who are vegan and vegetarian to meet the recommendations for protein."
– *Top Foods High in Leucine*; WebMD; 2023

To those who tend to believe in the "vegans don't get enough protein" concept, I ask: Do you know what the term is for protein deficiency? It very much is likely that you don't. Stop asking the protein question, pretending you are a protein expert, or being concerned about protein intake when you hear someone is vegan.

169

You know what contains more protein *per calorie* than meat, milk, or eggs? Lettuce. You may have heard iceberg lettuce doesn't contain any nutrients. The claim is nonsense. Iceberg lettuce – and all types of lettuce – contains amino acids, vitamins, minerals, enzymes, micronutrients, antioxidants, anti-inflammatories, and what you will not get from meat, milk, or eggs: fiber. Including fiber the microbiome of your digestive tract needs to function on a healthful level.

Red meat

If you have read this book up to here, you likely already understand this: Red meat can promote kidney disease, and end-stage renal disease (ESRD), because ingesting red meat produces waste products, and red meat contains chemicals that are stressing and damaging to, and cause renal hypertension, and overwhelm the kidney's filtration system. Red meat and animal protein also negatively impacts the intestinal organisms, decreasing helpful microbes, and increasing the presence of harmful microbes – leading to the formation of substances that then increase inflammation and promote various chronic and degenerative diseases, including cardiovascular disease, liver disease, kidney disease, autoimmune disorders, and colon cancer, and other types of cancer.

The breakdown of red meat protein releases the urea compound, which can build up in the tissues, and damage the kidneys. If someone already has compromised kidneys, the process magnifies the damage red meat ingestion can do to the kidneys.

"The pathophysiology of the association of animal protein with chronic kidney disease remains unclear. Our proposed mechanism is the link between animal protein consumption and hypertension, which observational studies and controlled trials have repeatedly demonstrated. Conversely, plant-based foods have been shown to have the opposite effect, so much so that emphasizing plant-based foods over animal-based foods is one of the principles of the Dietary Attempt to Stop Hypertension (DASH) diet. Animal protein consumption also may lead to weight gain, which might be another predisposing factor for kidney disease. Additionally, studies have demonstrated that, compared with intake of plant protein, intake of animal protein causes an imbalance in the composition of the gut microbiome by producing more ammonia and sulfur-based materials and having a proinflammatory profile, which may result in reduced kidney function and an increased risk of cardiovascular disease. Finally, high red meat intake has been associated with an increase in inflammation and oxidative stress."
– The Effects of High-Protein Diets on Kidney Health and Longevity; *Journal of American Nephrology*; July 15, 2020.

Meat and the kidneys

Red meat isn't the only problem meat for the kidneys. All mammal meat contains the cholesterol and saturated fat that promotes cardiovascular disease, and increase the risk of renal artery disease (R.A.D.), and inflammation, and cancer. Even fish can increase the liver's production of TMAO.

Consuming meat (including from mammals, birds, fish, reptiles, etc.) and other animal protein (dairy, eggs, rennet, etc.) can bring more blood to the kidneys, this can increase bleeding in already compromised kidneys. The result can be blood clots, slower kidney function, reduced kidney capillaries, and damage to already compromised kidneys.

Because meat is so problematic for the kidneys, can play a role in other degenerative and chronic health problems, and is not needed for human nutrition, cutting meat and other animal protein from the diet is a good choice for the long-term health of the heart, kidneys, liver, bones, blood, intestinal tract, immune system, lymph system, blood system, and other systems.

Amino acids: the building blocks of protein

Proteins are made of sequences of amino acids. It doesn't matter if the protein is from an animal or a plant. Proteins usually consist of a combination of amino acids, and are about 50 to 2,000 amino acids in length.

"There are 20 types of amino acids in proteins, each with different chemical properties. A protein molecules is made from a long chain of these amino acids, each linked to its neighbor through a covalent peptide bond. Proteins are therefore also known as polypeptides. Each type of protein has a unique sequence of amino acids, exactly the same from one molecule to the next. Many thousands of different proteins are known, each with its own particular amino acid sequence."
– The Shape and Structure of Proteins; *Molecular Biology of the Cell*, 4th edition

Fruits, vegetables, sprouts, herbs, nuts, beans, legumes, seeds, and seaweeds contain the amino acids our bodies need to obtain from food to form protein structures.

When you get enough calories from plants, you get more than enough amino acids for your body to make protein. But make sure it is quality plant material, not potato chips and other fried stuff, and beer, and other junk drinks, and cake, cookies, candy, and other such stomach filler – which can all be "vegan," but deplete health.

"The benefits of plant-based diet may include: Protection against heart disease. A review of eight studies found that people who followed a vegan or vegetarian diet were 30% less likely to die from ischemic heart disease than people who ate meat.

What you actually need from protein are the amino acids. You need 20 different ones. Your body makes some of them, but you must get nine from your diet. These are called *essential amino acids*.

People who follow plant-based diets have lower levels of type 2 diabetes than people who eat animal protein. People on plant-based diets are also less likely to be overweight. But the reduced risk of type 2 diabetes held up even among people of the same weight."
– The Difference Between Animal Protein and Plant Protein, WebMD; Oct. 2024

You can research the nine amino acids you need to get from food. The body does not synthesize them. You easily can get all of them on a plant-based diet.

Plants for protein

Excellent sources of protein are green leafy vegetables, other vegetables, and fruit, beans, legumes, nuts, sprouts, seeds, and seaweeds.

There are healthier choices, including whether or not the beans, legumes, nuts, seeds, and grains were raw and then soaked to enliven them. Depending on which food it is, this could mean being activated, germinated, sprouted, or what people call bloomed. (As explained in other parts of this book.) All of these plant-sources of food have more bioavailable – and less troublesome – protein, and fewer problematic substances in them than do meat, milk, and eggs, and other animal proteins, including bone broth, lard, whey, casein, and rennet*.

(*Rennet is the stomach lining of slaughtered calves used in cheese.).

Protein powders

The quality of the dietary protein needs to be monitored for people who have compromised kidneys.

A person with kidney disease should NOT be relying protein powders, including soy, pea, whey, casein, collagen, egg, or bone protein, or bone broth. Or, other isolated proteins as these increase the amount of nitrogen in the blood.

"Dietary casein promotes a progressive decline in the glomerular filtration rate (GFR) of remnant kidneys associated with metabolic acidosis and an endothelin-mediated increase in renal acidification."
– Dietary protein causes a decline in the glomerular filtration rate of the remnant kidney metabolic acidosis and endothelin receptors; *Kidney International*; Jan. 2008

"A nonprofit group called the Clean Label Project released a report about toxins in protein powders. Researchers screened 134 products for 130 types of toxins and found that many protein powders contained heavy metals (lead, arsenic, cadmium, and mercury), bisphenol-A (BPA, which is used to make plastic), pesticides, and other contaminants with links to cancer and other health conditions. Some toxins were present in significant quantities. For example, one protein powder contained 25 times the allowed limit of BPA."
– The Hidden Dangers of Protein Powders; Harvard Health Publishing; Aug. 2022

Through the animal protein shakes, it will spur their liver to produce TMAO. This increases the risk of cardiovascular disease, and the possibility of experiencing a heart attack or stroke. TMAO can reduce kidney filtration processes, and increases the risk of other kidney disease factors. TMAO can increase acidity and inflammation, and play a role in metabolic acidosis, autoimmune issues, and various forms of cancer. With all of those matters as risks, do you think it is wise to ingest concentrated animal protein shakes?

"Higher dietary protein intake is increasingly recommended for the elderly; however, high protein diets also have been linked to increased cardiovascular disease risk. Trimethylamine-N-oxide (TMAO) is a bacterial metabolite derived from choline and carnitine abundant from animal protein-rich foods. TMAO may be a novel biomarker for heightened TMAO risk.

High protein diets are also associated with an increased prevalence of diabetes and impaired kidney function."

172

– Protein Intake at Twist the RDA in Older Men Increases Circulatory Concentrations of the Microbiome Metabolite Trimethylamine-N-Oxide; *Nutrients* journal; Sept. 2019

A person can skip the animal protein, and instead go with plant-based sources of protein. This avoids the situation of consuming animal protein with all of its negative health impacts. Greens, sprouts, beans, legumes, and nuts are all excellent sources for the amino acids we need to form protein.

You might believe in the marketing claims of the companies selling protein powder products, or the labels of various commercialized products pushing their protein claims. What those marketing claims are is just that: wording meant to help sell products. Not wording aligned with science, or your body chemistry, or your nutritional needs. It's not about the companies caring about your health. The goal of the companies is to make money.

I don't use isolated protein products. I sometimes do use Infinity Greens powder blended into green juices or smoothies, or used in hummus, guacamole, or salad dressings. It isn't an isolated protein powder. It is a combination of a variety of plants, and contains a wide assortment of nutrients. I don't use the protein powder sold by that same company.

IF you do insist on taking a protein powder, use plant proteins, including because plants are acid neutral, and won't lead to taxing your kidneys by having to work harder to excrete acids, or other substances more prominent in – or only contained in – animal protein.

Be aware of the ingredients of the protein powder. Many protein powders tested have been found to be contaminated with industrial chemicals (including pesticides, and chemicals used in making plastics) and heavy metals (including arsenic, cadmium, mercury, and lead).

"Concerns have recently been raised about the presence of heavy metals in protein powder supplements following a *Consumer Reports* analysis of 15 protein powder products. The study found that the average amounts of heavy metals in three servings of protein powder per day exceeded the maximum limits of dietary supplements proposed by U.S. Pharmacopeia. In a follow up to the *Consumer Reports* analysis, another study reported that 40% of the 133 protein powder products they tested had elevated levels of heavy metals."

– A human health risk assessment of heavy metal ingestion among consumers of protein powder supplements; *Toxicology Reports Journal*; Aug. 2020

I recommend you don't take protein powders, but do eat a variety of greens, sprouts, other vegetables, beans, legumes, and other edible plants.

"Several observational studies have noted the source of dietary protein intake in relation to chronic kidney disease incidence, finding a strong association between intake of animal protein, especially processed and red meat consumption, and incidence and progression of chronic kidney disease. The Atherosclerosis Risk in Communities Study showed an increased risk of incidence of chronic kidney disease among participants consuming the highest quintile of red/processed meat compared with those consuming the least. Similarly, in the Singapore Chinese Health Study, consuming red meat strongly associated with end stage kidney disease risk in a dose-dependent manner. Data from these

studies also demonstrated that red meat, processed meat, or both associated with an increased risk of albuminuria, rapid eGFR decline, or both. Substituting one serving of red meat with plant-based protein such as legumes was associated with a 30%-62.4% reduced risk of chronic kidney disease."
– The Effects of High-Protein Diets on Kidney Health and Longevity; *Journal of American Nephrology*; Jul 15, 2020

Read elsewhere in the book about metabolic acidosis. Know what it is, the signs of it, what it does to your kidneys, and ways to avoid it.

Animal proteins, free radicals, heat-related chemicals, Neu5Gc, casomorphin

By consuming animal protein, you are also consuming tissue-damaging, inflammation-promoting free radicals, which exist and form in meat, milk, and eggs, and in other foods cooked to heat levels that form the chemicals known as AGEs.

Free radicals are more present after the animal proteins have been cooked, baked, grilled, fried, seared, sauteed, broiled, microwaved, or otherwise highly heated with dry heat, rather than wet heat (boiling, steaming, stewing).

Even if you are consuming some trace amounts of certain antioxidants in the animal protein, you are countering it by also consuming the damaging free radicals and AGEs in the animal flesh, dairy, or eggs. This is in addition to the other substances in meat, dairy, and eggs best not to ingest if you want to experience the most vibrant health.

The scenario of eating meat, dairy, and eggs to get antioxidants does not equate with excellent nutrition – especially considering that meat, dairy, and eggs also contain saturated fat, cholesterol, and a variety of other substances. For instance, the Neu5Gc in dairy and in mammal meat, and also the obesogens, casomorphins, cholesterol, and other substances in the various types of animal protein. Additionally, there are various health concerns involving whatever residues of farming and pharmaceutical chemicals the farmed animal was exposed to.

"Eating more plant-based foods, such as vegetables and grains in place of animal-based foods – such as red meat – can help prevent and slow kidney disease, diabetes, high blood pressure, and heart disease.

Studies show that eating whole grains, nuts, fruits, and vegetables is one of the most important ways to keep kidneys healthy."
– Plant-Based Diet and Kidney Health; National Kidney Foundation; 2025

Neu5Gc in dairy and meat makes cancer aggressive

"Neu5Gc is a common sialic acid type of sugar in mammals. It is a nine-carbon negatively charged monosaccharide that can be synthesized by most mammals and found at the tips of carbohydrate chains (glycans), glycoproteins, and glycolipids. Humans cannot synthesize Neu5Gc due to a deletion in the CMAH gene that encodes the cytidine 5'-monophosophate-Neu5GC hydroxylase. Yet, dietary Neu5Gc can be consumed then incorporated at low levels onto human cell surfaces, particularly in cancer, consequently displaying a broad assortment of immunogenic Neu5Gc-glycans. In face all humans examined thus far have a diverse collection of polyclonal anti-Neu5Gc antibodies. Thus, circulating anti-Neu5Gc antibodies continuously encounter Neu5Gc-containing epitodes on human tissues, and have been proposed to lead to xenosialitis, which in mice have been shown to exacerbate cancer and cardiovascular disease.

In human studies, glycan microarray analysis revealed that certain anti-Neu5Gc antibodies can serve as a carcinoma biomarker, and that high levels of total anti-Neu5Gc IgG are associated with increased colorectal cancer risk."
— Association between Neu5GC carbohydrate and serum antibodies against it provides the molecular link to cancer; *BMC Medical Journal*; Sept. 2020

The Neu5Gc molecule increases inflammation, and the aggressiveness of cancer. It is in cow and goat dairy products, and in mammal meat.

The Neu5Gc molecule isn't produced by humans, but is found on human cancer cells – only because the person ingested dairy products or mammal meat.

Humans have an immune antibody response when Neu5Gc-containing foods are ingested (cow and goat milk, and mammal meat), and create anti-Neu5Gc immunoglobulins.

"Neu5Gc was mainly found in red meat and liquid dairy products. The contents of Neu5gGc in beef, lamb, and pork were (30.32±2.84), (20.39±4.73), and (5.58±1.04) mg/kg, respectively, and in liquid milk and yogurt were (10.87±1.54), and (6.91±0.24) mg/L, respectively.

Dietary Neu5Gc intake is mainly from red meat and liquid dairy products, and its intake level is positively correlated with chronic inflammatory state of body."
— Study on the correlation between dietary N-glycolylneuraminic acid intake and chronic inflammation state of body; *Chinese Journal of Preventive Medicine*; June 2020

"A positive correlation between massive red meat consumption with colorectal cancer has been reported.

In 2015, the International Agency for Research on Cancer published the results of a study on the association of cancer with red or processed meat consumption, including the link of red meat consumption with human colorectal cancer and the 'probably carcinogenic to humans' classification of red meat. These growing research suggests a connection of the consumption of red meat-derived non-human Neu5Gc and various diseases, including cancer progression, cardiovascular disease, inflammation, and several autoimmune diseases."
— Overdose intake of Neu5Gc triggers colorectal inflammation and alters liver metabolism; Taylor & Francis online research article; Sept. 2023

"As brands like Yoplait continue to don the pink lids in support of finding a cure for breast cancer, the mounting research is constantly leading back to animal products as a major cancer culprit. Oh, the irony. A recent French study analyzed the link between Neu5Gc consumption (a compound only found in non-human animals) and cancer risk, and found a correlation between the two that cannot be ignored.

Neu5Gc is a sialic acid with a charge, meaning it has 'meet and greet' properties that allow it to bind to cell surfaces, lipids, and other biological structures. It is common in many mammals, but humans do not have the ability to form Neu5Gc. When ingested (IE by consuming meat or dairy), the human body develops an immune response against this foreign compound. This causes

inflammation – one of the precursors to chronic disease."
– The Link Between Dairy, Cancer, and Neu5Gc; Switch4Good.org; Feb. 2021

Eliminate the Neu5Gc molecule from your diet by avoiding all dairy and mammal meat. Doing so will be reducing your risk of a variety of inflammatory, degenerative, and chronic diseases.

Urea nitrogen

A blood test done in relation to kidney function is to check the blood urea nitrogen (in addition to potassium and other minerals). It is the Blood Urea Nitrogen (BUN) test.

Urea nitrogen is a waste product of the liver breaking down protein. The blood in a healthy person contains about 7 to 20 mg/dl of urea. A person on a high-protein diet would have more – which also involves the liver and kidneys doing more work.

A diet high in animal protein is harder on the digestive and cardiovascular system, including because of the cholesterol, saturated fat, and chemistry of meat, dairy, and eggs, as well as animal protein triggering the liver to create TMAO.

"Vegans had significantly lower leukocyte, lymphocyte, and platelet counts, and lower concentrations of complement factor 3 and blood urea nitrogen, but higher serum albumin concentrations.
– Dietary intake and biochemical, hematologic, and immune status of vegans compared with nonvegetarians; *The American Journal of Clinical Nutrition*; Sept. 1999

"Healthy adult vegetarians have better renal function than omnivores, and the higher dietary fiber intake associated with vegetarian diets may contribute to the protective effect on renal function.
– Healthy adult vegetarians have better renal function than matched omnivores: a cross-sectional study in China; *BMC Nephrology* journal; July 2020

Meat-heavy keto diet

Some people follow what they *think* is a healthful diet, but it might be largely centered on eating meat, dairy, eggs, and higher-fat foods, and concentrated protein powders, as in the trendy, meat-heavy keto diet promoted on the social media pages of manly posey gym bros – who often also sell products.

One trend I looked into was of social media "influencers" saying you can experience ideal health by eating lots of meat, dairy, eggs, and butter, bone broth, tallow, and even lard.

There are also the people who eat whatever is sold in packaging that features claims the product is "healthy" and nutritious. Food packaging is designed to sell products, not to improve your health.

Many people consider the keto diet as ideal, and companies are using that to promote their products, featuring the word "keto" on their labels. It's the whistle to trigger sales.

An animal protein-heavy, high-fat diet is not the diet a person should follow if they want to protect their kidneys and colon, and liver, spleen, pancreas, digestive tract, or brain, and is an especially harmful diet choice for anyone already with any level of kidney or heart disease.

Read some of what the *Journal of the American Society of Nephrology* has said about the keto diet.

"Although the ketogenic diet has recently received a disproportionate amount of attention because it is purported to help treat obesity and type 2 diabetes, evidence that it actually offers such benefits is limited. Long-term randomized trials have failed to show a clinically significant benefit over comparative diets. Worse, the diet it not without consequence: it may produce adverse effects in the average dieter, such as hyperlipidemia, vitamin and mineral deficiencies, and fatigue. For patients with or at high risk of kidney disease, the ketogenic diet may further tilt the risk/benefit ratio unfavorably by producing kidney-specific risks.

For patients with existing kidney disease, the diet's high protein intake may accelerate the progression of their kidney disease...

Data from several prospective studies show that animal protein – an integral part of many ketogenic diets – may increase the risk of developing chronic kidney disease."

– The Effects of High-protein Diets on Kidney Health and Longevity; *Journal of the American Society of Nephrology*; July 2020

The way many people find out about the keto diet is by following people who are popular on social media. "Social media influencers" may have absolutely no education in science, nutrition, or medicine.

Would you rather listen to six-pack Joe the keto guy on social media give you nutritional advice, or would you rather listen to people who studied the science behind nutrition, medicine, and disease processes?

Vegan keto and seizure prevention

For those with seizure issues, there might be benefits in following more of ketogenic vegan diet. The original ketogenic diet is credited to Dr. Russel Wilder of the Mayo Clinic. He developed it in the 1920s, and called it an "anticonvulsant diet," using it in combination with fasting as a way of reducing seizures in children. Wilder's version of the diet was 4% carbohydrates, 90% fat, and 6% protein. But it increased the risk of other health problems.

Yes, vegan keto is possible. It reduces the incidence of some of the complications of an animal protein-based keto diet. Among those complications are renal fibrosis, nephrolithiasis, glomerulosclerosis, glomerular hyperfiltration, interglomerular hypertension, proteinuria, albuminuria, high acid load, high lipid count, fatty liver, leaky gut, kidney stones, pre-renal azotemia, increased inflammation and cholesterol levels, and heightened TMAO production, cardiovascular disease, neural degeneration, bone loss, macular degeneration, and other matters.

With that said, you likely want to consider those issues relating to an animal-based keto diet, and investigate the possibilities of vegan keto.

Avocados*, olives**, hemp seeds, chia seeds (never eat dry chia seeds, always mix them with a liquid for at least ten minutes), flax seeds, tahini, coconut milk, and fermented coconut yogurt (like the fermented CoCoYo yogurt by GTsLivingFoods.com), and fermented cashew and/or pine nut cheese, and soaked raw nuts, all can be part of the vegan keto diet. Also look into the benefits of a high-fiber diet to prevent seizures, including vegetables, sprouts, and berries.

(*Avocadoes are high in potassium. One cup of avocado contains about 700 micrograms of potassium. The recommended potassium in a meal is 200 micrograms. Those with kidney disease may want to limit their consumption of avocados to what amounts to about a ping pong ball-sized amount per meal. Mix guacamole with an equal amount of oil-free, low-salt hummus, as garbanzo beans are much lower in potassium.

(**Olives could be high in salt. Rinse or soak them in water to remove some of the salt.)

Lemons and limes are included in vegan keto.

Protect the teeth enamel: Always rinse the mouth with water after drinking a daily morning shot of apple vinegar, or drinking water that has had lemon squeezed into it.

Raw, unheated, unfermented, sauerkraut is keto, and great for the gut microbiome. Sauerkraut is easy to make. In addition to cabbage, raw sauerkraut can also be made to include other vegetables. I like to include kale, fennel, garlic, horseradish, burdock root, ginger, lemon, thyme, oregano, nettle leaf, black pepper, and cayenne.

Keto-friendly berries include acai, blackberries, blueberries, raspberries, and strawberries. Some berries like bananas, blackcurrants, cranberries, goji berries, and mulberries are too high in carbs to be considered keto.

Infinity Greens powder can also be used in vegan keto. The company also sells Infinity Keto Bars.

Bear Bars are keto, and can be purchased online through BearBar.com (I happened to be eating a Bear Bar while typing this).

Research: vegan keto.

In addition to vegan keto, also, look into the benefits of CBD and the indica strain of marijuana and delta-9-THC for reducing and preventing seizures.

Research the benefits of vitamins B6 (pyridoxine) and E, and magnesium.

Be sure to include ample amounts of vegan sources of omega-3 fatty acids, including chia, flax, and hemp seeds, as well as edamame, walnuts, seaweeds (like nori), and algae. Have some – but not an abundance of – pumpkin and sunflower seeds, and be sure to get them raw, and to soak them before use. Broccoli sprouts, Brussels sprouts, sunflower sprouts, and basil are also sources of omega-3s.

A healthy gut biome can also play a role in reducing seizures. See the information in this book about improving the gut microbiome.

Stay hydrated, as dehydration can also be a risk factor for triggering seizures.

Certain breathing and meditation techniques can also help to reduce or prevent seizures.

Consider all options for preventing seizures, and reducing their intensity. Long-term health is key, including to protect your brain. Do what is right for your health.

"The term 'ketogenic diet' was created by Russel Wilder in 1921, and was initially utilized to treat epilepsy. It was popular for about 10 years as a treatment for pediatric epilepsy, but lost favor when antiepileptic drugs came on the market.

The idea of a ketogenic diet making a comeback as a quick weight-loss strategy is very recent."
— Is Losing Weight Wroth Losing Your Kidney: Keto Diet Resulting in Renal Failure; *Cureus* journal; March 2023

Ketogenic diet

To be kidney-safe, following a diet high in animal protein is too problematic. Including because too much fat can be a problem for cholesterol level, cardiovascular health, the gut microbiota, endothelium cell function (cells lining the walls of the cardiovascular and lymph systems), liver and lung function, energy issues, what it does to the vascular system in the kidneys (glomerulosclerosis), the increased risk of kidney stones, and other matters. There are the Neu5Gc concerns, the increased production of TMAO by the liver, and the risks of fatty liver disease, the inflammation and autoimmune issues, and the cancers, including of the colon, sex organs, bladder, and kidneys.

"High dietary acid load generated by the consumption of high animal fat and protein is associated with albuminuria (losing protein in the urine), and the onset of chronic kidney disease. In addition to increasing your chances of developing chronic kidney disease, research has linked the keto diet to an increased decline in kidney function for those who already have chronic kidney disease.

When you eat a nigh protein diet, the kidney must work harder because of increased blood flow to the filtrating unit of the kidney called hyperfiltration, which leads to the progression of chronic kidney disease. A keto diet potentially worsens metabolic acidosis, which is a common complication of chronic kidney disease, which ultimately affects bone and muscle health as well."
— The Keto Diet: Helping You Lose Weight, or Hurting Your Kidneys; MyTPMG.com; 2025

A keto diet can increase the risk of experiencing prerenal azotemia, a condition of the kidneys not filtering the blood of waste products. It can be caused by a variety of situations, including heart failure, a stroke, a heart attack, blood loss, dehydration, or otherwise decreased blood flow to the kidneys.

"Prerenal azotemia is the most common form of reduced kidney function in hospitalized people. Any condition that reduces flood flow to the kidney may cause it, including: burns, conditions that allow fluid to escape from the bloodstream, long-term vomiting, diarrhea, or bleeding."
— MelinePlus.com

"The ketogenic diet is becoming more popular as a weight loss regimen; however the evidence has failed to show clinically significant benefits over comparator diets. Even worse, it may cause hyperlipidemia, vitamin and mineral deficiencies, fatigue, and kidney damage, among other complications. Increased acid production from a ketogenic diet may cause metabolic acidosis and related issues, including weakened bone health. Studies show that people with chronic kidney disease and those without prior kidney problems are experiencing a decline in kidney function.

The proposed mechanisms of high protein dietary intake for kidney damage include mediators including acid load, high phosphate content, gut microbiome

dysbiosis, and inflammation."
– Is Losing Weight Wroth Losing Your Kidney: Keto Diet Resulting in Renal Failure; *Cureus* journal; March 2023

Those following the high-fat ketogenic diet have higher rates of hyperlipidemia (elevated cholesterol and triglycerides in the blood [increasing risk of atherosclerosis, peripheral artery disease, strokes, and heart attacks]), nutrient deficiencies, stress, and fatigue. None of those conditions are good for the kidneys, and will only increase the risks of experiencing and advancing kidney disease.

"In individuals with diabetes, low-carbohydrate diets may cause an initial reduction in blood glucose values, but these benefits are often largely gone by 12 months.

There may be some safety concerns with a low-carbohydrate diet. They often elevate plasma LDL cholesterol concentrations, with widely varying effects between individuals. Because low-carbohydrate diets restrict or eliminate fruits, whole grains, legumes, and other healthful foods, and are often high in saturated fats, they raise concerns about long-term risk of cancer, Alzheimer's disease, and other conditions. Long-term use of low-carbohydrate diets is associated with increased all-cause mortality."
– Perspective: Plant-Based Eating Pattern for Type 2 Diabetes Prevention and Treatment: Efficacy, Mechanisms, and Practical Considerations; *Advances in Nutrition* journal; June, 2021

High-protein diet and ketones, urea, and ammonia

The high-protein diet increases protein byproducts, including ketones, urea, and ammonia. The kidneys and liver play roles in clearing these from the system. But damaged kidneys don't do a good job of it, nor does a liver continually burdened by an unhealthful diet.

Ketosis

By restricting carbohydrates, the goal of being on a ketogenic diet is to go into a state of "ketosis," as the body then breaks down fat into molecules called ketones as it uses fat for fuel, instead of glucose from carbs from fruit and starches.

In a ketogenic diet, meat, dairy, eggs, and fatty foods like avocadoes and coconut are encouraged, along with some greens, certain berries, and other foods. But carbs are extremely restricted.

As mentioned earlier, some people follow the keto diet as a way to reduce epileptic seizures. Some put their children with pediatric epilepsy on a keto diet.

Some reports are that a keto diet slows certain types of cancer by restricting glucose, depriving the cancer cells of energy. Other studies identify the keto diet as promoting tumor metastasis.

"Our lab studies show metabolic stress regulates tumor growth and metastasis. How the ketogenic diet affects tumor growth has been reported by several groups, but we wanted to look at how it affects tumor metastasis, and we got a very surprising result.

We did indeed see that the ketogenic diet suppressed tumor growth. But we also saw that it promoted tumor metastasis.

Cancer cells detect that this place deprived of glucose is not nutritionally comfortable, so they want to escape. They don't want to stay in the wrong place. The consequence of that is metastasis."

– Wei Gu, PhD, who led a study conducted at the Herbert Irving Comprehensive Cancer Center finding that the keto diet increased cancer in the breasts and lungs.

"So far, no major cancer group recommends keto diets for either prevention, or treatment of cancer.

A ketogenic diet may worsen your cancer. Some keto-friendly foods like red meat can raise your chances for cancer."

– Cancer and the Keto Diet; WebMD; Dec. 2024

"Just looking at the [weight] scale, the ketogenic diet seems like a success, but what happens inside bodies tells a different story. On the keto diet, rates of body fat loss may slow by more than half, so most of what is lost is water. The reason less fat is burned on a ketogenic diet is presumably the same reason people who start fasting may start burning less fat: Without carbohydrates, the preferred fuel, our bodies start burning more of our own protein.

Inadequate intake of 17 micronutrients has been documented in those on ketogenic diets. Children have gotten scurvy, and some have even died from deficiency of the mineral selenium, which can cause sudden cardiac death. Bone fractures disproportionately plague children on ketogenic diets, along with growth stunting and kidney stones, and constipation is a frequently cited side effect. Keto diets have also been shown to reduce the richness and diversity of our gut flora, and all of that saturated fat can have a profound impact on the heart: a meta-analysis of four cohort studies following the diets, diseases, and deaths of more than a quarter million people found that those who eat lower-carb diets suffer a significantly higher risks of all-cause mortality, meaning they live, on average, significantly shorter lives.

Dieting is a particularly important time to make sure you're meeting all of your essential nutrient requirements, since you may be taking in less food. Ketogenic diets tend to be so nutritionally vacuous that one assessment estimated you'd have to eat more than 37,000 calories a day to get a sufficient daily intake of all essential vitamins and minerals.

Not surprisingly, constipation is very common on keto diets. As I've reviewed before, starving our microbial self of prebiotics can have a whole array of negative consequences. Ketogenic diets have been shown to 'reduce the species richness and diversity of intestinal microbiota,' our gut flora. Microbiome changes can be detected within 24 hours of switching to a high-fat, low-fiber diet. A lack of fiber staves our good gut bacteria. We used to think that dietary fat itself was nearly all absorbed into the small intestine, but based on studies using radioactive tracers, we now know that about 7 percent of the saturated fat in a fat-rich meal can make it down to the colon. This may result in 'detrimental changes' in our gut microbiome, as well as weight gain, increased leaky gut, and pro-inflammatory changes. For example, there may be a drop in beneficial Bifidobacteria and a decrease in overall short-chain fatty acid production, both of which would be expected to increase the risk of gastrointestinal disorders.

Based on the famous Harvard cohorts, eating more of an animal-based, low-carb diet was associated with higher death rates from cardiovascular disease, and

a 50 percent higher risk of dying from a heart attack or stroke, but no such association was found for lower-carb diets based on plant sources."
— Dr. Michael Greger, NutritionFacts.org; DrGreger.org

Dr. Michael Greger did a series detailing the health risks of the keto diet. He covers a broad spectrum of nutritional concerns relating to the diet. You can find his series on the NutritionFacts.org site.

One of my best friends for 17 years followed the ketogenic diet for more than a decade. I addition to eating mostly meat, dairy, and eggs, he regularly drank whey and casein protein smoothies. He'd ask me about the keto diet. I would send him studies about how it is not a good choice, as it increases risks of cancer, cardiovascular disease, kidney disease, liver dysfunction, and other health issues, including E.D. I strongly encouraged him to switch to a more plant-based diet. He was afraid he would lose his muscle definition, as he was very much into a lean, muscular appearance, and was into extreme fitness and martial arts. He worked as a photo double and stunt performer for actor Jean-Claude Van Damme in some of those action films. He spent his final month in a hospital. He told me they found cancer, and it had spread to his liver, a kidney, one ureter tube, his intestines, lungs, and heart, and there were two "floating" tumors in his torso.

As I mention elsewhere in the book, many of those protein smoothie products being used by people on the keto diet have tested positive for heavy metals (arsenic, cadmium, lead, mercury), farming chemicals, and industrial pollutants. These include both the animal protein and plant protein smoothies.

"The International Agency for Research on Cancer has long classified arsenic as 'carcinogenic to humans,' specifically, ingestion exposure of arsenic has been associated with skin, lung, bladder, kidney, and possibly liver and prostate cancer."
— A human health risk assessment of heavy metal ingestion among consumers of protein powder supplements; *Toxicology Reports Journal*; Aug. 2020

Meat-heavy diet: the shattered myth of the Massai tribe

People sometimes repeat the myth that men of the Massai tribe in Africa survive on beef, blood, and milk, and they are healthy.

George V. Mann, M.D. studied the men of the Massai tribe. His report was published in the September 22, 1977 edition of *The New England Journal of Medicine*, and is titled *Diet-Heart: The End of an Era*. He found the people of the Massai tribe had more arthrosclerosis than the average American men. His study is one of many revealing the meat-heavy diet as having a direct link to heart disease, and specifically a diet rich in animal protein. The study helped to spur the "heart healthy" diet plans.

Animal protein keto diets and kidney disease

Consider what Dr. Michael Greger says here about the keto diet, diabetes, and kidney disease:

"There is a keto product company that claims ketogenic diets can reverse diabetes. But they are confusing the symptom: high blood sugars, with the disease, which is carbohydrate intolerance.

People with diabetes can't properly handle carbohydrates, and this manifests as high blood sugars.

Sure, if you stick to eating mostly fat, your blood sugars will stay low, but you may be making the underlying disease worse at the same time.

We've known for nearly a century that if you put people on a ketogenic diet their carbohydrate intolerance can skyrocket – within just two days.

One week on an 80% high-fat diet and you can quintuple your blood sugar spike in reaction to the same carb load, compared to a week on a low-fat diet. Even a single day of excessive dietary fat intake can do it.

If you're going in for a diabetes test, having a fatty dinner the night before can adversely affect your results.

One meal high in saturated fats can make the cause of diabetes – carbohydrate intolerance – worse within four hours.

A true diabetes-reversal diet is practically opposite of a ketogenic diet: Diabetics off their insulin within a matter of weeks while eating 300 grams of carbs per day.

One of the reasons diabetics suffer such nerve and artery damage is due to an inflammatory metabolic toxin known as methylglyoxal that forms at high blood sugar levels.

Methylglyoxal is the most potent creator of advanced glycation end products – so-called AGEs – which are implicated in degenerative diseases, from Alzheimer's disease and cataracts, to kidney disease and strokes.

You get AGEs in your body from two sources: eating them pre-formed in your diet, or making them internally from methylglyoxal if you have high blood sugar levels.

On a keto diet, one would expect high exposure to pre-formed AGEs, since they are found concentrated in animal-derived foods high in fat and protein. But we would expect less internal new formation due to low levels of methylglyoxal given lower blood sugars [while] not eating carbs.

Dartmouth [University] researchers were surprised to find more methylglyoxal, though [in people following a high-fat diet]. A few weeks on the Atkins Diet lead to a significant increase in methylglyoxal, and those in active ketosis did even worse, doubling the level of this glycotoxin in their bloodstream. It turns out, high sugars may not be the only way to create this toxin [methylglyoxal].

One of the ketones you make on a ketogenic diet is acetone, known for its starring role in nail polish remover. Acetone does more than make keto followers fail breathalyzer tests, and develop what is described as 'rotten apple breath.'

Acetone can oxidize in the blood to acetol, which may be a precursor to methylglyoxal. That may be why keto dieters can end up with levels of this glycotoxin as high as those with out-of-control diabetes – which can cause the nerve damage and blood vessel damage you see in diabetics. That's another way keto dieters can end up with a heart attack. So the irony of treating diabetes with a keto diet may extend beyond just making the underlying diabetes worse, but by mimicking some of the disease's dire consequences."

> – Dr. Michael Greger in his video *Does a Ketogenic Diet Help Diabetes, or Make it Worse?* See his series about the Keto diet on NutritionFacts.org

Sexual region vascular dysfunction

Men may want to know a diet rich in dairy, meat, and eggs can play a role in experiencing E.D. Instead of looking to a pill as the solution, they may want to consider what they are putting into their system through food.

Artery-clogging foods also clog veins and capillaries throughout the body, not only in people with the male parts, but also in the people with the lady parts.

"Erectile dysfunction is a sign of narrowed arteries throughout the body, including to the penis, and can be an indication of heart disease. A meta-analysis of 25 studies found that men with E.D. have a 59% higher risk of coronary heart disease or atherosclerosis, a 34% higher risk of stroke, and a 33% higher risk of dying from any cause – compared with men without symptoms of E.D.

But a healthful plant-based diet can help unblock arteries, improving blood flow to the heart and brain, as well as to the penis. In fact, a plant-based diet is associated with reduced risk of erectile dysfunction, according to research recently published in the *Journal of Urology*. Previous research has found that men with the highest intakes of anthocyanins, flavones, and flavanones – compounds found in fruits such as strawberries, applies, blueberries, and citrus – lowered their risk of E.D. by 14% when compared to those who consumed the least."

> – Fight Erectile Dysfunction, Physicians Committee for Responsible Medicine; Nov. 2021

"In a well characterized national database, it was shown that a healthful plant-based diet is associated with less chance of having erectile dysfunction."

> – Plant-based diets are associated with decreases risk of erectile dysfunction; *The Journal of Urology*; Sept. 2021

"The plant-based diet is a safe and effective prophylaxis and treatment for hypercholesterolemia and atherosclerosis.

The Mediterranean diet is a plant-strong diet that results in better female sexual function in a dose-dependent manner, regardless of menopausal and metabolic syndrome status. The plant-based diet has the potential to be at least as good a treatment of FSD [Female Sexual Dysfunction].

A plant-based diet has the significant advantage of having no contraindications or adverse reactions, and is an affordable prophylaxis for all patients over long-term."

> – Female Sexual Dysfunction and a Plant-based Diet; *Journal of Gynecology and Women's Health*; Sept. 2023

Creatinine, creatine, and the amino acid methionine

People with kidney disease can have excessive amounts of urea in their blood. They also have creatinine in the urine, which is a waste product from the body using creatine, which is a chemical naturally synthesized by humans.

Creatine is a molecule stored as phosphocreatine, and this helps synthesize adenosine triphosphate (ATP), which is used by the brain and muscles during intense activities, and for recovery.

Creatine is synthesized by the body with the precursor being the amino acids arginine, glycine, and especially methionine.

Methionine is in both animal protein and in plants. Some people claim vegans should take methionine supplements. Vegans get methionine as they do other amino acids: by eating a variety of foods. Methionine is stored in the liver. Methionine is in black eyed peas, Brazil nuts, cashews, chia seeds, edamame and soybeans, flaxseed, hemp, lentils, oats, peas, pine nuts, quinoa, sesame seeds (and tahini), spirulina, sunflower seeds, wheat, wild rice, and other edible plants.

Simply because plants have less methionine than meat does not mean vegans need to take methionine supplements. If a substance is abundant in meat doesn't equate to it being ideal for human nutrition in that quantity.

Taking methionine supplements can get complicated, and play a role in bipolar disorder and liver disease. Women who are planning on getting pregnant, or who are expecting, or are breastfeeding should not take methionine supplements (and should consult with their doctor, and/or a nutritionist).

Additional creatine can be in the diet from eating animal protein.

Unhealthy kidneys are associated with a high level of creatinine in the urine. An abundance of creatinine in the urine can also be a sign of liver damage.

Eating a high protein diet with a high sugar diet, taking certain heart medications, or doing heavy exercise can increase levels of creatinine in the urine. Some people also take creatine monohydrate supplements, especially if they are involved in sports.

Typically, a kidney patient will be questioned about any medications and/or supplements they are taking, their physical activity, and their diet, and will be screened for liver function, and have a physical exam. They will have both blood and urine analysis. All of this will help to determine if their creatinine levels are related to kidney damage or function.

Type and quality of carbs, proteins, and fats

The type and quality of carbs, proteins, and fats – including what condition they are in, and, with some foods: what is done to prepare them, and what substances are within them – including because of how they were grown, and also if they are raw, or have been cooked to high heat crating AGEs – makes a tremendous difference in how your gut microbiome and body tissues and systems react to what you eat.

A clean, plant-based diet free of extracts and clarified substances reduces exposure to harmful chemicals. This includes synthetic chemicals in processed foods, and the chemicals called AGEs created by highly heating foods in dry cooking (rather than the less problematic wet cooking: steaming, boiling, and stewing). The synthetic and heat-created chemicals can play roles in various diseases. There also are chemicals made by certain plants that can interfere with nutrient absorption, and also be part of health issues. For instance, as explained elsewhere, beans, legumes, nuts, grains, and seeds can be soaked or enlivened to rid them of problematic substances, before using them in foods. And fermented foods can be prepared in ways to create a healthful chemistry that both enhances nutrition, aids in digestion, and protects the intestinal lining.

Filtering proteins and protein byproducts

Kidneys are filters for what doesn't belong in the body. Among the things they filter out are excess proteins, and protein byproducts.

"Observational studies have supported health benefits of plant-based protein intake. A cross-sectional study in which participants were stratified by estimated glomerular filtration rate (eGFR) showed that with every 33% increase in the ratio of plant protein to total protein, there was a 19% lower mortality risk intake with eGFR <60 mL/min/1.73 m. In a different study of 5,316 adults, each 20-g increase in plant protein intake was associated with a 16% decrease in chronic kidney disease incidence, suggesting that plant-based protein consumption may play a role in kidney function preservation."
    – Effects of Plant-Based Protein Consumption on Kidney Function and Mineral Bone Disorder Outcomes in Adults With Stage 3-5 Chronic Kidney Disease: A Systematic Review; *Journal of Renal Nutrition*; Nov. 2023

If you have read this far, you know diets high in animal protein can harm the kidneys in a number of ways, and increase the risks of experiencing cancer, diabetes, arthritis, and high blood pressure, and cardiovascular disease, and liver disease, among other maladies.

Clean plant-based diets free of junk, fried foods, clarified sugars, and overly processed foods, and synthetic chemicals can improve and preserve kidney and cardiovascular function.

If you are already diabetic, have kidney issues, or high blood pressure, or cardiovascular disease, and you follow a diet rich in animal protein, you are increasing your risk of health problems, including experiencing kidney failure, heart problems, and stroke. And cancer. And a variety of autoimmune disorders.

Dairy protein, casein, whey, and disease

Switching to casein or whey protein powders is also not the answer for getting protein. Those are extracts of milk, and may contain a variety of contaminants, including heavy metals (arsenic, cadmium, mercury, and lead) and industrial chemical residues.

"Milk whey (the main ingredient in whey protein powder supplements, and one of the main ingredients in weight gainer protein powder supplements) is a byproduct of cheese production, and although a direct link has not been established, it is likely that contaminated milk is one of the primary contributors to heavy metal contaminated why protein."
    – A human health risk assessment of heavy metal ingestion among consumers of protein powder supplements; *Toxicology Reports Journal*; Aug. 2020

You can learn about the problems of consuming cow milk by searching a list of health issues dairy consumption can increase the risk of:
- casein, whey, cancer
- casein, prostate cancer
- Neu5Gc, milk, cancer
- milk, allergies
- milk, Alzheimer's

- milk, appendicitis
- milk, arthritis
- milk, asthma
- milk, autoimmune conditions
- milk, back pain
- milk, breast cancer
- milk, cancer
- milk, cardiovascular disease
- milk, casein allergy
- milk, clogged arteries
- milk, colds and ear infections
- milk, colon cancer
- milk, COPD patients
- milk, dark circles beneath eyes
- milk, dermatitis
- milk, D-galactose and bone health
- milk, diabetes
- milk, eczema flare-ups
- milk, erectile dysfunction
- milk, facial swelling
- milk, flaring acne
- milk, headaches
- milk, heart disease
- milk, hives (urticaria)
- milk, increases risk of bone fractures
- milk, inflammation
- milk, irritable bowel syndrome
- milk, joint pain
- milk, kidney disease
- milk, lactose intolerance
- milk, liver disease
- milk, ovarian cancer
- milk, phlegm and mucus production
- milk, pneumonia
- milk, prostate cancer
- milk, psoriasis
- milk, rectum varicose veins
- milk, rosacea
- milk, tendonitis
- milk, testicular cancer
- milk, under-eye bags
- milk, varicose veins
- milk, vegan options

You don't need to consume cow or goat milk for your nutrition.

For nutrients, including minerals like calcium, eat a variety of greens, sprouts, and sea vegetables. And other foods rich in calcium, including apricots, chia seeds, flax seeds, oats, oranges, peas, pistachios, pumpkin seeds, sesame seeds and tahini, sunflower seeds, and others. (Research: sources of calcium in vegan diet.)

"Over the 20 years during which the women were tracked, 17,252 (28%) had sustained a fracture, and 15,541 (25%) died. Women who consumed at least three glasses of milk per day had a higher risk of fracture, and mortality compared with women who drank less than one glass per day.

Over the eleven years during which the men were followed, 5,066 (11%) had sustained a fracture, and 10,112 (22%) died. While less pronounced than the female group, men also had a higher mortality risk with increased milk consumption.

The researchers concluded that high milk intake was found to be associated with increased risk of fracture in women, and greater risk of mortality in both sexes."

– Fact or Myth: Does Drinking Too Much Milk Increase the Risk for Osteoporosis?, by Tom Greenhalgh; *Rheumatology Advisor*; May 2019

"Milk and other dairy products are top sources of artery-clogging saturated fat in the American diet. Milk products also contain cholesterol. Diets high in fat, saturated fat, and cholesterol increase the risk of heart disease, which remains America's top killer."

– Health Concerns About Dairy: Avoid the Dangers of Dairy With a Plant-Based Diet, by Roxanne Becker, MD; Physicians Committee for Responsible Medicine

Research, read, and learn.

Cow milk is the perfect chemistry for turning a baby cow or a baby bull into a huge animal, in a matter of months. It's not any sort of ideal nutritional chemistry for humans.

As mentioned elsewhere, read up on the science-based nutrition information – including about dairy – presented on NutritionFacts.org.

Breast milk and protein

In their most natural state, soon after birth humans begin consuming unheated, unprocessed food in the form of breast milk. Breast milk from their mother is the natural food for a human. Per calorie, breast milk is less than 4% protein.

As other mammals do, humans stop breast feeding at a young age. It is only their parents or caretakers who introduce toddlers to unhealthful foods – and unnecessarily feed them dairy products.

Cow and goat milk are not for adults. Adult humans have no nutritional need for breast milk, or milk from another species.

"The human body has no more need for cows' milk than it does for dogs' milk, horses' milk, or giraffes' milk."

– Dr. Michael Klaper

Dairy

Dairy is harsh on the kidneys. It also plays a role in a variety of other health problems, including asthma, skin issues, cancers, insulin-dependent diabetes, arthritis, varicose veins, cardiovascular disease, macular degeneration, weakened bones (osteoporosis), dental problems, stroke, back aches, headaches, colds, and inflammation.

Dairy contains no fiber. It can play a role in damaging the gut microbiota, including by reducing the numbers and varieties of beneficial microorganisms in the digestive tract, and increasing the number of damaging microorganisms.

Dairy can play a role in leaky gut, and otherwise intestinal inflammation and diseases involving it, including bowel inflammation and cancer.

I know someone awaiting a kidney transplant and he mentioned he drinks the produce called *Ensure*. I would not advise anyone to drink the product. While the various *Ensure* products have different ingredients, it contains ingredients those with kidney, cardiovascular, and autoimmune disorders, and cancer would do better without. Ingredients include dairy, corn syrup, various oils, artificial flavors, and other ingredients I suggest people avoid.

"For patients with chronic kidney disease, coconut milk compares favorably with dairy milk based on the lowest sodium, potassium, and oxalate levels. Macadamia milk is another option for patients who are restricting potassium and oxalate, but has a higher sodium content than coconut milk.

Calcium content is highest in macadamia followed by soy, almond, rice, and dairy milk; it is lowest in cashew, hazelnut, and coconut milk. Almond milk has the highest oxalate concentration, followed by cashew, hazelnut, and soy. Coconut and flax milk have undetectable oxalate levels; coconut milk also has comparatively low sodium, calcium, and potassium, while flax milk has the most sodium. Overall, oat milk has the most similar parameters to dairy milk (moderate calcium, potassium, and sodium, with low oxalate). Rice, macadamia, and soy milk also have similar parameters to dairy milk.

Oat, macadamia, rice, and soy milk compare favorably in terms of kidney stone risk factors with dairy milk, whereas almond and cashew milk have more potential stone risk factors. Coconut milk may be a favorable dairy substitute for patients with chronic kidney disease based on low potassium, sodium, and oxalate."
 – Plant-based milk alternatives and risk factors for kidney stones and chronic kidney disease; *Journal of Renal Nutrition*; May 2021

Dairy casein, and whey

There are no necessary nutrients in dairy you can't get in a better form by eating a variety of plants. The animal gets the nutrients by eating plants. You can skip the cow, and eat the plants.

There are substances in dairy damaging to health, and those do not exist in fruits, vegetables, sprouts, nuts, beans, legumes, seeds, grains, or seaweeds.

Canada re-evaluated the situation of cow's milk being a source for human nutrition, and they instead removed dairy from being a separate food group.

"A substantial proportion of the world's adult population (65%-70%) exhibits lactose nonpersistence, a reduced ability to metabolize lactose to glucose and galactose. Shifts in the US population, including a greater proportion of African Americans and Asians, are of key important because several studies have shown a markedly higher prevalence of lactase nonpersistence and, consequently a lower dairy intake among these groups. While cow's milk alternatives are available, families who used them will pay up to an additional $1,400 per year compared with those who are able to consume dairy products. Dietary guidance also contains downstream effects for government assistance, such as the U.S. Department of Agriculture's National School Lunch Program and School Breakfast Program. For reasons like these, Canada has recently removed dairy as a separate food group in national dietary guidance. The results of the present review suggest that consideration of this modification when developing population-level guidelines in the United States is warranted."

— Re-examination of dairy as a single commodity in US dietary guidance; *Nutrition Reviews, Nutrition Science*, Oxford Academic; Feb. 2020

As mentioned elsewhere, the casein protein in dairy increases cancer risk. It also can play a role in the reduction of capillaries in the nephrons of the kidneys. These are some of the reasons a person wanting to have healthy kidneys should avoid all dairy, including milk, cheese, butter, cream, yogurt, kefir, whey, and casein.

"Dietary casein promotes a progressive decline in the glomerular filtration rate of remnant kidney associated with metabolic acidosis and an endothelin-mediated increase in renal acidification."

— Dietary protein causes a decline in the glomerular filtration rate; *Kidney International*, journal of the International Society of Nephrology; Jan. 2008

Simply stop ingesting dairy. It isn't necessary for human nutrition.

"Milk is a dietary staple for many people, but its relationship with breast cancer has been a topic of controversy. Some studies suggest that consuming cows' milk may increase the risk of breast cancer, while others report no significant association. One possible explanation for the conflicting results is the presence of hormones in milk, such as estrogen and progesterone, which can stimulate the growth of hormone-sensitive breast cancer cells.

Therefore, it is advisable for breast cancer patients to avoid consuming cow's milk, or any other dairy product that contains hormones. Instead, they can choose plant-based milk, such as soy or almond, which do not contain hormones."

— The Best Diet for Breast Cancer Patients; CurieOncology.com.sg

"During the study period 29,277 new cancer cases were recorded, with the highest rate being for lung cancer, followed by female breast cancer, stomach cancer, colorectal cancer, and liver cancer.

People who consumed dairy products regularly had significantly greater risks of developing liver and breast cancer.

Regular dairy consumption was associated with an increased risk of lymphoma."

— Dairy products linked to increased risk of cancer: First major study to investigate dairy consumption and cancer risk in Chinese adults has found that greater intake was associated with higher risks of liver cancer and female breast cancer; Oxford University; May, 2022

"When it comes to cancer, leading experts expressed concern that the hormones in dairy, and other growth factors, could potentially stimulate the growth of hormone-sensitive tumors. Experimental evidence also suggests that dairy may also promote the conversion of precancerous lesions or mutated cells

into invasive cancers in vitro."
– Casein; NutritionFact.org; 2025

Casein allergies can also be a problem, as can the whey protein in dairy.

Dairy can also play a role in the liver producing the problematic TMAO that increases the risk of cardiovascular and kidney disease, and certain cancers, including of the colon.

The solution is to stop ingesting dairy.

There are plenty of easy-to-make dairy alternatives, including fermented coconut yogurt, fermented nut cheeses, non-dairy ice cream, and non-dairy milks.

Lactose intolerance

"Lactose intolerant" is a label placed on a person with the condition of their body not making adequate amounts of the lactose enzyme that digests the sugar (lactose) in milk. It is also known as lactose malabsorption.

Being lactose intolerant is not the same as a dairy allergy.

Being lactose intolerant also is not the rare, inherited metabolic condition called galactosemia, which is a person's inability to process the sugar called galactose in milk, and turn it into glucose. Galactosemia is usually detected as an infant, as they are given a screening test. It can cause a variety of health problems, including cataracts, convulsions, lethargy, jaundice, sepsis, weight loss, and vomiting. An infant with the condition needs special and urgent attention.

When people who are lactose intolerant ingest dairy, they can experience bloating, diarrhea, severe gas, stomach rumbling, cramps, abdominal pain, and vomiting. Ignoring the intolerance by continuing to ingest dairy can lead to weight loss, malnutrition, and anemia. Those conditions can lead to more health problems.

The lactose intolerant condition can begin at any age, and be triggered by food poisoning, or other infection, or by diabetic enteropathy, celiac disease, Crohn's disease, ulcerative colitis, inflammatory bowel disease, chemotherapy, radiation treatments, or a medical procedure on the bowels.

Some people with lactose intolerance use lactase enzyme powder in their milk, or eat lactose-reduced dairy products.

The solution to being lactose intolerant is to stop ingesting dairy.

It is completely normal for the human to naturally slow their lactose enzyme production. Those who go vegan may find out they can no longer eat dairy, as their body has adjusted to not having it in their system.

Humans don't have any nutritional need for cow's milk, or goat milk, in any form. Just as human breast milk is for baby humans, and pig breast milk is for piglets, and cat breast milk is for kittens, and goat milk is for a kid (baby goat), cow milk is for baby bulls (boys) and baby cows (girls).

"People don't understand that the majority of adult humans on planet Earth are unable to digest cow's milk. Throughout childhood, the enzyme you have that breaks down the milk sugar lactose begins to decline in most individuals throughout the world, which makes sense since milk is for babies. Why would we need to digest it after weaning from the breast? And so most people experience symptoms like bloating, abdominal pain, intestinal gas, and watery stool, or even nausea and vomiting."

– Is Soy Milk the Most Nutritious Non-Dairy Milk, Dr. Michael Greger; NutritionFacts.org, 2024

Cow's milk anaphylaxis

A milk allergy is a different issue than being lactose intolerant.

A person with a milk allergy who ingests milk can experience a variety of symptoms, including breathing issues, coughing, hives, vomiting, wheezing, itchy lips and/or mouth, and swelling of the lips, tongue, and throat.

A test for milk allergy involves a skin test done by an allergist. A small amount of milk protein is a applied to an area of the skin that has been pricked. Those with an allergy will develop a hive.

Some people with milk allergies take antihistamines. A doctor may advise the patient to carry an epinephrine injector pen, in case of a sever reaction to ingesting milk.

The solution to a milk allergy is to stop ingesting milk. As is mentioned earlier, there is no human nutritional need for cow or goat milk. There is no such thing as having a dairy deficiency. That's as real as having a chocolate or coffee deficiency.

"Casein allergies, or milk allergies, are a relatively common health concern, particularly among those with dairy sensitivities. This type of allergy stems from the body's immune response to casein, a protein found in milk and dairy products.

Casein allergy symptoms can vary widely and often include digestive issues, skin rashes, respiratory problems, and more. In severe cases of casein allergy, anaphylaxis, a life-threatening allergic reaction, may develop. Symptoms of anaphylaxis include: shortness of breath, and/or wheezing.

Whey is another protein in milk that commonly causes allergic reactions. To determine which protein a milk allergy patients is allergic to, allergy testing is required. Often times a patient can be allergic to both casein and whey."

– Milk/Casein Allergy Symptoms and Treatment, Food Allergy Institute

Dairy is a foreign material for humans

Dairy is a foreign material to the human system.

Ingesting dairy products can slow both cellular waste disposal and nutrient absorption. It can increase the work the body has to do to reduce inflammation, and for maintaining health. It makes the system more sluggish, and with decreased energy, including because of the fat in dairy slowing the function of the endothelial cells lining the cardiovascular and lymph systems.

Dairy contains the saturated fat, cholesterol, and inflammatory molecules that play into cardiovascular disease, heart attacks, strokes, and autoimmune disorders.

Similar to meat and eggs, dairy ingestion also encourages the establishment of a pro-inflammatory gut biome, leading to the liver converting TMA into problematic trimethylamine N-oxide (TMAO). As mentioned earlier, this increases the risks of experiencing cardiovascular and kidney disease, strokes, and certain types of cancer.

Casein protein in milk can play a role in leaky gut. This increases the risks of inflammation, autoimmune disorders, cardiovascular and kidney disease, and neurodegeneration.

Casein can also increase the risk of prostate cancer.

"**Conclusions: The milk protein, casein, promotes the proliferation of prostate cancer cells such as PC3 and LNCaP.**"
– A Milk Protein, Casein, as Proliferation Promoting Factor in Prostate Cancer Cells; *World Journal of Men's Health*; Aug. 2014

Dairy calcium and phosphorus and kidney disease

The buildup of calcium and phosphorus from dairy also contributes to kidney disease.

The minerals from dairy can accumulate in the blood, taxing the kidneys, increasing not only the state of kidney disease, but also heart disease. An increased rate of acidity increases calcium secretion from the bones into the blood, and then the urine. This leads to stressed kidneys, weakened bones (osteoporosis), spine and hip issues, back pain, and bone fractures. This is so especially in combination with leaky gut playing a role in autoimmune diseases, including arthritis, and in increasing the risk of kidney disease, which then can play into bone loss.

The dietary phosphorus that is most problematic is from animal protein.

Ulcer

I had a friend who was diagnosed with an ulcer. Her doctor told her to drink milk. He put her on prescription anti-inflammatory drugs, which carry the risk of causing ulcers.

The doctor was stuck in antiquated concepts mixed with outdated nutritional theory.

A person with intestinal issues – and especially with a damaged intestinal mucosa – should not be consuming animal products, in particular any sort of dairy. They would also be better off avoiding fried foods, oil sautéed foods, alcohol, clarified sugars, and foods containing synthetic chemicals. Gluten could also be a problem for them. A focus on improving the gut microbiome is key.

Osteoporosis

The dairy industry formerly marketed their products as good for bone health. They stopped, but the myth persists, with people believing ingesting milk, yogurt, kefir, cheese, and other dairy products will improve bone health.

"A study published in *The Journal of Nutrition* in 2015 found that eating dairy foods increased low-grade inflammation in a small sample of German adults. And a study of more than 40,000 people with osteoarthritis found that those who ate more dairy products were more likely to need hip replacement surgery."
– Is Dairy Arthritis-Friendly: Understanding the link between dairy and inflammation, by Amy Paturel; Arthritis Foundation; 2025

"Although some studies have reported the beneficial effects of milk and dairy product consumption on osteoporosis and risk of fracture, the findings are conflicting. We summarized earlier data on the association between milk and dairy intake and risk of osteoporosis and hip fracture through a meta-analysis.

Given the advantages of the cohort over case-control studies, we concluded that a greater intake of milk and dairy products was **not** associated with a lower risk of osteoporosis and hip fracture."

– Consumption of milk and dairy products and risk of osteoporosis and hip fracture: A systematic review and Meta-analysis; *Critical Reviews in Food Science and Nutrition* journal; Mar. 2019

"Women who reported drinking three or more glasses of milk each day nearly doubled their risk of death in relation to women who drank less than one glass each day. Men were not as affected as women, but those who drank three or more glasses of milk each day showed a significant increase in mortality."

– Can Drinking Too Much Milk Make Your Bones More Brittle?: High milk consumption linked to higher mortality, hip fractures; *Cleveland Clinic Health Essentials*; Jan. 2021

"The bone-thinning condition called osteoporosis can lead to small and not-so-small fractures. Many people believe dairy products, like milk and cheese, are a good source of calcium. However, this is not the whole story. In fact, in a 12-year Harvard study of 78,000 mostly white women, those who drank milk two or more times a day had a higher incidence of hip fractures than those who rarely drank milk. Similarly, an observational study out of Sweden found that higher milk intake was associated with greater incidence of bone fracture. Although the overall results are mixed regarding milk and bone health, most research shows no benefit to drinking milk for bone health.

Bone health is incredibly important, and cannot be overlooked. Getting calcium from plant-based products is optimal, as these sources will allow you to meet the daily recommended amounts while also providing you with other essential nutrients."

– Calcium and Strong Bones; Physicians Committee for Responsible Medicine; 2025

Milk proteins are acidic and increase calcium secretion through the kidneys, which can damage the kidneys. To neutralize the acidity, the body takes calcium from the bones, weakening them. Countries with the highest consumption of dairy also have higher rates of osteoporosis, and hip fracture.

Of course, the dairy industry had something to do with studies concluding consuming dairy is good for you. It's like the tobacco industry studies from decades past saying smoking tobacco is good for you.

For nutrients, rather than from dairy

For vitamins and minerals, and other nutrients, consume a variety of fruits, and vegetables, including sprouts, and green leafy and other green vegetables. Sea vegetables like nori – which can be purchased as a powder, flakes, or a roll – are particularly rich in minerals and other key nutrients. (I do use pinches of nori flakes in smoothies, salads, wraps, soups, stews, hummus, and guacamole.)

Vitamin D, lichens, mushrooms, and fortified foods

People with kidney disease are often found to have low levels of vitamin D.

Low levels of vitamin D can impact the health of everything from the bones to the heart, kidneys, brain, nerves, and other tissues and their functions.

In combination with lack of daily exercise, and an unhealthful diet, a consistently low level of vitamin D can play a role in weakening the bones, causing them to release calcium into the blood, which can then impact kidney function.

Depending on what your blood test reveals, your doctor might prescribe pharmaceutical vitamin D to get your system up to a healthful level of this nutrient.

As a person with kidney and/or heart or liver disease, study up on vitamin D.

Know the sources of vitamin D, how to get it, and what can be too much vitamin D.

Research: What are the health benefits of vitamin D?

Research: How does sun exposure result in vitamin D?

Research: Mushrooms and vitamin D.

Research: Lichen and vitamin D.

Research: What are the health risks of taking too much vitamin D?

Research: Vitamin D and kidney disease.

"Abnormalities in vitamin D metabolism play a major role in the pathogenesis of secondary hyperparathyroidism in chronic kidney disease. The gradual and progressive decline in 1,25-dihydroxyvitamin D in the course of chronic kidney disease is the result of several mechanisms that limit the ability of the failing kidney to maintain the levels of 1,25-dihydroxyvitamin D despite increasing levels of parathyroid hormone. Recent observations have indicated that chronic kidney diseases seems to be associated with a high incidence of nutritional vitamin D insufficiency or deficiency as manifested by decreased levels of 25-hydroxymivamin D. This contributes to the inability to maintain the levels of 1,25-dihydroxymitamin D; therefore, current practice guidelines suggest repleting vitamin D status by the administration of native vitamin D as a first step in the therapy of the abnormalities of bone and mineral metabolism in chronic kidney disease. The efficacy of this therapy is extremely variable, and active vitamin D sterols may be required, especially as kidney disease progresses."

– Vitamin D and kidney disease; *Clinical Journal of the American Society of Nephrology*; Sept. 2008

"Chronic kidney disease is an emerging public health problems, and one of the most powerful predictors of premature cardiovascular disease. Emerging evidence suggests that the progression of CKD and many of the cardiovascular complications may be linked to hypovitaminosis D. Patients with CKD have an exceptionally high rate of severe vitamin D deficiency that is further exacerbated by the reduced ability to convert 25(OH)vitamin D into the active form, 1,25 dihydroxy-vitamin D. As new evidence has improved our understanding of classical, as well as non-classical, functions for vitamin D, it has become apparent that the autocrine role in vitamin D is an important modulator of several systems including the immune, renal, and cardiovascular systems.

It appears that adequate replacement of vitamin D I deficient populations could potentially reduce premature morbidity and mortality.

Vitamin D has emerged as a vital compound in CKD, with newly ascribed autocrine functions vastly different from its classical function in mineral homeostasis. To ignore the significance of this vitamin and its potential impact on morbidity and mortality in CKD patients is no longer appropriate."

– Vitamin D and chronic kidney disease; *Ethnicity and Disease* journal; May 2010

There are sides to what vitamin D supplementation does for kidney patients.

"Vitamin D, in the form of supplements or its activated analogues, is a standard of care in the treatment of chronic kidney disease-mineral and bone disorder (CKD-MBD), the systemic complication of bone disease, biochemical abnormalities, and extraskeletal calcification present in many of the 800 million people worldwide with CKD. Reasons long touted for vitamin D use in this population include that it may improve high-turnover bone disease, restore systemic pleiotropic benefits of vitamin D, reduce vascular osteogenesis at low doses, and temper rising concentrations of parathyroid hormone (PTH), which has been consistently linked to mortality and poor outcomes in observational studies. None of these reasons are based on data from conclusive randomized clinical trials showing evidence of clinical benefit.

Primary analyses combined the effects of vitamin D supplements and activated vitamin D analogues and found no significant effect on the primary outcomes of all-cause mortality, cardiovascular death, or fracture. This was despite presumed beneficial changes in biomarker outcomes, such as increased bone mineral density and reduced PTH. The absence of demonstrable clinical benefit was consistent in subgroup analyses that separated vitamin D supplementation from activated vitamin D analogues. Treatment with activated vitamin D analogues, but not vitamin D supplementation, was associated with hypercalcemia"

– Vitamin D in CKD: An Unfinished Story; *American Journal of Kidney Diseases*; Nov. 2023

"Hypercalcemia is a condition in which the calcium level in the blood becomes too high. Too much calcium in the blood can weaken bones and create kidney stones. It also can affect the heart and brain.

Most often, hypercalcemia happens after one or more of the parathyroid glands make too much hormone. These four tiny glands are in the neck, near the thyroid gland. Other causes of hypercalcemia include cancer, certain other medical conditions, and some medicines. Taking too much calcium and vitamin D supplements also can cause hypercalcemia."

– Hypercalcemia: Symptoms and causes; Mayo Clinic; 2025

Whether or not you have kidney disease, vitamin D does play a role in maintaining health.

Don't simply purchase vitamin D, and not know how much to take, or take too much.

I do take a vegan vitamin D supplement extracted from lichen.

For vitamin D, besides exposing your skin to sunlight, you can also eat mushrooms exposed to sunlight, because mushrooms synthesize vitamin D. There is also vitamin D-fortified orange juice*, as well as non-dairy milks, and cereals fortified with vitamin D. Or take a vegan vitamin D supplement, which likely is derived from lichen – which grow on rocks and trees. (If it is NOT vegan vitamin D, it likely has been extracted from sheep's wool.)

(*If you are watching your potassium intake, it is better to eat half a peeled medium-sized orange, rather than to drink orange juice.)

People on every continent have a history of using certain types of lichen as food and medicine. If you consider harvesting wild lichen, there are things to know. Some forms of it can be poisonous, including the varieties called ground lichen, powdered sunshine lichen, and wolf lichen.

"Vitamin D controls your body's use of calcium. Increasing vitamin D intake has been shown to reduce fracture risk. About 15 minutes of sunlight on your skin each day normally produces all the vitamin D you need. If you get little or no sun exposure, you can get vitamin D from a supplement or fortified foods. The recommended daily allowance is 600 IU (15 micrograms) per day. Cow's milk is not a natural source of vitamin D, as it [vitamin D] is added after production, and plant-based milks are fortified with comparable amounts."
– Calcium and Strong Bones; Physicians Committee for Responsible Medicine; 2025

Vegan options for dairy

While a nonvegan diet that is vegetarian may include milk products, including butter, ice cream, kefir, yogurt, and rennetless cheese, a vegan diet may contain nondairy, fiber-rich versions of these foods, including milk made from almonds, oats, macadamia nuts, cashews, bananas, or hemp seeds; kefir made from coconut; ice cream made from bananas, coconuts, or other plants; and raw vegan cheeses made of ingredients like pine nuts, almonds, cashews, walnuts, sunflower seeds, or other nuts or seeds. There are also vegan cheeses made from things like potatoes and beans.

There are many recipes for vegan forms of milk, cheese, butter, cream, ice cream, yogurt, and kefir. Look for those that do not contain oil extracts, or an abundance of salt (sodium). Many of the recipes are easy to make using simple, common ingredients.

Check YouTube for dairy-free vegan recipes.

Toddler nutrition

As babies grow, they are naturally attracted to fruit.

Sadly, many parents feed their children the lowest-quality foods from an early age.

Rather than going from breast milk to whole foods, many children are being fed fried foods, cola, and things saturated with corn syrup, other sugar extracts, and processed salts, MSG, chemical dyes and flavorings, and other ingredients that dull and degrade health. It all ends up playing into degenerative and chronic health conditions, and gut biome dysbiosis, as well as learning disorders, and psychological issues. Low quality infant and child nutrition plays out in culture and society, and the level at which humanity is existing.

If you are responsible for a child, please give them a good start in life by feeding them a clean diet free of clarified sugars, synthetic chemicals, and ultra-processed foods. Choose the plant-based diet.

(Search: NutritionFacts.org/topics/infants/)

"A vegetable-based diet for children is generally more healthful than a diet containing the cholesterol, animal fat, and excessive protein found in meat and dairy products. Children and adolescents will get plenty of protein as long as they eat a variety of whole-grains, legumes, vegetables, fruits, and nuts."
– Dr. Benjamin Spock

Iodine

"Iodine is an essential mineral used by your body to make thyroid hormones.

197

These hormones control how fast your cells work. They are also needed for growth and brain development during pregnancy and childhood."

In the U.K., the general iodine intake recommended for adults is 140 micrograms per day."
— Iodine; VeganSociety.com/nutrition

"Plant foods have a low iodine concentration, so individuals who follow a plant-based diet may be at risk of iodine deficiency; animal sources (e.g. milk, fish, and eggs) currently provide the majority of iodine intake in many countries, including the U.K. In some countries (U.K., Ireland, and Iceland), there is no iodized salt policy, so moving away from animals foods will have a negative impact on iodine intake to a greater degree than in countries where animal foods provide a lower proportion of total iodine intake, and where iodized salt policies exist.

Seaweed is often cites as a rich plant-based source of iodine; however, the iodine content is highly variable and unreliable as a source of iodine, and could even result in excessive iodine intake.

It is important to note that plant-based diets and iodine sufficiency do not have to be mutually exclusive. For those following a plant-based diet, there are ways to optimize iodine intake. For example, if avoiding milk, individuals should opt for iodine-fortified plant-based alternatives, or increase their iodine intake from other food sources. A suitable iodine-containing supplements would be a more consistent and reliable way of ensuring an adequate iodine intake, if this cannot be achieved through diet. If a supplement is considered, this should not be a seaweed supplement, instead, iodine should be in the form of potassium iodide or potassium iodate, with a dose that does not exceed 150 micrograms per day."
— Iodine and plant-based diets: a narrative review and calculation of iodine content; *British Journal of Nutrition*; Aug. 2023

The nutritional requirement for iodine is quite small, but important. I do use small amounts of seaweeds in my foods. Often nori flakes, or dulse powder. I regularly have nutritional blood panels done, and my iodine is a healthy level.

Many foods are fortified with iodine, including salt, vegan milk products, cereals, and others. Read nutrition labels on packaged foods. Notice which foods are fortified with iodine, and what the measurement of iodine is per serving.

If you test low in iodine, supplements you can use include those containing potassium iodate and potassium iodide.

"When purchasing iodine, avoid stand-alone potassium iodide supplements that are intended to block radiation; they're measured in milligrams rather than micrograms, and can be many times the U.S. upper limit.

The United States upper limit for daily iodine intake is 1,100 micrograms. Although most adults can safely metabolize 1,100 micrograms, and even more, it's prudent not to supplement beyond the Unites Sates recommended dietary allowance (RDA) for iodine, which is 150 micrograms for adults.

If an iodine tablet contains significantly more iodine than what's recommended, they can normally be broken into halves or quarters.
— Iodine, by Jack Norris, RD; VeganHealth.org

Too much iodine can also be a problem, and lead to iodine disorders.

If you have kidney disease, make see if your blood test reveals any concern with iodine, as well as potassium, and other nutrients.

"Iodine is essential for the synthesis of thyroid hormones that, in turn, regulate cell metabolism. Iodine deficiency can cause hypothyroidism and goiter, apathy, and mental disorders. The main source of iodine in vegans are salt and seaweed. For this reason, vegans can show deficiency of iodine, especially if they live in geographical areas poor in iodine. Iodine levels in vegans were found to be below the limits set by the World Health Organization, therefore oral food supplements rather than fortified foods such as salt, potatoes, carrots, etc. are strictly recommended in vegans."
– Vegan Diet Health Benefits in Metabolic Syndrome; *Nutrients* journal; March 2021

"As a rule of thumb, it is good to be selective about supplementation – it should complement a balanced and varied intake of plant-based foods. Most plants do not require iodine for their growth, so the contents of plant foods vary and tend to be low. A steady and adequate dietary intake of iodine is important for thyroid health. One reliable option is to top up your intake using a daily supplement containing up to 150 micrograms in the form of potassium iodide or potassium iodate – an approach recommended during pregnancy planning, pregnancy, and breastfeeding do to the critical role of iodine in early brain development. Some people choose to take a vitamin and mineral supplement designed for vegans, like The Vegan Society's VEG 1. Anyone taking medication for a thyroid condition should seek advice from their doctor, because the guidance on iodine is different."
– Vegan diets and iodine: A vegan dietitian's perspective, by Heather Russel, British Dietetic Association; VeganSociety.com; June 2021

Leucine and eggs

One of the amino acids you need from food is leucine. This amino acid is needed for building and maintaining muscles and strength, and repairing muscles and healing injuries. Leucine plays a role in the regulation of blood sugar. It also helps maintain both growth hormone and the leptin hormone central to appetite regulation.

Some people say you need to eat eggs, beef, tuna, and salmon, or you don't get adequate leucine. Wrong. But, yes, eggs and those meats contain leucine. They also contain cholesterol that contributes to cardiovascular disease, strokes, and heart attacks. Eggs, beef, and other meats increase the risks of cancers of the breasts, colon, rectum, and prostate. Raw salmon and tuna, and other fish may also be rich in parasites and heavy metals, which is why many people have stopped eating sushi, and other fish.

"Even just a few eggs a week may be associated with a 19 percent greater risk of colorectal cancer. But hit three of more eggs a week, and the increased risk may be as high as 71 percent. And finally, breast cancer: a significant increase in breast cancer risk once women get up to around five eggs a week."
– Eggs and Breast Cancer: The Latest Research; NutritionFacts.org; Jan. 2019

Leucine from plants

You can get leucine from brown rice, oats, chickpeas, soybeans, navy beans, black beans, split peas, lentils, hemp seeds, sesame seeds, and nuts like almonds, pine nuts, Brazil nuts, and cashews. And from peanuts, which are legumes.

Kidney and liver damage from leucine-rich diet and supplements

If anything, people who eat large amounts of animal protein rich in leucine, and those who take leucine supplements can end up damaging their kidneys. One study revealing this was done in relation to the antibiotic drug doxorubicin. It found that on a leucine-rich diet there was a reduction of glomeruli. Those are the clusters of capillaries at the ends of kidney tubules, where waste products are filtered from the blood, initiating urine production. Meaning, a diet abundantly rich in leucine, or taking leucine supplements can reduce kidney function. It also has negative impacts on the liver.

"Although some studies have indicated benefits of a diet rich in L-leucine for the muscle tissue of animals that received doxorubicin, our results showed the liver as the most affected organ by the L-leucine-rich diet since the diet reduced its antioxidant defenses and increased the deposit of collagen and fat in the hepatic tissue [of liver]. In the kidneys, the main alteration was the reduction in the number of glomeruli.

Excess branched-chain amino acids (BCAAs), including leucine, rapidly interfere with renal function, decreasing the glomerular filtration rate, and promoting renal fibrosis.

BCAA excess is associated with non-alcoholic fatty liver disease and oxidative injury. In addition, clinical studies suggest that BCAA excess may harm liver structure and function."

– Effects of an L-Leucine-Rich Diet on Liver and Kidneys in a Doxorubicin Toxicity Model; *Life* journal from MDPI/Multidisciplinary Digital Publishing Institute; Aug. 2023

Stay safe by sticking with the plant-based sources of leucine. Especially if you have already been diagnosed with kidney issues.

There are many types of vegan "egg" products on the market. Made from plants, the vegan egg products won't cause the kidney or liver issues, or allergy problems, caused by eating chicken eggs. Vegan egg substitutes are also easy to make at home. (See YouTube for recipes.)

Bones and blood production

The kidneys play a major role in bone health. Kidneys produce the erythropoietin (E.P.O.) hormone which triggers the bone marrow to make red blood cells (erythrocytes).

The red blood cells function for about 120 days, and carry oxygen from the lungs into the tissues.

In a healthy person, the spongey tissue in most bones – the bone marrow – is either red or yellow. The red bone marrow contains the stem cells that become blood platelets, red blood cells, or white blood cells.

By controlling the blood plasma volume through the excretion of salt and water, while also playing a role in the production of red blood cells (erythropoiesis), the kidneys control the ratio of the volume of red blood cells to the total volume of blood, which is called hematocrit.

Anemia

Weakened kidneys can play a role in anemia, which is the condition of having too few red blood cells. This situation is of not enough blood being carried to the tissues.

Some people think if you are anemic, you need to eat more red meat and/or dairy. Eating more meat and/or dairy can worsen kidney function, damaging the kidneys, the bone marrow, and the cardiovascular system – while also increases risks of cancers, and autoimmune disorders – including diabetes, arthritis, asthma, lupus, and other chronic and degenerative diseases.

Don't turn to meat or dairy for iron.

Where did the cows get their iron? Cows naturally eat greens, not grains, or meat. They stop relying on mother's milk by the time they are in what amounts to their toddler stage.

Vegan sources of iron include apricots, arugula, beet greens, blueberries, broccoli, chard, chickpeas, collards, currants, dandelion greens, dates*, dulse (seaweed), elderberries, figs, herbs, kale, kidney beans, lamb's lettuce, lentils, lima beans, nori (seaweed), oats, peaches, peas, pistachios, prunes, pumpkin seeds, raisins, strawberries, string beans, sunflower seeds, sweet potatoes, tomatoes, unhulled sesame seeds, watercress, whole grains, and other plants.

(*Dates are high in potassium. Limit them to one date in a meal.)

We grow strawberries in the garden. We eat the leaves. Their flavor is similar to paper – as in, there is not much flavor. Strawberry leaves contain iron, calcium, and other minerals, and vitamins including A, C, and K, and antioxidants. Include the strawberry leaves in smoothies and salads.

Research: vegan food sources of iron.

Polycythemia and erythrocytosis

The opposite of anemia is having too many red blood cells. This is polycythemia (an increase in both red blood cells concentration and hemoglobin [a protein in red blood cells that carries oxygen]) or erythrocytosis (the increase in red blood cells relative to the volume of blood). These can play roles in bleeding gums, blotchy skin, blurred vision, bruising, clots, confusion, enlarged liver, fatigue, headaches, heart attack, high blood pressure, itchy skin, nosebleeds, purplish skin tones of the hands and feet, shortness of breath, stroke, tiredness, weakness, and heavy menstrual periods.

"Polycythemia vera (PV) is one of a related group of blood cancers known as 'myeloproliferative neoplasms' (MPNs) in which the cells in the bone marrow that produce the blood cells do not develop and function normally.

The signs, symptoms, and complications of PV occur because there are too many red cells, and often, too many platelets in the blood. An increase in the number of white cells does not put the patient at higher risk of infection, or cause other significant effects.

Too many red blood cells can make the patient's blood more viscous (thick), so the blood does not flow efficiently. High platelet counts can contribute to the formation of clots (thrombi). Underlying vascular disease, common in older persons with PV, can increase the risk of clothing complications. The clots may cause serious problems, such as stroke, heart attack, deep vein thrombosis, or pulmonary embolism. Blood clots occur in about 30 percent of patients even before the PV diagnosis is made. During the first 10 years after a diagnosis of PV, 40 to 60 percent of untreated PV patients may develop blood clots."

– Polycythemia Vera Facts; Leukemia & Lymphoma Society; April 2015

Inflammation and an unhealthy gut microbiota play roles in polycythemia.

What reduces inflammation and improves gut microbiota? A clean, plant-based diet free of junk, processed foods, and damaged oils.

Gut microbiota and polycythemia vera

"We report the composition of the gut microbiota to differ between the treatment groups.

These observations are highly interesting considering the potential for pathogenetic importance of an altered gut microbiota for the development of other diseases, including chronic inflammatory diseases. Our observations call for further gut microbiota studies to decipher potential causal associations between treatment and the gut microbiota in polycythemia vera (PV) and related neoplasms.

Apart from digestion of food, the human gut microbiota assists in the development of the host immune system, protection against pathogens, and has a variety of additional functions. Changes in the gut microbiota have been linked to several autoimmune and inflammation-driven diseases, such as systemic lupus erythematosus, obesity, atherosclerosis, and diabetes, but also response to immunotherapy."

– The gut microbiota in patients with polycythemia vera is distinct from that of health controls and varies by treatment; *Blood Advances* journal of the American Society of Hematology; Oct. 2022

In the study mentioned above, those who followed an omnivorous diet had higher concentrations of the bacteria Ruminococcus torques and Bilophila wadsworthia, which are both associated with higher rates of colon cancer and irritable bowel syndrome.

A clean, plant-based diet encourages a healthy gut biome.

Garlic, allicin, manganese, and selenium

Be sure to include the vegetables rich in allicin, which is in vegetables of the onion family, including chives, garlic, elephant garlic, wild garlic, leeks, shallots, and, of course, onions. Bananas also contain allicin.

Garlic is the most potent source of allicin, with onions being second. Garlic also contains vitamins B6 and C, and the minerals selenium and manganese.

"In chronic kidney disease, several trace elements are deranged. Adult and few pediatric studies demonstrated deficiencies in both elements (manganese and selenium) in dialysis-dependent patients.

Adult studies have shown low manganese levels in hemodialysis-dependent patients. Manganese deficiency results in poor growth and bone formation, skeletal defects, abnormal glucose tolerance, and altered lipid and carbohydrate metabolism in children, but is also detrimental for adults.

Deficiency of selenium may result in vascular disease, loss of hair and skin pigmentation, or nutritional cardiomyopathy. Adult studies associate worsening selenium deficiency with progressive chronic kidney disease. Selenium deficiency has been associated with mortality of adult hemodialysis patients."

– Plasma manganese and selenium levels in pediatric chronic kidney disease patients measured by high resolution sector field inductively coupled plasma mass spectrometry; *Bulletin of the National Research Centre*; 2023

"The kidney, where selenium is most distributed, absorbs selenium in plasma through renal tubular epithelial cells to synthesize GPx3 [a tumor suppressor gene] and maintain selenium homeostasis. Several studies have shown that selenium levels are associated with the severity of kidney disease. A selenium deficiency causes renal injury through increased oxidative stress and an impaired mitochondrial function.

The prevalence of diabetes and hyperlipidemia was not statistically associated with the selenium intake, but both hypertension and chronic kidney disease were found to be at low rates in the high selenium group.

In a randomized double-blind placebo-controlled prospective trial of 215 older adults, a significantly better renal function was found in the treatment groups with supplements of selenium and coenzyme Q10 [an antioxidant that also helps convert food to energy] than in the control group. Selenium supplements can protect the kidneys from renal ischemia [inability of oxygen and nutrients to be delivered to cells within the kidney tissues, as waste products also can't be taken away], heavy metals, and mycotoxins."

– Association between Selenium Status and Chronic Kidney Disease in Middle-Aged and Older Chinese Based on China Health and Nutrition Survey Data; *Nutrients Journal*; June 2022

"Selenium and manganese are essential micronutrients that are important elements of cell metabolism. They are involved in the composition of enzymes and regulate enzyme activity. Disturbances in the homeostasis of these micronutrients affect the development of many diseases and carcinogenesis, which can be linked to increased levels of oxidative stress and impaired antioxidant properties of many enzymes. Selenium has a very important function in maintaining immune-endocrine, metabolic, and cellular homeostasis. Manganese, on the other hand, is important in development, digestion, reproduction, antioxidant defense, energy production, immune response, and regulation of neuronal activity."

– The Role of Selenium and Manganese in the Formation, Diagnosis, and Treatment of Cervical, Endometrial, and Ovarian Cancer; *International Journal of Molecular Science*; June 2023

"Manganese is a trace mineral that is present in tiny amounts in the body. It is found mostly in bones, the liver, kidneys, and pancreas. Manganese helps the body form connective tissue, bones, blood clotting factors, and sex hormones. It also plays a role in fat and carbohydrate metabolism, calcium absorption, and blood sugar regulation. Manganese is also necessary for normal brain and nerve function.

Manganese is a component of the antioxidant enzyme superoxide dismutase (SOD), which helps fight free radicals. Free radicals occur natural in the body, but can damage cell membranes and DNA. They may play a role in aging, as well as the development in an number of health conditions, including heart disease and cancer. Antioxidants, such as SOD, can help neutralize free radicals and reduce or even prevent some of the damage they cause.

However too much manganese in the diet could lead to high levels of manganese in the body tissues. Abnormal concentrations of manganese in the brain, especially in the basal ganglia, are associated with neurological disorders similar to Parkinson's disease. Early life manganese exposure at high levels, or low levels, may impact neurodevelopment. Elevated manganese is also associated with poor cognitive performance in school children."

– Manganese information; Mount Sinai Health Library

Blood tests associated with kidney function should measure levels of manganese and selenium.

It is better to get your nutrients from whole foods, rather than from taking supplements. Unless you need a certain supplement, like CoQ10 if you are on statin drugs. Or if you are short on vitamin D, B12, zinc, iron, magnesium, and/or some other nutrients.

B12 is the nutrient people often mention as something vegans can be short in. It's easy to take a B12 supplement and quash those concerns. Nutritional yeast also has B12. I do take vegan B12.

B12 is important for all sorts of functions, including to keep homocysteine (an amino acid) levels in check, protecting against heart disease and stroke. B12 is important for healthy brain and motor function, and development. B12 helps to maintain the myelin sheath (an insulating layer of protein and fat surrounding each nerve cell) allowing for electrical impulses to travel along the nerves. B12 also protects against depression, and also vascular dementia, Alzheimer's, and other cognitive disorders, and otherwise neurodegenerative diseases.

I advise against taking supplements of manganese or selenium, unless, for some reason, you are doing so under the supervision of a nutritionist or doctor.

The trace amounts of manganese and selenium in garlic are not going to overdose you on the minerals. Besides garlic, these minerals also are in whole grains, nuts, legumes, and leafy green vegetables.

Allicin benefits

Allicin is a sulfur molecule that is an anti-inflammatory and anti-oxidant. It is helpful for the kidneys, liver, and heart.

The way allicin benefits the kidneys is especially because of its role as an antihypertensive agent. That is, it reduces hypertension. Doubly beneficial is that allicin also reduces oxidative stress.

"Hypertension is the leading cause of chronic kidney disease, and end-stage renal disease (ESRD), contributing to the disease itself, or, most commonly, contributing to its progression. Likewise, hypertension is reported as a consequence of kidney injury. In the United States, approximately 30% of incident ESRD cases are attributed to hypertension.

Recent studies suggest that allicin may play a role in chronic kidney disease, reducing hypertension and oxidative stress, and improving renal dysfunction.

The beneficial effects showed by allicin are similar, or even better, than those of losartan. In fact, the effect of allicin on blood pressure and renal function is comparable to reductions seen with losartan, a prescription drug commonly used as a first-line therapy.

Allicin treatment was as effective as losartan treatment in reducing the lipid oxidation in the cortex and medulla. Concerning the effects of allicin and losartan on oxidized proteins, both treatments reduced oxidation of protein in the cortex. This effect was not observed in the renal medulla, where only allicin showed antioxidant effects by decreasing protein oxidation.

Hypertension and oxidative stress in the kidneys is associated with an alteration in endothelial nitric oxide synthase (eNOS) expression. To address the issue was assessed the eNOS expression in immunoblotting. IN the CKD group, the expression of ENOS was decreased in comparison with the control group. However treatment with allicin or losartan increased the ENOS expression, with allicin being more efficient than losartan.

Allicin and losartan showed the same effectiveness to decrease hypertension, albuminuria, and urinary NAG excretion. The level of blood pressure reduction achieved with allicin was comparable to that of common antihypertensive medications.

Allicin may be a useful tool for the treatment of emerging diseases such as CKD."
– The Beneficial Effects of Allicin in Chronic Kidney Disease Are Comparable to Losartan; *International Journal of Molecular Sciences*; Sept. 2017

Allicin forms when compounds in garlic are mixed.

To get the most health benefits from your garlic, crush and dice it, let it sit for a minute, and then add it to raw/unheated to foods.

I simply crush and dice three cloves of garlic every morning, scoop them into a spoon, and drink them down with water.

Heat damages allicin, so include some raw, uncooked crushed and/or diced garlic in your foods. It can be added just before eating salads, hummus, and guacamole, and vegan soups, chili, bean dishes, and stews.

"Alliin is an organosulfur and defensive compound found in garlic and other Allium species. Its unique odor is easily detectable, and its effects on human health have been studied since ancient times.

Allicin has shown several therapeutic effects, such as cardiovascular disease protection, antioxidant, anti-cancer, antimicrobial, anti-asthmatic, immunoregulator, blood pressure lowering, and antilipidemic [lowers lipid levels in the blood].

Showing both antibacterial and antifungal activities, allicin also displayed an interesting potential in the prevention and treatment of several diseases, including diabetes mellitus, cardiovascular disease, and cancer. Indeed, its antioxidant and immunomodulatory effects are some of the mechanisms that may explain their biological activities.

Alliin and alliinase are enclosed in different compartments within the garlic clove. By cutting or crushing the clove, alliin and alliinase are brought in contact to produce allicin."

— Allicin and health: A comprehensive review; ScienceDirect; 2019

Coenzyme Q10 (CoQ10)

I take coenzyme Q10 (CoQ10), which is better to take in the morning, so it doesn't interfere with sleep.

CoQ10 is naturally found throughout the body, and especially in the heart, kidneys, liver, and pancreas.

In foods, CoQ10 is in legumes (lentils, peanuts, and soy beans), nuts (especially pistachios), and seeds (including sesame).

CoQ10 reduces inflammation and oxidative stress, and helps to maintain blood pressure.

Those with kidney disease likely could benefit from taking a CoQ10 supplement. It also can benefit those who experience migraines. As your doctor and/or nutritionist.

"CoQ10 helps generate energy in cells by making the antioxidant adenosine triphosphate (ATP), which is involved in cell energy transfer. It also serves as an antioxidant to protect cells against oxidative stress.

Your body produces less of it with age, but you can also get it from food supplements.

Low levels of COQ10 may be associate with diseases like cancer, type 2 diabetes, and neurodegenerative disorders."

— 9 Benefits and Side Effects of Coenzyme Q10; Healthline; Sept. 2024

People who take statin drugs may want to research what it is doing to their level of CoQ10. Their doctor likely advised them to take a CoQ10 supplement.

"Statins (30hyroxy-30-methylglutaryl coenzyme A deductase inhibitors) are widely used for the treatment of hypercholesterolemia and coronary heart disease and for the prevention of stroke. There have been various adverse effects, most commonly affecting muscle and ranging from myalgia to rhabdomyolysis. These adverse effects may be due to a coenzyme Q10 (CoQ10) deficiency because inhibition of cholesterol biosynthesis also inhibits the synthesis of CoQ10.

Even brief exposure to atorvastatin causes a marked decrease in blood CoQ10 concentration. Widespread inhibition of CoQ10 synthesis could explain the most commonly reported adverse effects of statins, especially exercise intolerance, myalgia, and myoglobinuria."

— Atorvastatin Decreases the Coenzyme Q10 Level in the Blood of Patients at Risk for Cardiovascular Disease and Stroke; *Journal of the American Medical Association*; June 2004

Heart health, the endothelium, oils, and nitric oxide

Adenosine, which is synthesized within and released by our cells, plays a role in heart health, including heart rhythm, blood pressure, and the function of the endothelial cells lining both the blood and lymphatic vessels.

The endothelial cells produce nitric oxide that plays into coronary vasodilation and vascular tone – keeping your veins, arteries, and capillaries open for easy blood flow.

Fatty foods decrease nitric oxide production, which results in narrowing the blood passageways, slowing blood flow, and decreasing energy. This is why some athletes follow a low-fat diet – especially for peak performance.

For you, if you want to be at peak performance, and to maintain a healthy cardiovascular system, follow a low-fat diet free of extracted oils. Especially avoid fatty foods during the morning and afternoon hours.

Extracted oils

As mentioned elsewhere, humans are the only animal that extracts oils and adds them to their foods.

The only fats you need are contained in every cell of fruits, vegetables, sprouts, and other edible plant matter. Consider those to be your essential fatty acids.

There is no nutritional need for adding bottled oils to your foods, and especially oils that have been highly heated.

Omega-3 fatty acids

While there are omega-3 fats in all raw fruits and vegetables, they are especially present in raw green leafed vegetables, raw hemp and flax seeds; sprouts (including sunflower and broccoli sprouts); and germinates or "soaks" – including soaked buckwheat, chia, and quinoa. (However, buckwheat and quinoa are listed as high in oxalates – not that we absorb many oxalates from food.)

Omega-6 fatty acids

A diet rich in omega-6 fatty acids can be problematic for those with celiac, gluten intolerance, leaking gut, arthritis, and other inflammatory diseases.

Omega-6 fatty acids are more present in packaged and processed foods, and in bottled oils, such as canola oil, safflower oil, corn oil, and sunflower oil. I encourage eliminating all of those from the diet.

For better health, simply avoid all heated oils (including fried foods and oil sautéed foods), and all bottled oils, including olive oil, flax oil, sesame oil, sunflower oil, canola oil, corn oil, and other oils.

If you do use oils, use them <u>sparingly</u>, such as raw, unheated organic coconut oil, hemp seed oil, or avocado oil (store them in the refrigerator or freezer).

Arginine, endothelial cells, and nitric oxide

The amino acid arginine helps the endothelial cells lining the veins, arteries, capillaries, and lymph system to produce the nitric oxide that keeps those passageways open.

"Nitric oxide is produced by nearly every type of cell in the human body and one of the most important molecules for blood vessel health. It's a vasodilator, meaning it relaxes the inner muscles of your blood vessels, causing the vessels to widen. In this way, nitric oxide increases blood flow and lowers blood pressure."
– Dr. Caldwell Esselstyn of ForksOverKnives.com

In addition to dilating the cardio and lymph systems, arginine plays a role in the immune system, in hormone function, in wound healing, and in kidney function.

Arginine is made by your body. It also is in almonds and other nuts, chickpeas, lentils, oats, corn, buckwheat, and other grains, peanuts, pumpkin seeds, sesame seeds, sunflower seeds, and other seeds, and soybeans,

Some people claim you need to eat animal protein to get arginine. Arginine is in legumes, whole grains, nuts, and seeds. These plants don't contain the cholesterol and saturated fat of meat, dairy, and eggs. The plants also don't contain the Neu5GC in dairy or mammal meat, and which makes cancer more aggressive. Plants also don't contain the substances in meat, dairy, and eggs that play roles in the development of cancer, Alzheimer's, varicose veins, macular degeneration, kidney disease, bone degeneration, or autoimmune disorders like diabetes and arthritis. Plant matter also contains other nutrients, and fiber – which help maintain healthy tissues, including of the digestive tract and cardiovascular system.

The production of nitric oxide by the endothelium cells helps the blood to flow more freely, increasing energy and muscle activity, including for sports and highly active physical activities. The low-fat, no oil vegan diet advised by ForksOverKnives and this book is especially helpful for the endothelium.

Some people are advised to take an arginine supplement to help reduce high blood pressure, and protect the fine blood system in the kidneys, eyes, and other tissues. This is the microvascular system consisting of arterioles, capillaries, and venules that mainly consists of endothelial cells, and works in combination with the macrovascular system consisting of arteries and veins. People with diabetes, often have problems with both the eyes and the kidneys.

For those who have been advised to take an arginine supplement, there are vegan versions available on the market.

Athletes and the plant-based, low-fat diet

A low-fat vegan diet is something many athletes are discovering helps them to perform better. As described above, fat slows the production of nitric oxide, and this results in narrower blood passageways. Fat in the diet also ends up in the blood, and slows it.

Fat can also interfere with the flow of blood in part of the blood system. It is one reason why heart attacks and strokes often happen after someone has consumed a high-fat meal. (Last year, a friend of mine ate a particularly fatty meal, and ended up in the hospital with a stroke he is still recovering from.)

Exercise every day

Exercise first thing in the morning, to the point of breaking a sweat. This stimulates hormonal and cholesterol balance, and helps to improve kidney function. It benefits the heart, adrenal glands, lungs, brain, nerves, liver, eyes, muscles, and bones all the way to the marrow. It helps to flush toxins and waste products from the system, and oxygenate the skin, giving you a healthful glow. It helps the digestive, lymph, and immune systems. It benefits metabolism, helping to level weight. It kickstarts the production of neurotransmitters, helping brain and nerve health, and improving mental clarity. It reduces stress and improves mood.

The energy and intention of exercising first thing in the morning will carry on into the rest of your day.

Getting to bed early enough to then exercise in the morning will also be a benefit. Exercising in the morning will help you to sleep better at night.

You don't need to join a gym to get adequate exercise. Everything from vinyasa yoga, stretching, calisthenics, isometric resistance band exercises, and weights are beneficial, as is cardiovascular exercise like running, speed walking, biking, jumping rope, and other non-gym activities.

If you want home gym equipment, look for used equipment, which is less expensive. I bought a used Versaclimber at a tenth of the original cost from a retired wrestler.

Exercise on a regular schedule, especially first thing every morning. And stay active throughout the day, perhaps with a lighter exercise session later in the day.

Stomach size and meal size

The stomach is part of the gastrointestinal tract. Its cells produce enzymes and acids that break down food assisted by contractions of the primary muscle of the stomach, the muscularis extrema. The stomach lining is called the *mucosa*. The submucosa lines the mucosa and has blood and lymph vessels, and nerve cells.

Whatever unhealthful substances your foods contain are exposed to the blood, lymph, and nerve systems within the stomach, and then also in the rest of your gastrointestinal tract. Anything that makes its way into the blood and lymph also makes it into your other organs, including your spleen, pancreas, liver, kidneys, and bladder, and the reproductive organs, and other parts of you, including your brain. Whatever you eat becomes a part of you, and can either help maintain good health, or can damage your health.

Conditions the stomach can experience include:

- Cancer
- Gastric ulcers: which can cause bleeding and pain
- GERD: gastroesophageal reflux disease, which can cause heartburn and coughing – especially at night
- Indigestion: dyspepsia, leading to burning in the upper stomach
- Inflammation: gastritis
- Nerve damage: gastroparesis
- Peptic ulcers: sores that can also be in the small intestine (duodenum)

Food choices can help prevent, or trigger – and make worse – all of the above conditions. A clean, plant-based diet surely will help.

To avoid stomach problems, get away from the low-quality SAD diet (standard American diet) – consisting of junk foods, highly processed foods, and foods rich in animal proteins, damaged oils, synthetic chemicals, and AGEs.

Make a loose fist as if you are holding a golf ball, and consider the size of your loose fist as about what a reasonably-sized meal would be. The stomach can expand to accommodate more – even, for some people, as much as what is the size of a gallon of water. But how much more than the size of a loose fist is overeating? It depends on what sort of foods you are eating, high calorie (heavily cooked and oily), and animal protein – or fresh fruit, or a raw salad with lots of greens free of added oils.

Toxic drinks, including sodas, colas, energy drinks, alcohol, and drinks containing clarified sugars, extracted oils, synthetic chemicals, and other low-quality ingredients degrade the stomach tissues, and expose your blood, lymph, and nerves to those ingredients.

Smoking or chewing tobacco can also play a role in stomach issues, including cancer.

I knew a woman who basically ate and drank whatever she felt like eating or drinking, with no apparent concern with contents, or nutrition. Fast foods, fried foods, microwaved foods, ultra-processed foods, dairy, meat, eggs, and toxic drinks were common. Her appearance reflected her diet. She looked like a toxic waste dump. When the stomach and intestine problems started, and she kept mentioning them, I suggested cleaning up the diet. Instead, she chose whatever prescription and over-the-counter meds she or her doctor thought would help. The very same medications she was taking carry the risks of damaging the lining of the stomach and intestinal tract, increasing the risk of experiencing – and worsening a variety of – health conditions. She took the drugs, and kept eating the garbage, and mentioning how much her stomach and intestines bothered her. She'd drink cow milk, thinking it would help her stomach and intestines. Even though milk can increase the production of stomach acids, worsening conditions like ulcers. Eventually, she had part of her stomach and small intestine removed. Then she had complications from the surgery. Only after going through all of that misery was when she chose to get strict about following a clean diet.

If you eat raw fruits and vegetables, know they are high in water content, and you can eat more of those than if you were eating something cooked down to enhance the flavor, or heavier foods, like grains and beans, or anything with high-fat.

The amount you eat also depends on how active you are. It's good to remain active, including because daily exercise benefits the gastrointestinal tract, heart, kidneys, nerves, brain, muscles, tendons, skin, eyes, and all parts of you.

Physical neglect and overeating: self-violence

Lack of exercise and neglecting physical activity, along with overeating, and consuming low quality foods lead to the accumulation of fat and toxins in the tissues, and often to other health matters damaging to the tissues of the body.

Overeating, choosing to eat low-quality foods, and lack of exercise can be so damaging to the body some have equated them as forms of self-violence.

Overeating overworks your system, stressing it and causing it to become less vibrant and more susceptible to degradation, distortion, weakness, inflammation, injury, an acidic state, and disease. This is magnified by inadequate exercise. And even more by choosing toxic foods.

On the other hand, eating an adequate amount of calories, following a clean diet, and maintaining a daily exercise practice creates a situation in which you are less likely to experience acidosis, inflammation, other gastrointestinal issues, oxidative stress, weight gain, and cardiovascular and kidney disease, and other issues, but are more likely to thrive in health.

"By including a higher proportion of foods with natural alkali, such as fruits and vegetables, a vegan diet is nearly acid neutral. Plant-based foods can be used to reduce both the dietary acid load, and the severity of metabolic acidosis. Similarly, a low protein intake in patients with advanced non-dialysis chronic kidney disease has also been shown to attenuate the severity of metabolic acidosis. NHANES III data have shown that, among 1,486 adult participants with chronic kidney disease, higher dietary acid load ascertained by 24-hour dietary recall was strongly associated with development of end stage kidney disease (ESKD) over a median follow-up of 14.2 years. Compared with participants whose dietary acid consumption was in the lowest tertile, those with dietary acid consumption in the highest tertile had triple the risk of incident ESKD, even after accounting for differences in sociodemographics, nutritional factors, clinical factors, baseline eGFR, proteinuria, and serum bicarbonate levels."

– The Effects of High-Protein Diets on Kidney Health and Longevity; *Journal of American Nephrology*; July 2020

Emotional eating

Overeating is often associated with emotions. It is said to be like shoving the emotions down in an attempt to block yourself from feeling them.

Unfortunately, people are more likely to eat low-quality foods when they are stressed – while also not getting adequate exercise, which magnifies the consequences – including dulling brain function, decreasing energy, gaining weight, and reducing vibrancy.

Chewing and the mood inhibitor: serotonin

Eating may be a natural response to stress because chewing increases serotonin, a mood inhibitor also involved with maintaining liver health.

Serotonin is naturally present in fruits and vegetables. It is also found in the gastrointestinal tract, and is stored in the blood platelets.

Serotonin is synthesized from substances found in food, and the receptors for it are on nerve cells.

Low levels of serotonin are associated with anger. Thus, a healthful diet containing plentiful amounts of fresh greens and fruits helps to regulate mood and balance emotions.

If you aren't eating quality nutrition your body is also not getting the serotonin it seeks from foods.

Stress nutrition

People often eat not for nutrition, but to deal with emotions. As always, especially when working to improve both physical and mental health conditions, it's better to select healthy foods – and to avoid junk foods.

Sometimes a glass of water and light exercise will help you to deal with stress better than food would.

Staying hydrated is important, especially for those with kidney issues. It helps the kidneys to filter waste products, acids, and excess minerals. It helps prevent a buildup of the myoglobin proteins (from injuries), and helps you to avoid forming kidney sediment, sand, or stones.

When you find yourself to be stressed, choose greens. Besides lettuce and spinach, greens include everything from cilantro to parsley, collards, chard, kale, broccoli, asparagus, cucumber, celery, zucchini, and herbs, and wild greens like purslane (but purslane is high in oxalic acid, which you might be avoiding), and dandelion.

Dice a variety of greens, mix with hummus, and/or avocado, or beans, or rice. Use as filler in a collard leaf wrap (of a collard leaf that had been wilted by putting in hot water). This is an easy way to get a variety of raw greens in your diet.

As has been revealed through various studies, the consumption of animal protein, and foods containing clarified sugars, and synthetic chemicals, and also alcoholic drinks all can degrade the gut microbiome, and the intestinal tract, where molecules of emotion originate. This plays out in mental health, including increased stress and anxiety, sleep disruption, and degraded nerve and brain function. It results in an imbalance of various systems, hormones, nutrients, and electrolytes.

"One of the metabolites produced by the intestinal microflora is TMAO. Researchers pay a lot of attention to the intestinal microbiome because of its possible role as a promotor of chronic diseases, cancers, and even neurological disorders. Intestinal microflora is connected with new age disorders like obesity, insulin resistance, atherosclerosis, cardiovascular disease, as well as type 2 diabetes, kidney failure, neurological disorders, and cancer (stomach, colon). TMAO was also associated with mortality and hospitalization for cardiorenal disorders, including atrial fibrillation, heart failure, acute myocardial infarction, and chronic kidney disease."
– Trimethylamine N-oxide (TMAO) in human health; *Experimental and Clinical Sciences Journal*; Feb. 2021

As is pointed out elsewhere, eliminating animal protein from the diet also eliminates the problematic TMAO (trimethylamine N-oxide) produced by the liver from TMA (trimethylamine) metabolized by gut bacteria chiefly from eating animal protein.

Following a clean, plant-based diet reduces inflammation, stress, anxiety, and neural decline. It improves blood flow, the gut microbiome, the production of short-chain fatty acids, and protects the nerves and brain. It is helpful for maintaining the homeostasis and cell energy production throughout the body, which is good for mental health.

What weakens the body

When a person's diet is lacking in raw plant matter, the digestive enzymes degrade and begin to draw on the metabolic enzymes. This series of events dulls and weakens the body, causes sluggishness, and helps to pave the way for illness to set in.

The standard American diet of low quality, overly processed, and highly heated, fried, and junk foods lacking in fiber, enzymes, antioxidants, and anti-inflammatories creates a situation far below peak health.

For many people, because of their horrid diet, the body is alive, but the system is weak, and is susceptible to limited physical and mental abilities, to increasingly consist of unhealthful, distorted, and damaged body tissues, and to varieties of illness.

You can weaken your enzyme potential by following an unhealthful diet.

Just as a houseplant may display damage from a time period of being neglected, the body may also be damaged by a low quality diet. Just as a plant can regain vigor when it is supplied with the right nutrients, so too can the human body.

Sleep

Many people overeat, or otherwise consume too many calories, including because they eat before they go to bed.

It is good to avoid eating anytime within a few hours before bedtime. It is a time best for the body to be shutting down for the night, and not for the organs to get busy digesting more food. Give your digestive system the rest it needs at night.

If food is desired before bedtime, consider an herbal tea. Avoid getting into the habit of eating before bed. To help shut down for the evening, also avoid looking at electronic screens. Do mild stretching, calisthenics, and yoga poses to help you to relax.

"Changes in sleep duration and time of sleep onset may have detrimental effects on renal function. Short sleep duration and shift work are associated with risk factors for chronic kidney disease, including hypertension, diabetes, and cardiovascular disease. As examples, individuals who report sleeping 5 hours or less per night are 20% more likely to develop hypertension, 34% more likely to develop diabetes, and 45% more likely to develop cardiovascular disease, compare with those sleeping 7 hours per night. A variety of cross-sectional studies have found that patients with kidney disease have shorter average sleep duration overall, and in a single prospective study of 6,834 Japanese adults, those who slept 6 or fewer hours per night were 70% more likely to develop proteinuria than individuals who slept for 7 hours per night."
– Association of short sleep duration and rapid decline in renal function; *Kidney International* journal; March 2016

Circadian rhythm and the sleep-wake cycle

The time of day you eat plays a role in being in tune with the natural nighttime circadian rhythm, which also plays a role in melatonin production, metabolism, fat/muscle balance, hormone levels, and autoimmune and nerve function. These are more reasons to avoid eating for a few hours before sleep.

A good night's rest is extremely important to your overall well-being and, it turns out, your kidneys. Kidney function is regulated by the sleep-wake cycle, which helps coordinate the kidneys' workload over 24 hours."
– 10 Common Habits That May Harm Your Kidneys; National Kidney Foundation; June 2016

Darkness and melatonin

Melatonin plays a role in better sleep, and in regulating your system in tune with your internal clock, and the circadian rhythm.

To sleep better, place a dark cloth over your eyes. Having your eyes in dark as you sleep helps you to produce melatonin, and balances your hormones. This process also occurs in blind people as their cells contain the mechanisms that respond to light and darkness.

It is best to sleep at night – before 10 p.m. – to keep in line with the circadian rhythm. Your body produces a different balance of chemicals at night, and part of it is because of how the kidneys help to regulate the sleep-wake cycle.

These patterns in tune with the processes of dark/sleep and light/awake are present in animals, plants, fungus, and microbes. In nocturnal animals, the process is reversed.

To learn more about circadian rhythm, research: chronobiology.

See the section of this book about the pineal gland.

Coffee

If you are a coffee drinker, to prevent interfering with body's reset of your circadian rhythm, and natural cortisol production that starts when you are exposed to morning light, wait at least 90 minutes to two hours after you awake to have coffee. But not much longer.

Drinking coffee too soon after you awake can block the purinergic adenosine receptors throughout the body. Then, you end up feeling more tired – and experience the afternoon energy crash.

Avoid caffeinated drinks and chocolate after the noon hour.

Those with IBD may be avoiding coffee. If they do drink it, they might want to try organic coffee NOT treated with ripening agents.

If you do drink coffee, don't put dairy in it. Avoid using commercial "creamers" as they usually contain a variety of unhealthful ingredients. Use non-dairy milks, such as coconut milk.

It is better if you make your own plant-based milks, to avoid some of the low-quality ingredients in packaged milks, and the chemicals leached from the lining of the container.

If you sweeten your coffee, try organic stevia, or the mild natural sweetener lucuma fruit powder. Get away from using clarified sugars, including white sugar, brown sugar, corn syrup, "simple syrup," and agave. Don't use synthetic chemical sweeteners.

If you feel as if coffee – or another caffeinated drink – negates your health, eliminate caffein from your routine.

Dandelion root latte

If you are taking antibiotics, diabetes or blood sugar meds, diuretics, or lithium, dandelion lattes, teas, and tinctures may need to be avoided. Ask your doctor or dietician if it is okay to drink.

Dandelion root latte is a non-caffeinated, natural, hot or warm drink some people have at any time of the day. Made vegan, it is of dried and ground dandelion root, and might contain chicory root, nutmeg*, cinnamon**, and carob. It could contain soaked and blended hazelnuts (as the form of milk), or oat milk. Sweetened with stevia.

(*Avoid using large amounts of nutmeg. A little nutmeg here and there is good, but it does contain myristicin, which is a psychoactive compound. Large amounts of nutmeg can increase the risk of dizziness, irregular heartbeat, nausea, and seizures, and even hallucinations.

**Cassia cinnamon – also known as Chinese or Saigon cinnamon – is the most common, and contains a compound called coumarin, which can be harmful to the liver if cassia cinnamon is used too often. Ceylon cinnamon contains only trace amounts of coumarin.)

Dandelion root contains the prebiotic fiber inulin, which feeds gut bacteria. It also has various vitamins, minerals, anti-inflammatories, and antioxidants, including beta-carotene and polyphenols. The flavonoids and hydroxycinnamic acid in dandelion may be helpful in maintaining blood lipid levels. The chicoric and chlorogenic acids in dandelion can help improve insulin sensitivity by helping to regulate the absorption of glucose into the muscles, and the secretion of insulin.

Dandelion root latte or tea is something people with pre-diabetes and diabetes might drink.

There are also dandelion leaf and root tinctures, or powders in capsules that can be taken, and that include the beneficial nutrients.

Side effects to dandelion could include contact rashes for those with sensitive skin.

There also may be allergic reactions to dandelion among those who also have allergies to burweed marsh elder, eupatorium, groundsel, mugwort, rabbit brush, ragweed, and/or sage.

Yerba mate, matcha, green tea

Some people say yerba mate tea gives them a more steady energy than coffee. Yerba mate does contain caffeine. Some say the same things about green tea, which also contains caffeine.

Matcha is also a drink some people have instead of coffee. Matcha is made from green tea leaves that had been shade-grown during the weeks before harvest. Matcha usually is blended or mixed into water, milk, or non-dairy milk.

Some people put matcha powder in their coffee. That seems like a recipe for the caffeine shakes, and bad sleep. I'm not a fan of matcha.

Awakening

Avoid being a person who puts caffeine in your system within the first hour of awakening.

To help your body awaken, within a half hour of waking go outside, or stand by a window, to expose yourself to daylight as this will help kick in your cortisol production.

Also to awaken, engage in stretching, yoga, calisthenics, isometric resistance, and other exercise. Use movement to help your body awaken your cardiovascular, lymph, hormonal, nerve, digestive, and other systems. All parts of you benefit from morning movement.

Yoga

The August 2009 issue of the *Journal of the American Dietetic Association* contained a study conducted by researchers at the Fred Hutchinson Cancer Research Center and the University of Washington. The study found those who practiced yoga for at least one hour per week had an average body mass index (BMI) of 23.1. Those in the study who didn't practice yoga were found to have an average BMI of 25.8, which is considered overweight. The researchers concluded that those who practice yoga are less likely to overeat, are less likely to overeat when stressed, and are more likely to practice what they called "mindful eating," which is eating only until full. Researchers concluded that the mental focus involved in practicing yoga helps to maintain more control over eating.

Sleep patterns and kidney health

Part of maintaining kidney health is a regular sleep pattern.

"Kidney function is regulated by the sleep-wake cycle. It helps to coordinate the kidneys' workload over 24 hours. We also know that nocturnal patterns can affect chronic kidney disease, and that people who sleep less usually have faster kidney function decline."
– Dr. Ciaran McMullan, Brigham and Women's Hospital

"A poor sleep profile is associated with increased risk of chronic kidney disease development. Therefore, sleep duration and quality should be considered when developing strategies to improve sleep and thus prevent CKD."
– Sleep and the Risk of Chronic Kidney Disease: A Cohort Study; *Journal of Clinical Sleep Medicine*; March 2019

"Sleep disorders are highly prevalent in chronic kidney disease, but are often underrecognized. Restless legs syndrome, which is common in CKD owing to issues with dopamine metabolism and is exacerbated by iron deficiency and uremia [high levels of waste products in the blood], can lead to poor sleep quality and increased daytime fatigue. Insomnia is also prevalent in CKD, particularly in patients requiring dialysis, with increased sleep latency and sleep fragmentation being reported. The cause of insomnia and CKD is multifaceted – poor sleep habits and frequent napping during dialysis, uremia, medications and mood disorders have all been suggested as potential contributing factors. Sleep apnea and CKD are also now recognized as having bi-directional relationships. Sleep apnea is a risk factor for accelerated progression of CKD, and fluid overload, which is associated with kidney failure, can lead to both obstructive and central sleep apnea. The presence of obstructive sleep apnea in CKD can exacerbate the already heightened cardiovascular morbidity and mortality in these patients, as well as leading to daytime fatigue and reduced quality of life. Increased awareness, timely diagnosis, and appropriate therapeutic interventions are essential to reduce the negative impact of sleep disorders in patients with kidney disease."
– Sleep disorders in chronic kidney disease, by Owen D. Lyons; *Nature Reviews Nephrology*; May 2024

"There is growing evidence that changes in sleep duration and time of sleep onset may have detrimental effects on renal function. Short sleep duration and shift work [working all night] are associated with risk factors for chronic kidney disease (CKD), including hypertension, diabetes, and cardiovascular disease.

The kidney is influenced by circadian rhythms, and entrained to the sleep-wake cycle allowing anticipation of the metabolic and physiological demands of the kidney throughout a 24-hour cycle. Although sleep disruption has been studied extensively in cardiovascular and metabolic disease, its association with chronic kidney disease has not been shown. We examined this in a prospective cohort study of 4,238 participants from the Nurses' Health Study and analyzed the association of self-reported sleep duration with decline in renal function over an 11-year period (1989-2000). Individuals who reported shorter sleep duration were more likely to experience a rapid decline in estimated glomerular filtration rate (30% or more). Compared with sleeping 708 hours per night, the adjusted odds ratios for rapid decline in renal function were significant 1.79 for 5 hours or less of sleep per night, a significant 1.31 for 6 hours sleep per night, but an insignificant 0.88 for 9 or more hours of sleep per night. Similarly, there was a significant trend in the adjusted annualized decline in estimated glomerular filtration rate for individuals sleeping 5 hours or less per night, 6 hours per night, 7-8 hours per night, and nine hours or more per night, respectively. Thus, shorter sleep durations is prospectively and independently associated with faster decline in renal function."

– Association of short sleep duration and rapid decline in renal function; *Kidney International journal*; March 2016

Sleep is important for kidney health, and what is good for kidney health is good for heart health, liver health, and all other areas of health.

"Unhealthy sleep, unhealthy heart. Simple and true. Take the results of a 2011 study that tracked 474,684 men and women of varied ages, races, and ethnicities across eight different countries. Short sleep was associated with more than a 45 percent greater risk of fatal and nonfatal coronary heart disease within seven to twenty-five years from the start of the study. A similar relationship was observed in a Japanese study of 2,282 male workers. Over a fourteen-year period, sleeping less than six hours a night was associated with more than a three times greater risk of suffering a cardiovascular or coronary event, such as a sudden cardiac death. This was relative to those sleeping 7 to 7.9 hours a night. I should note that in many of these studies, the relationship between short sleep and heart failure remains strong, even after controlling for other known cardiac risk factors, such as smoking, physical activity, and body mass. A lack of sleep more than accomplishes its own, independent attack on the heart."

– Matthew Walker, MD, in his book *Why We Sleep: Unlocking the power of sleep and dreams*; Scribner; 2017

Antioxidants and free radicals

Beneficial substances in plant matter include natural chemicals called antioxidants. These chemicals exist in animal protein only in trace amounts, relating to what the animals ate.

Antioxidants shield us from free radicals that naturally occur in our bodies, and also that are introduced to our systems through low quality foods, including meat, dairy, eggs, and processed foods, and also by way of drug abuse, smoking, and drinking alcohol.

Free radicals damage body tissues, including the muscles, bones, tendons, ligaments, and fascia, and the cardiovascular system, and everything from the skin to the brain to the DNA. A diet rich in free radicals increases the risk of experiencing cancer, and diseases of the heart, kidney, liver, and other tissues.

Eyes, free radicals, inflammation, diabetic retinopathy, and type 2 diabetes

Free radicals are harsh on the mechanisms within the eyes. This is one reason why antioxidants called carotenoids found in carrots, and in other vegetables, and in fruits help the eyes. Foods rich in free radicals, AGEs, damaged oils, and synthetic chemicals and other low-quality ingredients can damage the eyes.

Those with diabetes – who often also have some level of cardiovascular and kidney disease – likely have been told one reason they need to follow a diet along the lines of the fiber- and plant-rich, low-sugar Mediterranean diet is because it also protects the microvascular network in the eyes, and protects the eyes from diabetic retinopathy (damage to the blood vessels of the retina).

"A plant-based eating pattern is associated with a reduced risk of developing type 2 diabetes, and is highly effective in its treatment. Diets that emphasize whole grains, vegetables, fruits, and legumes, and exclude animal products improve blood glucose concentrations, body weight, plasma lipid concentrations, and blood pressure, and plan an important role in reducing the risk of cardiovascular and microvascular complications."
– Perspective: Plant-Based Eating Pattern for Type 2 Diabetes Prevention and Treatment: Efficacy, Mechanisms, and Practical Considerations; *Advances in Nutrition* journal; June 2021

Even in people who do not have diabetes, or cardiovascular or kidney disease, the eyes benefit from a diet containing what it takes to prevent inflammation. That is, a plant-based, low fat diet free of processed foods rich in salt, and containing damaged oils, clarified sugars, and synthetic chemicals.

Spectrum of nutrients

Antioxidants are so centric to high-quality nutrition they are a basic key to maintaining vibrant health and a strong immune system.

A diet lacking in plant matter doesn't include the spectrum of beneficial antioxidants, anti-inflammatories, and fiber obtained through the consumption of plants.

Go for stronger antioxidant-rich foods

Someone may say there are some antioxidants in meat. They are not incorrect. But it is like comparing a raindrop to a lake, with a piece of meat being the raindrop, and salad of raw vegetables and fruit being a lake of beneficial nutrients. Any antioxidants in the meat are related to what the animal ate.

Photosynthesis and spectral nutrients

Animals, including humans, do not conduct photosynthesis, which is the process that takes place in plant cells when they absorb sun energy and store it in a combination of that has been gathered from the air, water, and soil, forming the colors in the plants.

Antioxidants in the natural colors of plants are more available in edible, raw plant substances. These are among nutrients you will not get from meat, dairy, eggs, whey and casein, bone broth, and processed foods.

Consuming animal protein to try to access antioxidants is less effective than licking the juice from a knife that just cut through a piece of fruit, instead of simply eating the fruit itself.

No matter what type of kidney disease you might have, the spectrum of nutrients in plants will benefit you.

Polycystic kidney disease

Polycystic kidney disease is not what I have, but, because anything you ingest ends up going through the kidneys, any kidney condition benefits from a clean diet free from animal protein, clarified sugars, high sodium, bleached grains, synthetic chemicals, and from clarified, processed, and highly heated – or otherwise damaged – oils.

Polycystic kidney disease is an inherited condition causing cysts to form in the kidneys to the extent that the cysts take over the kidney tissue. A goal is to keep the remaining kidney tissue functioning healthfully.

Burdening polycystic kidneys with the condition of renal hypertension that happens when following a high animal protein diet – or through substance abuse – is not wise.

Blood urea nitrogen from the liver breaking down protein

A high protein diet increases the blood urea nitrogen (BUN), which is a waste product made by the liver breaking down protein. This needs to be filtered from the blood by the kidneys. As is mentioned earlier, this is another way in which a high protein diet taxes – and can damage – the kidneys.

A consistently high BUN can increase inflammation, oxidative stress, cardiovascular disease, and dysfunction of the endothelial cells lining the vascular and lymph systems.

Metabolic acidosis, inflammation, and fibrosis

One way a diet rich in animal protein is harmful is that it can increase metabolic acidosis, a condition involving the digestive and urinary systems, and the pH balance of the blood being too acidic. Alcoholic drinks, smoking, and a high-salt diet can worsen the condition.

The metabolic acidosis situation happens because the kidneys aren't removing enough acids from the blood. The more acidic the blood, the lower the rating, down to zero. The more alkaline it is, the higher the rating, up to 14. A normal range is 7.35 to 7.45.

The more damaged your kidneys are, the more likely they will not be able to remove acids from the blood.

Diabetes and/or kidney disease are part of the mix of experiencing metabolic acidosis. Blood and urine tests help to diagnose the condition. In the blood the bicarbonate and ketone levels will be considered. In urine, the ketones, pH, and the presence of albumin protein will be tested. (Albumin in the urine is also a sign of kidney damage).

Symptoms of metabolic acidosis include breathing difficulties (rapid breathing when the condition is in the early stages, or long, deep breaths when the condition worsens), confusion, dizziness, fatigue, headache, loss of appetite, nausea, tachycardia (racing heartbeat), vomiting, weakness, and a sweet, fruity scent to the breathe.

"Contemporary diets in Western countries are largely acid-inducing, and deficient in potassium alkali salts, resulting in low-grade metabolic acidosis. The chronic consumption of acidogenic diets abundant in animal-based foods (meats, dairy, cheese, and eggs) poses a substantial challenge to the human body's buffering capacities and chronic retention of acid wherein the progressive loss of bicarbonate stores can cause cellular and tissue damage. An elevated dietary acid load has been associated with systemic inflammation and other adverse metabolic conditions.

Plant-based diets are most effective at reducing dietary acid load. Results from clinical studies and recommendations in the form of expert committee opinions suggest that for a number of common illnesses, wherein metabolic acidosis is a contributing factor, the regular inclusion of plant-based foods offers measurable benefits for disease prevention and management."
– Observational and clinical evidence that plant-based nutrition reduces acid load; *Journal of Nutritional Science*; Oct. 2022

Metabolic acidosis can lead to more kidney damage, including by increasing inflammation and fibrosis. Severe cases can lead to kidney failure, and death.

Long-term (chronic) acidosis is also a chronic acid-stress condition that can be part of numerous health problems, and worsen them.

Foods that can play a role in worsening acidosis include meat (including fish and poultry), dairy (specifically cheese), eggs, acidifying grains, drinks containing alcohol, and soft drinks. These foods – which increase "diet acid load" (DAL) – have all been identified as playing roles in increasing the risks of experiencing not only chronic and degenerative physical diseases, including autoimmune, cardiovascular, kidney diseases, and various types of cancer, and neurodegenerative conditions like Alzheimer's and Parkinson's, but also mental health issues, including anxiety and depression.

While the amino acids arginine, histidine, and lysine are essential nutrients as building blocks of protein, the abundance of them in animal protein can help lead to an acid state as the metabolization of them in the liver produces hydrochloric acid, and with too much of that, the blood can get out of balance – especially when the person has compromised kidneys. The abundance of the amino acids cysteine, homocysteine, and methionine in animal protein can result in the production of sulphuric acid, also being a problem. The type of phosphates used in processed meats like bacon and sausages, and in dairy products like cheese, and also in soft drinks, are acidic phosphates, and can raise the blood acidity level – especially in someone who has kidney disease. These are more reasons for people who have kidney disease to follow a plant-based diet as it will help balance the pH of the blood, and protect the kidneys.

Foods that help maintain an alkaline blood level include: whole fruits, vegetables, and legumes. And water.

"Plant foods (vegetables, legumes, and seeds), contain phosphorus in the form of phytate, which has a significantly lower bioavailability and neglectable acidizing effect. Instead, most plant-based foods have alkalizing effects due to their high availability of potassium salts of organic anions."
— Observational and clinical evidence that plant-based nutrition reduces acid load; *Journal of Nutritional Science*; Oct. 2022

The short-chain fatty acids acetate, butyrate, and propionate metabolized by fermentation of plant fiber and carbohydrates are a source of organic anions, and help to protect against metabolic acidosis.

Certain health conditions, or reactionary situations, can also bring about, and/or worsen metabolic acidosis. These include food poisoning, ingesting antifreeze (ethylene glycol), taking too much aspirin, dehydration, severe diarrhea (removing too much sodium bicarbonate from the system), and methanol poisoning (an alcohol),

Lactic acidosis involves the buildup of lactic acid in the body. Causes of lactic acidosis include liver failure, low blood sugar, alcohol consumption, carbon monoxide poisoning, hypoglycemia (low blood sugar), seizures, cancer, asthma, and situations causing prolonged lack of oxygen to the tissues, including heart failure, anemia, and shock (metabolic acidosis can also cause shock).

Over the long-term, chronic metabolic acidosis can worsen osteoporosis (bone loss), and weaken the muscles. In children, chronic metabolic acidosis can slow and stunt their growth because metabolic acidosis interferes with growth hormones.

If you have kidney disease, have the blood and urine tests done to determine if you are in a stage of metabolic acidosis, and what your risks are of experiencing it. The doctor or nutritionist can help you lower your risks.

A clean, plant-based diet can reduce your dietary acid load, decreasing risks of metabolic acidosis, as well as lowering your risks of experiencing cardiovascular, autoimmune, liver, spleen, pancreas, and kidney diseases, and cancer.

Protecting the brain, and neurological well-being through a plant-based diet

Among the many benefits of a clean, plant-based diet and how it protects the gut microbiome and the gut-brain axis, is that it that reduces neuroinflammation. This protects the brain from cognitive decline and mood disorders.

"The systemic anti-inflammatory effects of vegan and vegetarian diets further contribute to their neurological benefits. Chronic low-grade inflammation is a well-established driver of neurodegenerative diseases, including Alzheimer's and Parkinson's, as well as mood disorders like depression. A meta-analysis by Tansey et al. (2022) demonstrated that individuals adhering to vegan and vegetarian diets consistently show lower levels of pro-inflammatory markers such as C-reactive protein (CRP) and interleukin-6 (IL-6). This reduction in systemic inflammation is likely attributed to the high intake of antioxidant-rich foods, such as fruits, vegetables, and whole grains, which counteract oxidative stress and mitigate the effects of aging on the brain. For instance, polyphenols found in berries and green tea have been shown to inhibit the production of reactive oxygen species, a key factor in the pathogenesis of Alzheimer's disease.

Another dimension of neurological health influenced by vegan and vegetarian diets is their impact on mood and mental well-being. Psychological studies have increasingly highlighted the link between dietary patterns and mental health outcomes. Vegan and vegetarian diets, due to their nutrient-dense composition, may support the production of mood-regulating neurotransmitters such as serotonin and dopamine."

– Impact of Vegan and Vegetarian Diets on Neurological Health: A Critical Review; *MDPI* journal of the Multidisciplinary Digital Publishing Institute; Feb. 2025

Amyotrophic lateral sclerosis (ALS) is an extremely dreadful, debilitating, neurodegenerative disease of the central nervous system and lower motor neurons. The current trend in ALS points toward a global 70% increase in the disease by 2040. Like Alzheimer's and Parkinson's, ALS responds to a diet rich in antioxidants and anti-inflammatories. Those are richly present in a clean, plant-based diet.

"A vegan diet has gained attention in the context of ALS for its potential role in both preventing the onset of the disease and slowing its progression. While ALS is a complex neurodegenerative disorder with multiple contributing factors that prove challenging to tackle, several key health benefits of a vegan diet make it a dietary choice of interest in the prevention and fight against this devastating condition. In a neuroepidemiology study conducted in Japan, the researchers examined the relationship between dietary habits. More specifically, they looked at the intake of vegetables, fruits, and antioxidants alongside the risk of developing ALS. Their findings indicated that individuals with a higher consumption of fruits and vegetables had a statistically significant reduction in the risks of ALS. There was also a beneficial association between the intake of various types of vegetables and ALS risk. The study suggests that a diet rich in antioxidants found in fruits and vegetables may offer protection against the development of ALS."

– Exploring dietary approaches in the prevention and management of Amyotrophic Lateral Sclerosis: A literature review ; *AIMS Neuroscience* journal; November 2023

Reducing phosphorus and potassium

With the advanced stages of kidney disease, under medical care, the amount of sodium, phosphorus, potassium, and protein in the diet will be limited. This is the reason it is suggested – if bread or rice are eaten – to use white bread (such as white sourdough bread), and white rice instead of whole grain, as these bleached foods contain far less of both phosphorus and potassium. Greens like Swiss chard, spinach, and beet greens are high in potassium, and will need to be reduced, or eliminated. Bananas are high in potassium, and it may be suggested they be limited (perhaps only a fourth of a banana, rather than the whole thing), or eliminated from the diet. Rather than drinking orange juice, only eat half of a peeled orange, which greatly reduces potassium intake, but improves both fiber and vitamin C intake. Rather than eating dried fruits (apricots, dates, prunes, and raisins, and dried tomatoes), which are high in potassium, eat whole, fresh fruits. Avocado consumption could be reduced, or eliminated. Potatoes should be sliced, soaked in water, strained, and then boiled, which is a process of greatly reducing their potassium content. Relish, pickles, and pickled olives are high in potassium, and therefore greatly reduced, or off the menu. So are processed, smoked, and cured meats (simply eliminate all meat from the diet). And all processed foods, chips, pretzels, and crackers. Alcohol consumption and energy drinks are a bad idea. Beer and cola drinks might have added phosphorus, so it is wise to eliminate those from the diet. Beer isn't your friend. Cow and goat milk contains phosphorus and potassium, and also increases the amount of TMAO metabolized in the liver, which are some of the reasons it is best to avoid dairy. Unsweetened coconut milk free of additives is a safer milk choice for those with advanced kidney disease.

Read food labels, and learn about the potassium and phosphorus content of foods. Consult with your doctor and nutritionist about what foods are okay on renal diet.

Saturated fat

With kidney disease, you want to reduce saturated fat in the diet. This is one of the reasons why we avoid bottled oils. Even olive oil contains saturated fat, and we also don't use olive oil at home.

As mentioned elsewhere, you get enough oil by eating a variety of vegetables, fruits, and sprouts, as every cell of every plant contains oil.

Signs of kidney problems, kidney stones, and nephropathy (kidney disease), include:

• Anemia

The kidneys play a role in the production of blood, and balancing of the minerals. This is in combination with the kidney's ability to produce the erythropoietin hormone.

• Cancer of the kidney

Men are more likely to experience kidney cancer, and, in America, on average, African-American people have a higher rate of kidney cancer.

Everything from diet and weight to lifestyle and substance abuse, as well as high blood pressure, genetics, and kidney problems can play a role in raising your risk of experiencing kidney cancer. Kidney cancer is often discovered from the ages of 50 to 70.

A genetic disorder called von Hippel-Lindau disease (VHL) can cause tumors and cysts to grow in the kidneys, and other parts of the body. Although considered to be non-cancerous or benign, these tumors can lead to great health complications, especially when they cause renal cell carcinoma, or malignancies in the nerve system. Besides the kidneys, other areas where they form include the eyes, ears, brain, brain stem, spinal cord, pancreas, and adrenal glands, and, in females, the broad ligament, and, in men, the epididymis. Those with the condition are likely to be diagnosed in early adulthood – far earlier than those with kidney cancer. Those with VHL do have an increased risk of both kidney and pancreatic cancer.

Kidney cancer usually happens in one kidney, but can form in both. It is one of the ten most common types of cancer.

Sometimes only a part of a kidney is removed to eliminate cancer, leaving the healthy part of the kidney. Other times the entire kidney may be removed. Freezing or using radio waves to heat the tumor to kill it might also be considered. Immunotherapy may be part of the approach in fighting the cancer by boosting the immune system. One therapy also aims to block a protein called mTOR that can play a role in cancer cell growth. Radiation and chemotherapy are less likely to be used to fight kidney cancer.

Signs of kidney cancer can include blood in the urine, pain, a lump in the region of the kidney, unexplained tiredness and weight loss, anemia, and fever.

Kidney cancer can be diagnosed – or ruled out – in a variety of ways, including a urine test (to look for blood and cancer cells), a blood test (to do a blood count of red cells, white cells, and platelets), an ultrasound, a CT scan (computerized tomography), an MRI (magnetic resonance image), PET (positron emission tomography), and – less likely – by a biopsy.

A tumor might be small when it is found, which, if there is a tumor, is a good thing. Time can be taken to research what is best for the patient. The doctor may also want to wait and see if it is growing.

Things taken into consideration when being diagnosed with kidney cancer include your age, state of health, tobacco, drug, and alcohol use, past and current health conditions, your weight, and the size of the tumor, which will be given a stage grade. They may also consider your history of being exposed to anything from toxic industrial chemicals from job sites or professions, to environmental toxins. If you were in the military, the doctor likely will want to know what sorts of substances you were exposed to (such as burn pits, bomb residues, and radiation).

Stages of cancer are from one to four. Four means it has spread to other parts of the body.

A clean diet and healthy gut biome can help in the prevention of – and fight against – kidney cancer.

- **Erythropoietin hormone**

Kidney damage can result in the kidneys not producing adequate amounts of the erythropoietin hormone (EPO). This hormone signals the bone marrow to make red blood cells. The red blood cells bring oxygen to the organs, and to other tissues.

- **A foul taste in the mouth (dysgeusia)**

This can be accompanied by bad breath, a metallic taste in the mouth, loss of taste, and sudden changes in taste of foods, known as dysgeusia. Foods might suddenly taste acidic, bitter, bland, sour, or metallic. There may also be a loss of appetite, even when formerly "favored" foods are available. This could also be a condition more likely to accompany dialysis patients.

- **Concentration issues (diabetic hypoglycemia and the hyperosmolar hyperglycemic state)**

Experiencing sudden confusion and the inability to concentrate can be related to kidney and blood sugar issues. The situation could feel as if you were drugged, have brain fog, and you might become dizzy. This condition is diabetic hypoglycemia (low blood sugar). Symptoms include dehydration, concentration and confusion issues, abnormal behavior, and difficulty speaking clearly, or completing sentences. The condition known as hyperosmolar hyperglycemic state (HHS) is when blood sugar is too high, and can cause confusion and seizures, and can be life threatening. If you have experienced these symptoms, get tested for diabetes, kidney dysfunction, and nutrient deficiencies.

Also, if you have these types of symptoms, be careful about driving, operating heavy machinery, or making any important decisions. Be safe.

• **Dark urine**

Or the urine might simply look like pure blood. (As was often my case, before I switched to a plant-based diet.)

Could be a sign of kidneys releasing blood – a sign of kidney stones.

Blood in the urine is called hematuria.

All reasons to undergo a physical, see a urologist and/or nephrologist, clean up your diet, and seek treatment for any substance abuse issue you have. ASAP.

Both kidney and liver disease can cause urine to be dark, especially late-stage kidney disease. As can a urinary tract infection, and a condition called porphyria that has to do with the nerves and skin.

• **Diabetes**

Can cause micro vessel disease, including to the extent of causing blindness, and kidney failure, damage to the heart and other organs, and nerve damage, especially in the legs, feet, and toes (diabetic neuropathy).

• **Difficulty breathing**

This can be related to fluid in the lungs, low iron levels, high sodium levels, acidic blood (metabolic acidosis), and/or a kidney infection.

See a doctor. ASAP.

This is another reason to clean up your diet, and to stay away from junk food, fried foods, salty foods, dairy, and sugary snacks, foods, and drinks, and all sugar extracts. (These include cane sugar, beet sugar, agave, corn syrup, rice syrup, and other clarified sugars. Rather than drinking fruit juice, eat whole fruit. Etc.)

• **Edema (also spelled oedema)**

Fluid retention that can result in swollen feet, ankles, and arms that remain indented after you press a finger against them. Joint stiffness and heavy-feeling legs and arms are symptoms. These all are a sign the kidneys are not filtering liquids. The condition could also be a sign of other health conditions.

A person might also have puffy hands and wrists, and puffy upper and lower eye lids. All are signs the kidneys might not be filtering out liquids.

Again, see a doctor. Get a physical, including a blood nutrition test.

• **Estimated glomerular filtration rate is not at a healthy level: The stages of kidney disease**

Kidney tests include the eGFR = estimated glomerular filtration rate.

The eGFR helps to determine how well your kidneys are functioning. It involves a blood test measuring the creatinine in the blood, as a buildup of creatinine indicates likely kidney malfunction.

The eGFR measurement also takes into consideration your age, sex, weight, muscular body type, and hydration.

Pregnancy also effects the filtration rate of the kidneys.

Stage one kidney disease:
When the eGFR is 90 milliliters per minute, it is considered normal. This is also called stage one kidney disease (even though that is not a concerning disease state). No damage is likely to be occurring at this stage.

Stage two kidney disease:
When the eGFR goes down to 60-89 milliliters per minute, a person could be considered to be in stage two kidney disease. This is when issues start to become problematic. If not corrected, it leads to the next level. At this stage blood work should be done to determine if minerals are off balance, and to monitor the blood sugar and insulin levels. The blood pressure also needs to be monitored.

Stage three kidney disease:
When the eGFR drops to 60 milliliters per minute, it is an indication of more serious kidney disease. If this lasts more than 3 months, it is considered stage 3 chronic kidney disease. At that stage kidney damage can result.

Stage four kidney disease:
Stage four kidney disease is an eGFR of 15-29. This is when severe kidney damage can be present, including bone disease.

Stage five kidney disease:
Stage five is an eGFR of 15, or below. This is advanced kidney disease. The kidneys are failing. They are not adequately filtering excess fluids, they are not balancing blood pressure, and are having problems filtering phosphorus, potassium, nitrogen (a waste product from protein), and sodium.

The body needs the essential minerals phosphorus, potassium, and sodium to function healthfully, but the mismanagement of the minerals by damaged kidneys becomes the problem.

The inability to regulate the minerals will require medical attention – by a nephrologist.

At this stage, the kidneys are suffering more damage.

The person will likely be advised to be put on dialysis, and are on the path to potentially getting a kidney transplant. (If their health allows it, and if a kidney is found in time.)

• **Fatigue and lack of energy that can also seem unrelenting**

If you are experiencing these, get your blood and urine tested. See what is going on with your system. Take the steps necessary to protect your health. Do what is right for you.

Among other diabetes management practices, daily morning exercise, and a regular and adequate sleep schedule are important – as is a clean diet rich in unprocessed fruits and vegetables, and free of clarified sugars, bleached grains, high sodium, and junk ingredients.

Get your blood nutrition test, and see if your B12 and/or vitamin D levels are low.

• Foamy urine

This might be protein in the urine, and/or a kidney infection (glomerulonephritis).

With diabetes, foamy urine could mean the blood vessels and filtering units in the kidneys are damaged, causing protein to be in the urine. This deterioration of the kidney function is called diabetic nephropathy. Keys to treating this situation, and ending the deterioration of the kidneys are to clean up the diet and get daily exercise.

Nitrogen is a waste product of protein metabolism, the situation when proteins are turned into fuel.

If a person is eating a diet rich in protein, such as meat, dairy, eggs, and bone broth, it can increase the nitrogen in the blood to levels that damage the kidneys. This is especially likely if a person is in stage 3 – or worse – of kidney disease. And/or if they have issues with blood pressure and hypertension.

As mentioned elsewhere, the body makes proteins from amino acids. It needs amino acids from foods, and the body also makes certain amino acids.

The amino acids humans need from food easily can be obtained on a vegan diet, as the amino acids are in fruits, vegetables, sprouts, nuts, legumes, seeds, beans, and seaweeds. This way of "getting protein" is easier on the system.

• Gastric bypass surgery and kidney stones

Another thing that can increase the risk of forming kidney stones is gastric bypass surgery – which is usually performed for weight loss, but could be to repair an injury, or a birth defect, or because of infection, cancer, or other issue.

Because it could increase oxalates in the urine, those who have undergone gastric bypass surgery may be advised to follow a low-oxalate diet.

Maybe – for long-term health – those thinking of undergoing gastric bypass for weight loss may want to first consider taking the route of healthful eating combined with significant daily exercise. Perhaps avoiding the surgery table is the better choice.

I had a friend who had the surgery, and there have been what seem to be endless complications impacting her health. She deeply regrets it.

Just because a doctor agrees to perform a surgery on you – or even advises it – doesn't mean it is your solution. Explore your options. And get 2nd and 3rd opinions. See if there are YouTube videos of patients explaining what the surgery was like for them.

• Gout

In this condition, there is a buildup of uric acid in the system, resulting in crystals that inflame the joints – often of the big toes. It is related to how your body deals with urea, and the breakdown of proteins. This involves both the kidneys and liver. Gout is one sign of kidney disease, but gout can also lead to kidney disease.

- **High blood pressure**

Diabetes is the leading cause. This can also lead to even more kidney damage. Often related to consuming animal protein, salty foods, and a generally unhealthful diet, combined with lack of physical activity, and an unhealthful sleeping pattern.

The kidneys help to maintain blood pressure, red blood cell balance, and oxygen absorption, etc.

- **Increased sensitivity to cold**

This could be a sign of uremic wastes accumulating in the system, and a sign of anemia. These are symptoms of kidney disease.

- **Inflammation and metabolic acidosis**

As described earlier, a diet high in animal protein encourages inflammation, and the condition called metabolic acidosis.

Dairy, eggs, and meat, as well as fried and otherwise highly-heated (damaged) oils, are all pro-inflammatory. Highly-heated animal protein is even worse, as it contains heat-generated, pro-inflammatory chemicals.

Inflammation is one of the problems with brain diseases, including Alzheimer's, encephalitis, and CTE (chronic traumatic encephalopathy, which is common with football players, boxers, and people who have suffered repeated head impacts.).

It is wise to follow an anti-inflammatory diet, including to protect the blood vessels of the brain.

"Vegetarian and vegan diets offer significant neurological benefits, including reducing oxidative stress and inflammation, supporting cognitive function, and lowering the risk of neurodegenerative diseases. These diets also promote a health gut-brain axis, and improve vascular health, contributing to overall brain health.

However, careful planning and awareness of potential accessibility barriers are essential to prevent nutrient deficiencies, primarily in omega-3 fatty acids, vitamin B12, iron, zinc, selenium, and iodine."
– Does a vegetarian diet help or harm your brain? Here's what the science reveals, by Priyanjana Ptamanik, MSc; *News Medical Life Sciences*; March 2025

Fruits, vegetables, sprouts, raw veggie juices, and beans, legumes, nuts, seeds, and seaweeds are anti-inflammatory, rich in anti-oxidants, and are acid neutral. A plant-based diet naturally has a low dietary acid load.

"Although high-protein diets continue to be popular for weight loss and type 2 diabetes, evidence suggests that worsening renal function may occur in individuals with – and perhaps without – impaired kidney function. High dietary protein intake can cause intraglomerular hypertension, which may result in kidney hyperfiltration, glomerular injury, and proteinuria [elevated protein in the urine]. It is possible that long-term high protein intake may lead to de novo chronic kidney disease. The quality of dietary protein may also play a role in kidney health. Compared with protein from plant sources, animal protein has been associated with an increased risk of end-stage kidney disease in several observational studies, including the Singapore Chinese Health Study. Potential mediators of kidney damage from animal protein include dietary acid load, phosphate content, gut microbiome dysbiosis, and resultant inflammation.

In the United States, 60% of the population meets the criteria for being obese or overweight. In this context, growing interest in low-carbohydrate, high-protein diets has emerged over recent decades. The revived popularity of low-carbohydrate, high-protein diets may be partially fueled by their promotion across social media as an effective means for rapid weight loss and better glycemic control. For patients with chronic kidney disorder, or at risk of CKD, high intake of dietary protein, including animal protein, may have detrimental effects on kidney function, and long-term kidney health.

Although some instances of short-term glomerular hyperfiltration, such as that which occurs during pregnancy, may not be associated with a decrease in kidney function, it is possible that prolonged, recurrent glomerular hyperfiltration induced by consumption of a high-protein diet may lead to kidney damage through multiple pathways over time."

– The Effects of High-Protein Diets on Kidney Health and Longevity; *Journal of American Nephrology*; July, 2020

• Insomnia or poor sleep

There can be many causes for this, but it could also be part of kidney disfunction.

Morning exercise, and movement throughout the day helps sleep.

Avoiding caffeine and chocolate can help reduce sleep issues. If you have drinks or foods containing caffeine or chocolate, do so no closer than ten hours before sleep.

Taking a magnesium supplement at night can help with sleep. As can a dark room, a dark, natural fabric (such as hemp) cloth over the eyes, and a colder room. And avoiding food for at least three hours before sleep.

• Insulin resistance

The insulin rises to unhealthy levels. It relates to the pancreas releasing high levels of insulin, which is to get blood sugar to the cells. The condition happens when the cells stop responding to the insulin, keeping the blood sugar levels high, as the pancreas continues to produce insulin.

Symptoms include unusual thirst and hunger, even after drinking water and eating. The person might also feel unusually tired, and the need to urinate often. They are also more susceptible to infections, and have tingling feet and hands. A blood test can help to reveal this condition.

• Itchy skin (pruritus or uremic pruritus)

(Topics covered in other parts this book.)

This can be the result of inflammation, high parathyroid hormone levels in the blood, a buildup of toxins and cell waste, high aluminum and magnesium levels, low white blood cell count, and nerve cell opioid receptors being off balance.

This may also be due to an imbalance of electrolytes, including high calcium and phosphorus in the system causing dry skin. This itching could include the back, arms, and face. Overly hot or cold temperatures can increase skin itchiness associated with kidney failure.

One thing the kidneys do is balance the electrolytes, including phosphorus. In a kidney failure state, the electrolytes become unbalanced.

The phosphorus in plants is not a problem, especially if legumes and/or nuts are not abundant in the diet. Meat, including fish, and also dairy, and soft drinks (because of the phosphoric acid added to those beverages) should be avoided as the phosphorus in them is more easily absorbed.

• **Kidney stones or sand**

Stones and sand forming in the kidneys could be the result of a number of situations.

You might notice sand – or what appears to be dirt or sediment – in the urine. Or, a small stone. Urine should not contain any of these.

Years ago, when my kidneys were bad, I guzzled water and a quart of pure concord grape juice, and found this to clear stones, sand, and/or sediment from the kidneys and into the urine. I would do this once-in-a-while. It worked to help clean out my kidneys. I started doing this after one time drinking a lot of wine with friends, and noticing sand in my urine (I rarely drink alcohol). I then tried it with grape juice and water, and it worked. I didn't know the process of drinking an abundance of pure grape juice followed by water had been recommended for centuries as a natural solution to cleaning the kidneys.

Anchovies, bacon, organ meats, sardines, scallops, and even baker's yeast are purine-rich. Consuming them increases uric acid in the kidneys, and this can lead to the development of kidney stones. This scenario is magnified if the person also consumes dairy, which results in more calcium being excreted. The calcium and uric acid combine to form calcium oxalate stones. A high-fat diet also plays a role in stone formation, and especially fried oils, or otherwise highly-heated or damaged oils.

• **Lack of appetite and gastroparesis**.

Especially when accompanied by other symptoms on this list. This could be related to damaged nerves in the gastrointestinal tract causing digestion to slow. It's a condition called gastroparesis.

• **Leaky gut**:

Read the parts of the book about the gut biome, and nurturing a healthy digestive tract.

In diabetics, the intestinal flora can become out of balance (dysbiosis) in combination with a damaged tract (leaky gut). This condition allows undigested proteins to travel through the gut into the blood stream, where they can tax and damage the kidneys, or cause more damage to already compromised kidneys. The substances can also land in the joints and soft tissues, triggering inflammation, and playing a role in or complicating (autoimmune) conditions like arthritis, and the genetic disorder called Dupuytren's that causes scar tissue to form in the hands.

As explained earlier, leaky gut can play into everything from neurodegenerative diseases and mood issues, to cancer, and the wide variety of autoimmune disorders, and kidney and cardiovascular disease.

A clean, plant-based diet greatly reduces the risk of experiencing leaky gut.

Consider learning about building a healthy base of intestinal flora. Research vegan probiotics and vegan prebiotics. Read the parts of this book about dysbiosis, symbiosis, and short-chain fatty acids.

• Liver production of the albumin protein is insufficient.

This is in combination with a low level of albumin in the blood, and a high level of albumin in the urine. It causes an imbalance of water in the blood stream. The condition of having albumin in the urine is called albuminuria.

Insulin helps to stimulate the liver to produce albumin.

Low albumin is also a sign of liver disease, and also could be a sign of infection.

Problems with albumin production and excretion balance occur especially with stage 5 kidney disease, as the kidneys drain the albumin. This can play a role in severe edema.

Albumin is given to dialysis patients, because dialysis also filters albumin from the blood.

• Muscle cramping

Could be related to mineral balance issues – especially of calcium and phosphorus.

The kidneys play a key role in balancing the electrolytes in the blood.

Symptoms of impaired kidney function include muscle cramps. The cramps likely will be in the legs, but can be in other muscles.

• Myoglobin protein in the urine

The urine test done to determine the health of the kidneys includes measuring myoglobin protein in the urine.

The myoglobin protein is released by damaged or worked-out muscles, and filtered from the blood by the kidneys. A buildup of myoglobin in the kidneys can damage them. This is another reason why it is good to stay hydrated with water during and after a workout, or any physically taxing activity.

Persons with muscle injuries, or who have experienced a drug overdose, heart attack, burns, crush injuries, or other catastrophic injuries, or a seizure with prolonged contraction can have a high level of myoglobin in the urine.

Too much myoglobin can trigger renal failure. This is one reason for placing certain patients on I.V. fluids (to help flush the kidneys).

• Nausea and vomiting

Especially accompanied by kidney pain, usually at the bottom back of the rib cage, and/or pain of a ureter tube (through which urine travels from the kidneys to the bladder). This could be a kidney stone.

Some who have experienced vomiting while passing a kidney stone say the vomiting is more likely to happen if the stone is in the right kidney. This does not mean you will experience the same situation.

Excessive vomiting can cause dehydration, and other issues. See a doctor.

• Thyroid issues

A blood nutrition panel will reveal if there is an issue with your iodine level. It is better to know it, and to not guess if you do or do not have adequate iodine. Then you will know if you need a supplement. See the iodine section in the book.

You likely can purchase a small bottle of organic kelp iodine at your natural foods store, or easily order some online. I also include pinches of nori flakes in my salads, soups, and veggie juices.

When I was first diagnosed with kidney disease, they also recommended the removal of my thyroid (thyroidectomy), and then, once I had that procedure, they would stick me on a prescription synthetic thyroid hormone (levothyroxine) and calcium supplements – for the rest of my life.

I refused to have my thyroid removed, which displeased a couple of my doctors. I was not an agreeable patient, always second guessing doctor advice, doing my own research, and not following medical advice. Some doctors refused to see me anymore as a patient. I didn't care.

I kept my thyroid, and my thyroid tests have been normal for many years.

• Urinalysis showing protein, albumin, myoglobin, minerals, blood infection

In addition to a blood nutrition panel test, kidney function tests often include a urinalysis (including urine protein content, the albumin protein level, the presence of myoglobin, and the mineral content, and also signs of blood and/or infection in the urine), ultrasound, and blood pressure measurement. The condition of the hands, wrists, arms, legs, ankles, feet, toes, teeth, and tongue are taken into consideration. A complete general physical might be ordered, including ultrasound images, and/or other images, and heart tests.

• Urinating too much, or too little

Especially if urinating more than a couple times at night. Waking up more than once or twice per night to pee is called nocturia – which could be problematic for the sleep cycle, and leave you tired and fatigued during the day. (Research: nocturia.)

• Urine smelling strongly of ammonia

The body is not converting the ammonia into urea. This can play a role in dementia, and other serious health issues. The urine can be concentrated, and is one sign the person is dehydrated. It also can be related to a urinary tract infection, bladder stones, and liver failure.

With diabetes, high blood sugar can cause the urine to have a sweet smell, but it can also be related to a genetic disorder named maple syrup urine disease. Tests would need to be done to factor the cause.

Ammonia is a byproduct of protein breakdown. When this is not filtered from the system, one of the long-term results is an increased risk of dementia.

A healthy liver and kidney system will turn the ammonia into urea, which then leaves the body through the urine, a product of the kidneys.

You may have heard people claim that drinking your urine is some sort of health elixir. However: **Drinking urine very much absolutely is NOT a wise**

thing to do.

Your urine contains what your body needs to get rid of. Don't put those substances back into your body, or you may suffer consequences, including diarrhea, nausea, vomiting, and infections. Drinking urine can worsen infections, and kidney and autoimmune issues you already have.

"Urine is a potent combination of salts and chemicals your body is attempting to remove. These chemicals can cause significant health problems if you consume them. Furthermore, urine provides no health benefits that cannot be found by consuming other foods and beverages.

By drinking urine, which contains a high concentration of sodium, you can quickly develop a negative feedback loop in which you feel thirstier despite drinking liquids.

The field manual for the US Army explicitly recommends avoiding drinking urine as a form of hydration, even in emergency situations.

Despite the common myth, urine is not sterile. It contains bacteria just like any other bodily excretion.

By drinking urine, you are consuming these toxins your body explicitly intended to remove. This can lead to kidney damage."
– Are There Health Benefits to Drinking Urine?; WebMD; Sept. 2024

• **Urine looks like pure blood, and/or has blood clots in it**

Could be a sign of kidney stones, or other problems. As above, see a doctor ASAP. The doctor likely will order a urinalysis, a blood test (including to check your mineral and other nutrient levels), and an ultrasound of your kidneys.

Blood red urine was an issue I had, until I switched to a clean, plant-based diet.

• **Vitamin D imbalance and the presence of hyperparathyroidism**

If you take a vitamin D supplement, consult with your urologist. Get a blood test to check your nutritional panel, including your vitamin D level. If vitamin D continues to be low, this can impact the absorption of calcium, impacting bone health, mood, and a variety of health issues.

I do take a vegan vitamin D supplement. I also live in a region with plenty of sunshine, which helps the skin to formulate vitamin D.

You both don't want to have too little, or too much vitamin D. Consult with your doctor, and/or a dietician about this matter.

"Abnormalities in vitamin D metabolism play a major role in the pathogenesis of secondary hyperparathyroidism in chronic kidney disease. The gradual and progressive decline in 1,25-dihydrogyvitamin D in the course of chronic kidney disease is the result of several mechanisms that limit the ability of the failing kidney to maintain the levels of 1,25-dihydroxyvitamin D despite increasing levels of parathyroid hormone. Recent observations have indicated that chronic kidney disease seems to be associated with a high incidence of nutritional vitamin D insufficiency, or deficiency as manifested by decreased levels of 25-hydroxyvitamin D. This contributes to the inability to maintain the levels of 1,25-dihydroxyvitamin D; therefore, current practice guidelines suggest repleting vitamin D status by the administration of native vitamin D as a first step in the therapy of the abnormalities of bone and mineral metabolism in chronic kidney disease. The efficacy of this therapy is extremely variable, and active vitamin D sterols may be required, especially as kidney disease progresses.

It has been well established that secondary hyperparathyroidism begins relatively early in the course of chronic kidney disease, and steadily progresses as GFR declines. The pathogenetic factors that contribute to the development and maintenance of secondary hyperparathyroidism are multiple but principally involve the closely related consequences of phosphate retention and abnormalities in vitamin D metabolism.

In-depth research in the past two decades has uncovered many of the potential mechanisms in which vitamin D is involved in the initiation and maintenance of the disturbances of bone and mineral metabolism in the chronic kidney disease population."
  – Vitamin D and Kidney Disease; *Clinical Journal of the American Society of Nephrology*; Sept. 2008

And so forth, and so on.

Do your research. Find out what's right for you.

Oxalic acid: oxalates

Many people hear of this, but know little to knighting about it, or have – and seem to maintain – a misunderstanding about it. Do some research, and learn for yourself. Especially if you have kidney problems.

"Oxalate, or oxalic acid, is a substance that can form insoluble salts with minerals, including sodium, potassium, calcium, iron, and magnesium. These compounds are produced in small amounts in both plants and mammals. All major groups of photosynthetic organisms produce oxalate. It is suggested that plants manufacture oxalate for a variety of functions, including calcium regulation, plant protection, and detoxification of heavy metals. In mammals, endogenous [created in the body] oxalate is a metabolite of ascorbate, glyoxylate, hydroxyproline, and glycine. Urinary oxalate mostly consists of endogenous oxalate, as opposed to exogenous [from outside the body, or…] dietary oxalate.

Absorbed dietary oxalates are believed to contribute to calcium oxalate kidney stone formation. Insoluble oxalates, on the other hand, are excreted in the feces. Due to their effects on nutrient absorption and possible role in kidney stone formation, oxalates are considered by some to be 'antinutrients.' Although events of toxicity have occurred in livestock chiefly grazing on oxalate-rich plants, a balanced human diet typically contains only small amounts of oxalates."
  – Is There Such a Thing as "Anti-Nutrients"? A Narrative Review of Perceived Problematic Plant Compounds; *Nutrients Journal*; Sept. 2020

The second common form of kidney stones are calcium phosphate stones, which tend to grow faster and larger than calcium oxalate stones.

Those who have a history of kidney stones are often advised to reduce their consumption of spinach. Some say that when it is eaten, it should be in a meal free of oily foods, and to drink additional water.

Learn about other foods high in oxalates. Not that you will avoid all oxalates, as they are in many types of foods, including beans, grains, greens, herbs, nuts, root vegetables, spices, and teas. An oxalate-free diet isn't recommended. Nor should you avoid all oxalate-rich foods, as they do contain a variety of compounds beneficial to health. Do eat a wide variety of plants to obtain varieties of nutrients.

Spinach and other foods rich in oxalates

As covered earlier, you also want to avoid a high-fat diet, and meat, dairy, and eggs, as they all increase the saponification in the gut that can lead to the formation of kidney stones.

Read up on what the medical literature says about oxalates and the risk of kidney stone formation. There are contradictions, and ongoing studies.

"For participants in the highest compared with lowest quintile of dietary oxalate, the relative risks for stones were 1.22 for men and 1.21 for older women. Risk was higher in men with lower dietary calcium. The relative risks for participants who ate eight or more servings of spinach per month compared with fewer than 1 serving per month were 1.30 for men and 1.34 for older women. Oxalate intake and spinach were not associated with risk in younger women. These data do not implicate dietary oxalate as a major risk factor for nephrolithiasis [kidney stones]."

– Oxalate intake and the risk for nephrolithiasis; *Journal of the American Society of Nephrology*; July 2007

"Findings suggest that total fluid intake, water, coffee, tea, alcohol, fruit, vegetables, dietary fiber, dietary potassium, magnesium, and calcium decreases the risk of kidney stones, whereas high BMI, total meat intake, animal protein, dietary sodium, spinach, oxalate, fructose, and soda increased the risk.

Fifty relevant articles with 1,322,133 participants and 21,030 cases in total were identified. Prominent risk factors for incident stones were body mass index, dietary sodium, fructose, meat, animal protein, and soda. In contrast, protective factors included fluid intake, a Dietary Approaches to Stop Hypertension (DASH) style diet, alcohol, water, coffee, tea, vegetables, fruits, dietary fiber, dietary calcium, and potassium. Vitamin D and calcium supplementation alone increased the risk of stones in meta-analysis of observational studies, but not in RCTs, where the cosupplementation conferred significant risk.

Several modifiable factors, notably fluid intake, dietary patterns, and obesity, were significantly associated with nephrolithiasis."

– Dietary and lifestyles factors for primary prevention of nephrolithiasis: a systemic review and meta-analysis; *BMC Nephrology* journal; 2020

Bok choy, instead of spinach

When speaking of kidney stones, people often mention spinach. This is because spinach is high in oxalate, which is a naturally occurring organic acid that can bind with calcium, iron, and magnesium, and lead to the formation of calcium oxalate kidney stones. However, humans also form oxalates, and much of what is in food is not absorbed. To be safe, many people choose to follow a low-oxalate diet.

Bok choy is a cruciferous vegetable lacking in the oxalates spinach contains. Bok choy contains potassium, which is protective of the kidneys.

However, if you have later stage kidney disease (less than 25% of kidney function), and/or have cardiovascular disease, you also have to be careful of your potassium intake. One third cup of cooked bok choy has about 200 milligrams of potassium, which is as much as you should get from one meal. Or, depending on your stage of kidney issues, too much.

With kidney and cardiovascular disease, you are likely already under the care of a doctor and dietitian. Follow their guidelines on potassium intake.

Like other cruciferous vegetables, bok choy contains chemicals called thiocyanates, which can interfere with iodine absorption. This is why it is good to not overdo it with cruciferous vegetables. Steaming, boiling, stewing, using them in soups, and non-oil sautéing, are ways of cooking that reduce the amount of thiocyanates. Eating some cruciferous vegetables every week is a good thing, but overdoing it can load your system with thiocyanates, and play into thyroid disorders. No need to have them in every meal.

Bok choy contains a variety of nutrients, including the minerals iron, magnesium, calcium, potassium, selenium, and vitamins A, K, and C, and folate, alpha-linolenic acid (omega-3 fatty acid), enzymes, amino acids, antioxidants (including carotene), anti-inflammatories (including quercetin), and (as all fruits, vegetables, beans, nuts, legumes, and seeds do) fiber (which works as a prebiotic, essential for the metabolization of vitally important short-chain fatty acids).

I grow bok choy. It is increasingly common for it to be sold in stores, often as "young" or "baby bok choy."

Bok choy can be chopped and used in salads and raw or steamed in bowl dishes, and as one of several ingredients in smoothies.

I don't "oil sauté" food, but many people do sauté bok choy.

For kidney health, I encourage you to avoid fried and oil sautéed foods. If you sauté, instead of using oil, use one of the following: vegan broth, apple vinegar, carrot juice, a fruit juice, or the brine water from jarred olives or raw sauerkraut (but also be careful of your sodium intake).

Because bok choy is low in FODMAPs (fermentable short-chain carbohydrates oligosaccharides, disaccharides, monosaccharides, and polyols), it is safe for people with Crohn's disease and IBS.

Because bok choy does contain salicylates, those with aspirin sensitivity might want to avoid it.

Those who have a hay fever reaction to mugwort pollen might experience a reaction to cruciferous vegetables, including bok choy.

Celery is your friend

One juice increasingly common among the health crowd is organic celery juice. You might have noticed stores selling single-serving bottles of it.

Why kidney patients eat more celery and have celery juice: Celery and celery juice help the system detoxify ammonia, filter urea from the body, and protect against kidney stone formation.

I grow celery. Sometimes I juice a bunch of it. I'll also dice it and use it in salads, in meal bowls, and as an ingredient in wraps, soups, and vegan stews. I'll make salt-free peanut butter from scratch, and spread that on a rib of celery as a snack.

Citrates help to prevent kidney stones

Urine tests done on people who have kidney stones often detect an abundance of calcium and uric acid oxalates. And, a lower than normal presence of citrates.

Citrates are formed by the body, but also are in lemons, limes, oranges, and grapefruits. They are also in broccoli, carrots, cucumbers, pineapple, tomatoes, watermelon, and some types of peppers.

Citrates bind with oxalates, preventing the binding of oxalates with calcium, and this lowers the risk of kidney stone formation.

I was told in my 20s that I would need to take a prescription to increase my citrates. A woman who ran a kidney organization told me I could simply have lemon every day to provide the chemical as it exists naturally in lemons. Learning this, I never took the prescription medication. I have plenty of organic lemons available from local trees.

Eventually, my doctors told me they no longer prescribe the medication I had been told to take. Instead, they said to squeeze lemon in my morning water.

Lemon juice is about 5% citric acid. A morning routine could include first drinking water with lemon squeezed into it. To protect the teeth enamel, some people drink lemon water with a straw. Then, rinse with water, and brush the teeth.

Citrus can also help to prevent gout.

Apple cider vinegar helps to prevent kidney stones

One way to help prevent kidney stones from forming is to take a shot of apple cider vinegar. As with lemons, also rinse the mouth with water. The acid in apple cider vinegar is protective of the kidneys, including by helping to balance blood sugar.

"Epidemiological evidence of over 9,000 people suggests that daily intake of vinegar whose principal bioactive component is acetic acid is associated with a reduced risk of nephrolithiasis [kidney stones].

We found individuals with daily consumption of vinegar compared to those without have a higher citrate and a lower calcium excretion in urine, two critical molecules for calcium oxalate (CaOx) kidney stones in humans.

Vinegar is a promising strategy to prevent CaOx nephrolithiasis occurrence and recurrence."

– Dietary vinegar prevents kidney stone recurrence via epigenetic regulations; EBioMedicine / *The Lancet*; June 2019

List of high-oxalate foods

This list doesn't mean you shouldn't eat these items. They contain many other beneficial nutrients.

Do avoid the junk ones – French fries, and low-grade chocolate.

Oily meals that also are high in oxalate are not a good idea. Ways to reduce oxalates include making oil-free dressings, avoiding fried and oil-sauteed foods, and taking other measures to reduce oil use. For instance, when making hummus, use water instead of oil. And when sautéing, use other things to sauté with, instead of oil – such as vinegar.

Do increase water intake, squeeze lemon in your morning water (then, to protect teeth enamel, rinse with regular water, and brush the teeth). Also, take a daily shot of apple vinegar (then drink water), and follow an unprocessed, low-fat diet.

The body also makes oxalates. It isn't something we can be free of. Simply choose a variety of plant-based, low fat foods.

- **Almonds**: An ounce has about 120 milligrams.
- **Beets**: About 150 milligrams per cup.
- **Buckwheat groats**: About 133 milligrams per cup.
- **Cocoa**: About 67 milligrams in four teaspoons.
- **Corn groats or grits**: About 97 milligrams per cup.
- **Corn meal**: About 64 milligrams per cup.
- **Dates**: One date can have about 24 milligrams. A different choice is figs, as they have a much lower oxalate content. Dates are high in potassium, so those with kidney disease may want to limit dates to about one per meal to avoid going over the recommended daily allowance for potassium on a renal diet.
- **French fries**: About 51 milligrams per 4 ounce serving, but also has damaged oils.
- **Navy beans**: About 150 milligrams per cup. Kidney beans have a much lower oxalate content.
- **Okra**: About 150 milligrams per cup.
- **Potatoes**: About 97 milligrams in a medium white potato. Sweet potatoes have about a third of the oxalate content as white potatoes.
- **Quinoa**: 54 milligrams per cup. If you choose to eat it, prepare it first by soaking it for a couple of hours, discard the water, and add new water before boiling. The soaking will help to break down the antinutrients, reduce the oxalates, and increase the amino acids (protein) content. Don't add oil to quinoa.
- **Raspberries**: 48 milligrams per cup. Blackberries and blueberries have lower oxalate content.
- **Rhubarb**: About the same as spinach.
- **Rice bran**: About 281 milligrams per cup.
- **Soy yogurt or soy milk**: About 336 milligrams in a cup.
- **Spinach**: A half cup of spinach can contain about 750 milligrams of oxalates.
  Because naturally calcium-rich foods can help prevent kidney stones: Dandelion greens, broccoli, collard greens, and kale, which are all rich in calcium, are a good mix with spinach. As is drinking extra water when eating spinach (or any foods high in oxalates), as dehydration can help to cause kidney stones. Avoid using oil on spinach (or other high-oxalate foods), as that can increase chances of kidney stones.
- **Tofu**: About 235 milligrams in 3 ounces.
- **Turmeric**: But turmeric can prevent the binding of calcium and oxalates. Turmeric also is rich in anti-inflammatories.
- **Wheat berries**: About 98 milligrams per cup.

Other problems with oxalates can include

- **Salt**: A high salt diet can also release calcium from the kidneys, and increase kidney problems.
  A high-oxalate diet also high in salt can cause gout-like symptoms with the

formation of crystals that inflame the tissues.

• **Digestive tract issues**: If a person already has a compromised digestive tract –
including because of an unhealthy gut biome, inflammation, celiac, Crohn's, or
otherwise irritable bowel issues, or they have undergone a gastric bypass, fat
absorption can be altered, and can bind with calcium – making the oxalates more
likely to end up in the blood, and then in the kidneys, where they can result in
kidney stones.

A clean, low fat, plant-based diet free from processed foods can help prevent
inflammation, celiac, Crohn's, leaky gut, and irritable bowel issues. It can help
prevent obesity, and kidney stones.

For those concerned about oxalates

Soaking and then steaming or boiling certain oxalate-rich foods – including
beans, sliced beets, sliced carrots, and also greens like chard and spinach – helps to
reduce their oxalate content.

Consuming calcium-rich foods with high-oxalate foods reduces soluble oxalate
absorption.

Reducing or eliminating oil extracts in the diet – including fried, oil sautéed,
and otherwise highly heated or damaged oils of all kinds – can help reduce kidney
stone formation. Including because oily foods can damage the gut flora, which you
need to help degrade oxalate. This is one of the reasons why reducing the oil
content of the diet is advised for those with a history of kidney stones.

"Dietary oxalate is thought to play a role in hyperoxaluria, a risk factor in the
formation of calcium oxalate kidney stones. Total dietary oxalate intake is only in
the range of 50-200 mg, though in some individuals could be as 1,000 mg. It has
been suggested that dietary oxalate may contribute up to 50% of total urinary
oxalate excretion, and that one-third of stone formers hyper-absorb oxalate at a
rate of more than 10% total oxalate consumed.

Dietary potassium, magnesium, and phytate all decrease kidney stone
formation through an array of mechanisms. Despite significantly more dietary
oxalates, and oxalate-containing foods such as nuts, vegetables, and whole grains,
participants with higher DASH [Dietary Approaches to Stop Hypertension]
scores have a 40-50% decreased risk of kidney stones. This is perhaps attributed
to the protective and synergistic effects of phytate, potassium, calcium, and other
phytochemicals all abundant in the DASH dietary pattern."
  – Is There Such a Thing as "Anti-Nutrients"? A Narrative Review of Perceived Problematic
  Plant Compounds; *Nutrients Journal*; Sept. 2020

A healthy gut biome decreases the incidence of calcium-oxalate stone
formation. A plant-based, low fat diet free of fried and oil sautéed foods
encourages a healthful base of gut bacteria.

Other stones are uric acid stones, but those only make up about 5 to 8 percent
of kidney stones. They are related to consuming animal protein.

A diet high in animal protein increases acidity of the system, and the excretion
of calcium. This increases the binding of oxalates with the calcium, and the result
is kidney stones.

Saponification and food oils

The risks of forming kidney stones is increased by consuming animal protein. This is because the fat in the animal foods – and if you eat a high-fat diet – frees the oxalates from the high-oxalate fruits and vegetables while in the gut, and this helps form calcium oxalate bindings in the gut, resulting in kidney stones. It's a process called saponification.

Those who follow a lower-fat, vegan diet free of processed foods are less likely to form stones, especially if they choose starches based on grains.

The fat you need is in every cell of fruits and vegetables. You don't need to be adding bottled oils to your foods. This includes avocado oil, coconut oil, hemp oil, olive oil, safflower oil, sunflower seed oil, and other oils being sold as health foods. They all contain saturated fat that can contribute to cardiovascular disease, and can play a role in the formation of kidney stones.

Humans are the only creature that extract oils from things, and then add those oils to foods.

A person continually bombarding themselves with high-fat meals is more likely to have degenerative health situations in alignment with that way of eating, including cardiovascular disease, heart attacks, strokes, and liver and kidney issues, dysbiosis of the gut biome, acidosis, and autoimmune disorders.

Vitamin A, E, and K

Be cautious or avoid taking vitamins A, E, and K, as these can build up in the system.

It is best to aim to get your vitamins by eating a variety of fruits, vegetables, sprouts, seaweeds, beans, legumes, and raw, activated nuts and seeds.

If your doctor or dietician suggests a nutritional supplement, it is likely good to follow the advice.

Itchy, dry, and discolored skin, and rashes

People on dialysis may experience a buildup of phosphorus in their tissues, which can lead to temporary or chronic itchy skin, and other problems, including of the heart and bones.

If you have any of those issues relating to kidney disease, being on dialysis, or have had a kidney transplant, consult with your doctor and dietician.

"Uremic pruritus, also known as chronic kidney disease-associated pruritus, is a common and debilitating symptom experienced by patients with CKD and end-stage renal disease. Uremic pruritus is characterized by itching that is not attributed to other causes, and can be either localized or generalized. Uremic pruritus significantly impacts patients' quality of life, affecting sleep and leading to poor clinical outcomes and adherence to treatment. Additionally, uremic pruritus is associated with poor adherence to treatments, and worse clinical outcomes. Therefore, it is essential to recognize and treat uremic pruritus promptly.
– Uremic Pruritus Evaluation and Treatment; StatPearls; Aug. 2024

Phosphorus

"Phosphate is a key element for several physiological pathways such as skeletal development, bone mineralization, membrane composition, nucleotide structure, maintenance of plasma pH, and cellular signaling. Phosphate is mainly stored in the bone, but the kidneys have a key role in phosphate homeostasis with two hormones playing important roles in renal phosphate handling: parathyroid hormone and fibroblast growth factor 23."

> – Physiology of FGF23 and overview of genetic diseases associated with renal phosphate wasting; *Metabolism* journal; Feb. 2020

Pruritus is one reason kidney patients, and especially those on dialysis, may be put on a diet limiting foods high in phosphorus. They also may be prescribed phosphorus binders to take at every meal. (Unless they are on dialysis or have terminal kidney disease. Consult with your doctor and dietician about these matters.)

"Dietary protein intake, which is also strongly correlated with phosphorus intake, may account for 84% of the variance in dietary intake. Hyperphosphatemia is a critical factor for morbidity or mortality in patients with chronic kidney disease. Several large epidemiologic studies have found higher phosphorus levels (even in those within the normal range) to be associated with an increased risk of cardiovascular disease morbidity or mortality, even in individuals with normal kidney function. Dietary phosphate loading increases expression of fibroblast growth factor 23 (FGF-23), which is a phosphaturic hormone. Elevated FGF-23 levels are associated with vascular calcifications among patients with chronic kidney disease, and left ventricular hypertrophy in experimental animals with uremia. In a long-term observational study over 10 years among an elderly community population, FGF-23 independently associated with all-cause mortality and incidence of heart failure. In addition, in the Ramipril Efficacy In Nephropathy trial, participants with higher serum phosphate levels had faster progression of kidney disease compared with those who had lower levels."

> – The Effects of High-Protein Diets on Kidney Health and Longevity; *Journal of American Nephrology*; July 2020

Reduce your risk of and intensity of kidney disease by eating a diet lower in phosphorus.

Reduce dietary phosphates to safe levels, decreasing risks of renal osteodystrophy and cardiovascular disease

Foods at the top of the list of those that increase phosphate levels in the blood (serum phosphate levels) are chicken, turkey, pork, organ meats, fish and shellfish, dairy, processed meats, dried meats, and egg yolk. The list also includes cola beverages, processed and fast foods, and frozen prepared meats and other packaged-to-cook meals that may have had added phosphates to both improve shelf life and speed cooking times. It is best to avoid all of those foods.

Plants contain phosphorus, but at much lower levels than any type of meat, dairy, or eggs, or processed foods containing added phosphates. Some seeds, including pumpkin and sunflower have phosphorus stored as phytic acid, which humans can't digest.

"Phosphorus from plants is thought to be poorly absorbed, because they majority of it exists as part of phosphorus storage molecules called phytates, which cannot be broken down by human digestive enzymes.

Hyperphosphatemia is a common complication in patients with chronic kidney disease, which is thought to contribute to renal osteodystrophy [bones weakened by kidney dysfunction] and cardiovascular disease."
– Examining the proportion of dietary phosphorus from plants, animals, and food additives excreted in urine; *Journal of Renal Nutrition*; Oct. 2016

"Your kidneys help regulate mineral levels of calcium and phosphorus in your blood. They also produce calcitriol hormone by activating vitamin D to keep your bones strong and healthy. When your kidneys fail or aren't functioning as well, they can't maintain proper levels of these minerals and calcitriol hormone. This can weaken your bones and lead to fractures."

Renal osteodystrophy is a complication of chronic kidney disease that weakens your bones. It's caused by changes in the levels of minerals and hormones in your blood. The main signs are bone pain and fractures."
– Renal Osteodystrophy; Cleveland Clinic; 2025

The kidneys have so many functions that those with kidney disease may experience a variety of health issues linking back to their kidneys, and also involving the cardiovascular, hormonal, and nerve systems.

In addition to maintaining mineral balance, including of calcium and phosphorus, as mentioned earlier, the kidneys play a role in blood pressure.

The kidneys also release the erythropoietin hormone, stimulating the bone marrow to create red blood cells.

Calcitriol

The kidneys also produce the calcitriol hormone, an active form of vitamin D.

Calcitriol plays into calcium absorption through the intestines into the blood (plasma calcium), and the release of calcium from the bones to balance minerals in the blood.

Calcitriol also plays a role in the function of the parathyroid glands in the neck. The parathyroid glands release the parathyroid hormone. This hormone helps to maintain levels of calcium in the blood, including the release of calcium stored in the skeletal system.

Osteodystrophy – bone loss related to kidney disease

If the hormonal and mineral balance continue to be an issue, too many minerals can leach from the bones, weakening them. In relation to kidney disease, this is called renal osteodystrophy, which is a weakening of the bones. This increases risk of bone fractures, and bone deformities – including rickets.

Most people with kidney disease, especially later stages, and those who are on dialysis also have some level of osteodystrophy.

Those with kidney disease who have bone pain may be experiencing a symptom of renal osteodystrophy. In more advanced cases, bone structure changes become noticeable – especially in children who may experience stunted growth. Speak with your doctor about any of these concerns.

Blood tests can help detect renal osteodystrophy, including by measuring levels of alkaline phosphates, calcium, parathyroid hormone, phosphorus, and vitamin D.

Diagnostic imaging, including a CT scan, and MRI, and X-rays are also used to help detect renal osteodystrophy. A bone density test called a low-radiation DEXA scan can also help to diagnose renal osteodystrophy. It is also used to diagnose osteoporosis. A DEXA scan also can detect arthritis, which is often also experienced by those with kidney disease.

A lesser-used test to help diagnose osteodystrophy is a biopsy to check the bone density.

The imbalance of calcium and phosphorus can be part of cardiovascular disease with calcium plaque forming in the blood vessels, which plays into to the condition called atherosclerosis, greatly increasing the risk of high blood pressure, heart attacks, and strokes.

Those with kidney disease may be given an echocardiogram and/or ultrasound to identify blood vessel calcium deposits, and other issues.

Renal osteodystrophy combined with hormonal and mineral imbalance, and cardiovascular disease are CKD-MBD (chronic kidney disease mineral and bone disorder). This can increase the risk of arrhythmias [problematic, erratic, irregular, or slow heart rate or rhythm], infections, strokes, and general muscle weakness.

"Chronic kidney disease-mineral bone disorder (CKD-MBD) is a complex syndrome characterized by disruptions in calcium, phosphorus, parathyroid hormone (PTH), vitamin D, and fibroblast grown factor-23 (FGF23) levels. These disruptions lead to alterations in bone morphology and systemic effects, with elevated mortality rates primarily due to cardiovascular complications. Critical aspects of CKD-MBD include serum imbalances of calcium, phosphorus, PTG, and vitamin D, effecting bone health and extraskeletal calcifications. Evidence suggests their associations with adverse outcomes such as increased fracture risk, and cardiovascular mortality.
– Chronic Kidney Disease-Mineral Bone Disorder; StatPearls; April 2024

Types of renal osteodystrophy include:

• **Adynamic bone disease**: The bone tissue is not being restored, as in calcium is not being stored. This raises blood calcium levels too high, as the kidneys are not doing their role in helping to balance calcium.

The parathyroid hormone is deficient.

Adynamic bone disease, is often present in combination with being on dialysis, having terminal kidney disease, or advanced kidney disease.

Vitamin D and calcium supplements may be prescribed, which then may result in deficiencies in parathyroid hormone.

Diabetes may also play a role in adynamic bone disease, as low levels of insulin and high levels of glucose can result in lower levels of the parathyroid hormone.

Those who receive dialysis through the abdomen (peritoneal dialysis) may experience lower levels of parathyroid hormone. It's another concern of dialysis that needs to be monitored and addressed.

• **Mixed renal osteodystrophy**: Includes the symptoms (an amalgam of) of both

243

osteitis and osteomalacia.

- **Osteitis fibrosa**: The bone tissue is releasing calcium into the blood too quickly, causing high levels of the parathyroid hormone (hyperparathyroidism that is often experienced in those with chronic kidney disease). One thing this can cause is the formation of fibrous cysts or lesions in the bones, structurally weakening them.

- **Osteomalacia**: This involves the bone tissue both breaking down and not being restored, which is one form of degenerative bone disease. Osteomalacia is related to vitamin D deficiencies, and the excretion of phosphate. It can also play into osteocytes in the bones releasing higher levels of the hormone fibroblast growth factor-23 (FGF23), which plays a role in some forms of cancer.

"Hyperphosphatemia has been studied as a cause of increased mortality, particularly in patients with nondialysis CKD. A notable meta- analysis involving nearly 5,000 patients with CKD highlighted a 35% increase in mortality per milligram rise in serum phosphate above the normal range. Achieving complete recovery from renal osteodystrophy usually requires a renal transplant. However, when assessing the overall prognosis of this condition, it is crucial to consider other factors, such as the bone-vascular axis. Vascular calcifications, arteriosclerosis of blood vessels, and subsequent cardiovascular events in patients with renal osteodystrophy are all components of this axis. Understanding and addressing these interconnected factors are essential to determining the outcome for patients with this condition."
– Chronic Kidney Disease-Mineral Bone Disorder; *StatPearls*; April 2024

It's all linked

Linked to all of this is bone health, kidney health, parathyroid health, blood health, cardiovascular health, intestinal health, nerve and brain health, hormonal balance, and on and on through the networks and systems throughout the body. Somehow, in one way or another it is all related to the health of the heart and kidneys, which is related to nutrition, exercise, sleep patterns, and other measures to maintain and protect health.

These are more reasons for kidney patients to get regular blood nutritional panels done, also called CMP (comprehensive metabolic panel). Your doctor will likely order as CMP at least once more per year.

With depleted vitamin D, you may be prescribed a vitamin D supplements. As mentioned elsewhere, there are vegan vitamin D supplements on the market, including vitamin D taken from lichen (the stuff that grows on rocks that is neither plant, nor animal, but is a combination of a structure of algae feeding off of a fungus.)

In relation to phosphorus and vitamin D, there is also the fibroblast growth factor (FGF) hormone produced by the bones, and which helps to balance both phosphorus and vitamin D.

With kidney disease, one thing that can be impacted is the level of FGF produced by the bones, often to higher levels than normal.

With damaged kidneys also producing decreased amounts of calcitriol, and not removing phosphorus, it leads to that mineral accumulating. The amount of parathyroid hormone is increased, also leading to damaged bones.

It should be of no surprise how nutrition plays a role in all of these cardiovascular and kidney issues.

Bread

Kidney patients could be advised to have white bread, instead of whole grain bread, and white pasta, instead of whole grain pasta, and white rice, instead of brown rice. This is to reduce potassium and phosphorus in the diet. However, there are healthier choices for loaf bread, rolls, bagels, and other grains in the diet.

If you have issues with gluten, it is another issue, and you'll need to stay away from breads and other foods containing gluten. There are numerous recipes you can find online for making gluten-free bread using whole-ingredients. There are also more and more gluten-free bread products being sold in stores. Read food labels to know what is in them.

Bread is rich in fiber, which is important for numerous nutritional reasons – including because it helps to control blood sugar. A fiber rich diet also decreases cancer risk, and improves brain and nerve function as it helps to keep the gastrointestinal tract healthy, which is where most of the emotional chemicals originate.

Bread is a carbohydrate (which the body needs), and contains a variety of nutrients, including amino acids the body uses for building protein.

As a kidney-safe diet is not heavy in protein, the calories need to come from somewhere, and complex, unprocessed carbohydrates are the choice.

Bread can be part of a healthy diet, IF…

High quality breads – in combination with a clean diet – can be part of a healthy diet for kidney patients.

Choose organic, vegan breads, and not ones containing preservatives, added sulfites, or synthetic chemical dyes, flavors, or scents, or clarified sugars, or dairy products, or other problematic ingredients. As mentioned elsewhere, avoid breads containing potassium bromate. (See information about potassium bromate elsewhere in the book.)

If you react badly to gluten, look for organic, vegan, gluten-free breads.

Learn how to make bread. It's not difficult. People have been doing so for thousands of years using the most basic tools. You don't need a fancy bread-making machine.

White bread

If you are going to have white bread, consider organic, real sourdough bread. And not low-quality white bread. It might be better to choose whole-grain sourdough.

The process of kneading the dough and letting it rise, then kneading it again before cutting it into loaves and allowing them to rise again before baking helps to break down proteins. The bread will then be easier to digest with the nutrients more bioavailable. It can also help to reduce or eliminate allergic reactions.

The thing about staying away from whole grain bread might not be realistic, as the phosphorus in grain is far less bioavailable as phosphorus is in animal protein. However...

This is important: If you stay away from low-quality bread and grain products, you also reduce your exposure to problematic phosphate additives, clarified sugars, and chemical additives. Low-quality breads, bagels, rolls, and other grain products are also likely to be higher in both sodium and sugar.

One clean brand of bread many people use is the Foods for Life brand Ezekiel sprouted grain bread. There is also the Dave's brand of bread that is organic, whole grain, and free of additives. Or any organic, whole grain, phosphate-additive free bread free of sugars, chemicals, oils, and potassium bromate.

Sugars

Sugars you might see listed on food labels when considering breads, bagels, rolls, and other grain products:
- Agave
- Barley malt syrup
- Beet sugar
- Brown sugar
- Cane sugar
- Coconut flower syrup
- Coconut sugar
- Corn syrup
- Date sugar
- Dextrose
- Erythritol
- Fructose
- Galactose
- Granulated sugar
- High fructose corn syrup
- Honey
- Maltose
- Malt syrup
- Maple syrup
- Molasses
- Monk fruit
- Rice syrup
- Sucrose
- White sugar (might be cane or beet)

Some of those sweeteners are the same thing, under different names.

Some labels might only simply list "sweetener" as an ingredient, and not detail the type of sugar. As a kidney patient, it likely would be good to avoid products with mystery ingredients.

Read food labels to know what you are eating, and what to avoid.

To sell foods across state lines in the U.S., the labels are to list ingredients and nutrition information. If you are purchasing foods made within your same state, the labels are not covered by the same laws.

246

If you do choose a sweetener, perhaps choose organic date sugar, molasses, monk fruit powder, or coconut sugar. Sparingly, and not daily. They are less clarified, and contain components giving a better spectrum of nutrients.

Get out of the habit of luxuriating your taste buds with added sugars.

Also avoid artificial sweeteners, as those are chemicals, and can trigger a variety of health issues, including nerve disorders, migraines, learning disabilities, autoimmune disorders, an increased risk of cardiovascular disease, stroke, and heart attack, and cancers of the blood, lymph system, and bladder.

Learn to make food from scratch using whole, unprocessed ingredients, free of chemicals and clarified substances.

Phosphorus and phosphate ingredients

Dietary phosphorus from plants is estimated to have about a 30-35% absorption rate. Animal sources are about 70-80%. Processed foods containing phosphate additives can be more than a 90% absorption rate.

According to the National Kidney Foundation, below is a list of inorganic phosphate additives in processed foods. These should be among what is listed on the nutrition ingredient label on the packaging. The added inorganic phosphates may be in baked goods, frozen foods, cake mixes, pancakes and waffles, colas (which is one of the reasons why colas are bad for the bones), processed meats, canned meals, bottled salad dressings, dressing mixes, sauce mixes, broth, fast foods, convenience foods, and snack foods. The phosphates often are added as preservatives, or to enhance the texture and/or flavor. In baked goods the phosphates could be part of the leavening. In meats the phosphates can be used to help keep the carcass bits moist and tender. In frozen items phosphates might be added to help them cook faster:

- Dicalcium phosphate
- Disodium phosphate
- Monosodium phosphate
- Phosphoric acid
- Sodium hexameta-phosphate
- Trisodium phosphate
- Sodium tripolyphosphate
- Tetrasodium pyrophosphate

These are more reasons why it is good to avoid ultra-processed food products.

High phosphorus foods

Foods high in phosphorus include meat, including beef, pork, lamb, bison, turkey, chicken, and seafood. Also, bone broth, meat jerky, "cold cuts," or any processed and smoked meats. Dairy is high in phosphorus, as are eggs. People who have kidney disease, stomach ailments, intestinal problems, cardiovascular disease, autoimmune disorders, or cancer would likely be better off avoiding all of those foods.

As a kidney patient, or dialysis patient, you will need to monitor your phosphorus intake. Part of this means getting used to reading food labels, and knowing which brands are more healthful, and which food company products to avoid.

"High levels of phosphorus can weaken your bones by pulling calcium out of them, and can lead to harmful calcium deposits in your blood vessels, lungs, eyes, and heart. Over time, this can increase your risk of heart attack, stroke, or even death. High levels of serum phosphorus are also directly linked with a risk of mortality in people on dialysis."
    – National Kidney Foundation; Oct. 2024

Bioavailability of phosphorus

As is mentioned earlier, phosphorus in animal protein is more bioavailable, which can be part of the problem with it overloading in the system of those with kidney disease.

The phosphorus in plants is less available as it is a component of phytates, and not as easily accessed by the digestive system.

Plant-based sources of phosphorus include everything from lentils to peas, oats, amaranth, seeds (pumpkin, sesame, sunflower, etc.), quinoa, nuts (almonds, Brazil, cashews, pine, peanuts [which aren't a nut, but a legume], pistachios, etc.), soy beans (soy milk, tofu, tempeh, natto, soy burgers, etc.), other beans (black eyed peas, black beans, chickpeas, great northern beans, kidney beans, navy beans, pinto beans, white beans, etc.), cauliflower, carrots, celery, corn, asparagus, and so forth – and foods made containing them.

Most of the phosphorus in seeds is in phytic acid, or phytate, and is not digestible. Once the raw, viable seeds are soaked to bring them out of their dormant state, or grown into sprouts, the phosphorus becomes more bioavailable as the phytate breaks down, but still isn't as absorbed as phosphorus from meat, dairy, eggs, or bone broth.

Soaking raw, viable, untoasted nuts also can make the phosphorus in them more bioavailable.

See the information in this book about soaking, germinating, blossoming, sprouting, or otherwise activating seeds, grains, legumes, and beans. (And advice on which beans to avoid sprouting.)

"The 2003 National Diet and Nutrition Survey found that average daily intakes of phosphorus from food were 1,112 milligrams for women, and 1,493 milligrams for men. That's 202 percent and 271 percent of the recommended amount for women and men respectively. Overall, no men and less than 0.5 percent of women had an intake of phosphorus below the lower recommended level. These intakes had increased since the previous survey in 1986/87. It seems likely intakes may have increased further given the prevalence of phosphorus in processed foods.

Typical Western diets tend to be high in phosphorus due to high content in meat, dairy, nuts, and other foods rich in protein. The amount of phosphorus in Western diets is further increased by its use in preservatives added to processed foods and fizzy drinks. Plant-based proteins may be richer in phosphorus compared to animal proteins, however, the phosphate in plant proteins is only 30-

50 percent bioavailable, while that in animal proteins is estimated to be 70-80 percent bioavailable."

— Phosphorus; Viva.com

Phosphorus is a necessary nutrient

Phosphorus isn't a bad thing. You need it. It is an important nutrient, including for maintaining the pH level of the body. The kidneys help to balance the phosphate in the blood. It is under conditions of kidney disease when the level of phosphorus in the blood can accumulate to problematic levels. This increases the risk of cardiovascular disease.

Phosphorus is highly present in your teeth and bones, and in cartilage, connective tissues, ligaments, muscles, and tendons. It binds to calcium, and plays a role in nearly all functions, including of the brain and nerves, and muscle contractions, and energy storage. Hemoglobin uses both iron and phosphorus to transfer oxygen throughout your body. Phosphorus is a component of cell membranes, and is a key in the formation of DNA and RNA.

Dialysis and phosphorus

Dialysis may remove some phosphorus, but additional measures to control phosphorus levels may be needed.

One sign of phosphorus building up in the system is the skin become itchy. Benadryl or other antihistamines, lanolin, witch hazel, or creams containing capsaicin (an extract of hot peppers) may be helpful. Exposure to sun could also offer some relief to itchy skin.

If the condition continues, consider it might be a reaction to the dialyzer, the tubing, or the type of heparin used in the treatment.

Consult with the medical staff about those issues.

Kidney disease and skin issues

Besides itchy skin, those with late-stage kidney disease, or who are undergoing dialysis, might also experience dry, rough, red skin rashes consisting of small bumps that may also crust, swell, and become quite painful. This is also a sign of phosphorus imbalance, an imbalance of magnesium and parathyroid hormone, and of waste products building in the tissues. Tests of the area might including applying patches to check for allergies, and a biopsy for lab testing. Treatments may include antihistamines, and the pain relievers gabapentin and pregabalin, and also medication to treat the imbalance of nerve signals. Sun exposure, or treatment with ultraviolet B phototherapy, can also help offer relief. As will avoiding soaps and skin products containing artificial chemicals, including fragrances, perfumes, and dyes.

If you are experiencing skin issues in relation to a kidney or other health condition, do what it takes to nurture a healthy gut biome. The gut biome is vitally important for all areas of your health.

Dry skin and dialysis

In addition to pruritus, dialysis and kidney patients may experience dry skin (xerosis). This is because of the changes to the oil and sweat glands. This may

249

increase skin infections, and slow healing.

Patients experiencing xerosis are advised to avoid long, hot baths or showers, and chemicals and synthetic perfumes in soaps, shampoos, moisturizers, and other skin and hair products. Also, use natural, compostable laundry cleaners, including both for clothing and bedding.

Even if you don't have kidney problems, look for natural, moisturizing soaps and skin products free of synthetic chemicals. Consider learning how to make your own from scratch using natural ingredients.

Discolored skin and nails

Discoloration of the skin (hyperpigmentation) also is a condition experienced by people undergoing dialysis, as are discolored nails. Often the skin discoloration results in a metallic or grayish tone to the skin. The nails can become reddish pink, or more brown. This is because the urochrome pigments can become out of balance, instead of being excreted by healthy kidneys.

Another skin condition that might be experienced by dialysis patients is a white, powdery substance on the skin called uremic frost left after sweat evaporates. This could be a sign of the dialysis session being too short.

Blisters may also form, especially on the hands, feet, and face, leaving scars.

Kidney tissues and microtubule function

The kidneys are filters. They contain veins and arteries interwoven with glomerular capsules and proximal convoluted tubules. The microtubules are small vessels that filter protein byproducts, excess sugars, excess minerals, heavy metals, and chemicals, including pharmaceutical drugs, food chemicals, and chemicals from tainted water. Environmental pollution and chemicals in cosmetic products absorbed through your skin are also filtered by the kidneys, and the liver.

As the kidneys help to regulate the fluid in the body, and play the key role in blood pressure.

The kidneys help to balance the blood sugars, and regulate the electrolytes (bicarbonates, calcium, chloride, magnesium, phosphate, potassium, sodium). This plays into the pH level – or acid-base balance – of your system.

The electrolyte balance is needed for many reasons, including the electrical charges among your muscle cells, nerve cells, and other cells.

The electrolytes are needed for every function throughout the body, from the digestive tract to the brain, from blood pressure and heart rhythm to water balance to the ability of cells to maintain pressure, absorb nutrients, and dispose of waste products. A healthy balance of electrolytes is needed to maintain the structures of everything from the bones to the teeth, ligaments, cartilage, and organs.

These are more reasons for those with cardiovascular, kidney, parathyroid, blood sugar, and other health issues to get their blood nutrients tested. Nutrition is key to maintaining electrolyte balance.

Renal hypertension and microvessel disease

High blood pressure and hypertension can damage the microvessels in the eyes (ocular hypertension) and kidneys (renal hypertension) as the increased pressure strains the vessels.

Microvascular disease can be in many parts of the body, from the brain to the heart, liver, kidneys, and other organs. It's unlikely to only be nowhere else but in the kidneys.

"Microvascular disease, or small-vessel disease, is a multisystem disorder with a common pathophysiological basis that differentially affects various organs in some patients. The prevalence of small-vessel disease in the heart has been found to be higher in women compared with men.

Small-vessel disease, or microvascular disease, refers to a group of pathological processes with various etiologies affecting the small arteries, arterioles, venules, and capillaries."
– Microvascular Disease and Small-Vessel Disease: The Nexus of Multiple Diseases in Women; *Journal of Womens Health*; June 2022

"Although microvascular dysfunction (MVD) has been well characterized in individual organs as different disease entities, clinical evidence is mounting in support of an underlying systemic process.

In the kidney, microvascular dysfunction manifests in the form of glomerular impairment leading to decreased kidney function, proteinuria, and eventually kidney failure.

Multiple mechanisms have been described in the pathogenesis of microvascular dysfunction of individual organs, ranging from increased inflammation, oxidative stress, adhesion molecule expression, activation of immune cells, endothelial dysfunction, impaired vasodilation, attenuated angiogenesis, and increased endothelial permeability."
– Is microvascular dysfunction a systemic disorder with common biomarkers found in the heart, brain, and kidneys?; *Microvascular Research* journal; March 2021

Again, when the kidney microtubules are damaged, it is called microvessel disease. This condition can also happen in the eyes, and other areas. People with diabetes are often identified as suffering from these two situations, with the advanced stages of the damage causing blindness and kidney failure.

"Diabetic retinal disease (DRD) includes all diabetes-related changes in the retina, including harm to retinal blood vessels (diabetic retinopathy or DR), swelling in the retina (diabetic macular edema or DME), and damage to retinal nerve cells that help us see (diabetic retinal neurodegeneration or DRN). Over the next few decades, growing rates of diabetes across the globe will put increasing numbers of people at risk for vision loss and blindness from DRD."
– Mary Tyler Moore Vision Initiative; MaryTylerMoore.org; 2025

If the microvascular systems in the eyes and kidneys show damage, it is more than likely to also be present in other areas of the body, including the brain.

"Since the kidney and brain share unique susceptibilities to vascular injury due to similar anatomical and functional features of small artery disease, kidney impairment can be predictive of the presence and severity of cerebral small vessel disease. Chronic kidney disease has been reported to be associated with silent brain infarcts, cerebral white matter lesions, and cerebral microbleeds, independently of vascular risk factors. In addition, chronic kidney disease effects cognitive function, partly via the high prevalence of cerebral small vessel diseases. Retinal artery disease also has an independent relationship with chronic kidney disease and cognitive impairment. Stroke experts are no longer allowed to be ignorant of chronic kidney disease. Close liaison between neurologists and nephrologists can improve the management of cerebral small vessel diseases in kidney patients.

CKD is an established risk factor for stroke.

In addition to the increase in the risk of incidence of stroke, CKD affects initial neurological severity and chronic outcomes of ischemic and hemorrhagic stroke."
– Cerebral Small Vessel Disease and Chronic Kidney Disease, by Kazunori Toyoda; *Journal of Stroke*; Jan. 2015

Here we go, again: A clean, low-fat plant-based diet free of synthetic chemicals, clarified sugars, fried and highly heated – or otherwise damaged – oils, and a diet rich in a variety of fruits, vegetables, sprouts, and other plant matter is rich in antioxidants and anti-inflammatories. It reduces inflammation and oxidative stress. It improves the endothelial function of the cardiovascular and lymph systems. It is protective of the liver, kidneys, heart, spleen, pancreas, adrenals, colon, and other organs and glands. It improves the microbiome and function of the digestive tract, and the production of molecules of emotion, helping to protect nerve and brain function. It decreases the risks of various types of cancers, including of the colon, reproductive organs, and other organs. It reduces the risks and expression of a variety of degenerative and chronic diseases, including diabetes, lupus, asthma, arthritis, and other autoimmune disorders.

Type 2 diabetes and microvascular disease

The number one cause of microvascular disease is type 2 diabetes as high blood sugar can cause swelling of the vessels, damaging them.

"Microvascular complications of diabetes are those long-term complications that affect small blood vessels. These typically include retinopathy [eyes], nephropathy [kidneys], and neuropathy [nerves]."
– Diabetes Mellitus: Management of Microvascular and Macrovascular Complications, by Robert S. Zimmerman; Cleveland Clinic for Continuing Education; Sept. 2016

Metabolic syndrome

Sugar and insulin resistance, which are synonymous with type 2 diabetes, can cause kidney damage. These are reasons why it is good to find out early if you have diabetes, hypertension, metabolic syndrome (which includes type 2 diabetes and hypertension), or high blood pressure, and to follow a diet helping prevent and reduce the damage.

"A vegan diet generally reduces the risk of developing chronic non-communicable degenerative diseases, such as metabolic syndrome and, in addition, requires fewer natural resources for food production than an omnivorous diet.

The latest evidence suggests that plant-based diets are associated with a significant reduction in the risk of cardiovascular disease and cancer onset. Subjects following a plant-based diet usually have a lower body mass index, and reduced total cholesterol, low-density lipoprotein cholesterol, triglycerides, and blood glucose levels compared to omnivores.

The main concern regarding these dietary approaches is the risk of developing nutritional deficiencies of proteins, omega-3 fatty acids, vitamin B12, iron, zinc, iodine, vitamin D, and calcium. However, plant-based diets are rich in fruits and vegetables, and they are characterized by a high content of fiber, antioxidant substances, phytochemicals, and omega-6 fatty acids. If well planned and balanced, plant-based diets can be appropriate for all age groups, even in pregnancy or breastfeeding women."

– Vegan Diet Health Benefits in Metabolic Syndrome; *Nutrients* journal; March 2021

Maintaining a healthful weight, including through nutrition, exercise, and a regular sleep pattern, is key to maintaining health, and avoiding many varieties of health problems.

Metabolic and kidney disease prevention through fecal microbiota transplantation

A growing focus on helping to fight metabolic disease – and other conditions – is the possible benefits of a fecal transplant.

The process is as it sounds, taking fecal matter from a tested person to "implant" in the receiver's colon. It may also be done through an oral application (frozen capsule), or nasogastrically (a tube inserted through the nose and into the stomach).

If you have been diagnosed with metabolic disease, bowel diseases, gut microbiome dysbiosis, or CKD, perhaps research the possible pros and cons of undergoing a fecal transplant.

As with any non-emergency medical procedure, take your time to research it, listen to a variety of opinions, read up on the studies relating to it, and get 2nd and 3rd opinions from medical professionals.

"The history of fecal microbiota transplantation (FMT) dates back even to ancient China. Recently, scientific studies have been looking into FMT as a promising treatment for various diseases, while in the process of teaching us about the interaction between the human host and its resident microbial communities. Current research focuses mainly on Clostridium difficile infections, however interest is rising in other areas such as inflammatory bowel disease (IBD) and the metabolic syndrome.

With regard to the latter, the intestinal microbiota might be causally related to the progression of insulin resistance and diabetes."

– Fecal microbiota transplantation in metabolic syndrome: History, present and future; *Gut Microbes* journal; Feb. 2017

"A relatively unexplored mechanism through which obesogen exposure might predispose exposed individuals to obesity is via alterations to the gut microbiome. It is well established that obesity is associated with composition of the gut microbiome. Transplant of the gut microbiome from obese individuals can induce obesity in germ-free mice. In contrast, transplant of the microbiome from a lean individual promoted a lean phenotype in similar experiments. Transplant of the microbiome from lean donors improved metabolic end points in recipients with metabolic syndrome."

– Environmental Obesogens and Their Impact on Susceptibility to Obesity: New Mechanisms and Chemicals, by Riann Jenay Eguquiza, and Bruce Bumberg; *Endocrinology Journal*; March 2020

Faecall microbiota transplantation (FMT) has attracted increasing attention as an intervention in many clinical conditions, including autoimmune, enteroendocrine, gastroenterological, and neurological diseases. For years, FMT has been an effective second-line treatment for Clostridium difficile infection (CDI) with beneficial outcomes. FMT is also promising in improving bowel disease, such as ulcerative colitis (UC). Preclinical and clinical studies suggest that this microbiota-based intervention may influence the development and progression of chronic kidney disease via modifying a dysregulated gut-kidney axis. Despite the high morbidity and mortality due to CKD, there are limited options for treatment until end-stage kidney disease occurs, which results in death, dialysis, or kidney transplantation. This imposes a significant financial and health burden on the individual, their families, and careers, and the health system. Recent studies have suggested that strategies to reverse gut dysbiosis using FMT are promising therapy in CKD."

– Faecal Microbiota Transplantation and Chronic Kidney Disease; *Nutrients* journal; June 2022

The following study used frozen oral capsules to administer the fecal transplantation.

"The gut microbiota has protective, structural, and metabolic functions that help maintain a healthy intestinal homeostasis. An imbalance in the microbiological community, also called dysbiosis, is involved in the progression of chronic diseases, including CKD, diabetes mellitus, and arterial hypertension, among others. Alterations in the gut microbiota (i.e. dysbiosis), particularly a decrease in bacterial diversity, can be associated with CKD. An increase in pro-inflammatory and uremic metabolite-producing bacteria and a decrease in anti-inflammatory-producing bacteria contribute to disease progression. In patients with CKD, uremia alters the composition and metabolism of the gut microbiota. Gut microbiota composition can also contribute to the development of other diseases such as immunological and metabolic disorders. Targeting gut microbiota at all stages of CKD can be used to restore gut microbiota to improve kidney function. Thus, restoring the health gut microbial community is an optimistic therapeutic strategy in diseases associated with gut dysbiosis.

Fecal microbiota transplantation (FMT) is the infusion of a fecal suspension recovered from a healthy donor directly into the gut of a recipient.

This study represents the first clinical trial of the administration of FMT in frozen capsules to patients with CKD secondary to diabetes and hypertension. CKD patients showed less disease progression at 6 months after FMT administration."

– Changes in the Progression of Chronic Kidney Disease in Patients Undergoing Fecal Microbiota Transplantation; *Nutrients* journal; Feb. 2024

Notice how the study above mentions that "an increase in pro-inflammatory and uremic metabolite-producing bacteria and a decrease in anti-inflammatory-producing bacteria contribute to disease progression."

What is clear is that a diet rich in animal protein and ultra-processed foods INCREASES pro-inflammatory bacteria, DECREASES ant-inflammatory-producing bacteria, and DECREASES the variety of bacteria in the gut.

A clean, plant-based diet free of ultra-processed foods DECREASES pro-inflammatory bacteria, and INCREASES anti-inflammatory-producing bacteria, as well as INCREASES the variety of bacteria in the gut.

Glomerulonephritis and glomerulosclerosis

Glomerulonephritis (kidney infection) is another thing that can damage the vessels of the kidneys.

Of course, following a clean, kidney safe diet can play a major role in avoiding and overcoming glomerulonephritis.

Depending on the extent of the glomerulonephritis situation, treatment could include blood pressure meds, corticosteroids (like Prednisone), diuretics, and, in severe cases, dialysis, or a kidney transplant.

I've had kidney infections, but not for many years. They stopped happening after I cleaned up my diet to be plant-based. But there are a variety of things that can cause kidney infections.

"Glomerulosclerosis is scarring of the tiny filtering units inside the kidneys (glomeruli). This causes a loss of protein into the urine. These proteins help fluids stay within the blood vessels.

Glomerulosclerosis may develop in children or adults and may result from many different causes. Glomerulosclerosis may be caused by infection, certain medicines, diabetes, sickle cell disease, or another glomerular disease.

Early stages of glomerulosclerosis may not cause any symptoms. The most important sign of this condition is protein in the urine (proteinuria). The loss of large amounts of protein could cause swelling in the ankles. It can also cause buildup in the abdomen, puffy eyes, or weight gain from widespread fluid buildup. Severe proteinuria could mean end-stage renal disease (ESRD) will develop."
– Glomerulosclerosis; Johns Hopkins Medicine; 2025

"When the kidneys' filters (glomeruli) become inflamed and scarred, it is called glomerulonephritis. The kidneys slowly lose their ability to remove wastes and excess fluid from the blood to make urine.

Glomerulonephritis can be caused by:
• Toxins or medicines.
• Viral infections, such as HIV, hepatitis C.
• IgA nephropathy, or Berger disease.
• Lupus-related kidney inflammation.
• Bacterial infections that commonly cause throat and skin infections, such as strep or bacteria.

The kidneys can be badly damaged before any symptoms appear. These are the most common symptoms: fatigue, high blood pressure, swelling of the face, hands, feet, and belly, blood and protein in the urine (hematuria and proteinuria), decreased urine output, nausea and vomiting, fever, and flu-like symptoms."
– Glomerulonephritis; Johns Hopkins Medicine; 2025

"With glomerulonephritis, damage to the glomeruli (kidneys' blood filters) by the immune system causes them to lose their ability to remove wastes and extra water. Blood can also be lost in the urine. Nephrotic syndrome means very high amounts of protein are being lost in the urine.

Glomerulonephritis is one of two main groups of glomerular diseases. The second group is glomerulosclerosis, which is damage to the glomeruli caused by hardening and scarring of blood vessels.

There are different types of glomerulonephritis: Acute, chronic, and rapidly progressive.

Sometimes, one type of glomerulonephritis can lead to another type. For example, the acute type can eventually become chronic. The acute or chronic types can become rapidly progressive glomerulonephritis. There are many reasons this can happen. Sometimes, it's due to a change in health. Other times, it's due to another infection or injury. It's important to keep on top of your health and let your healthcare team know if you notice any sudden changes in your health, or notice new symptoms.

Foamy urine can mean there is protein in the urine (albuminuria/proteinuria). Dark or cola colored urine can be a sign of blood in the urine (hematuria). Certain medicines and food colorings can also cause dark colored urine. Speak with a healthcare professional if you aren't sure of the cause.

Glomerulonephritis can have many causes. The acute (sudden) type is often caused by an infection, such as strep throat (caused by streptococcus, a type of bacteria). It can also be caused by other infections, including pneumococcus (another type of bacteria), chickenpox (varicella, a type of virus), malaria (a type of parasite), and others. This is known as post-infectious glomerulonephritis.

The acute type can also be caused by other illnesses, including membranoproliferative glomerulonephritis, immunoglobulin A (IgA) nephropathy, lupus, Goodpasture syndrome, and many others.

Many of these diseases are caused by changes in the body's immune system that can damage kidneys. The immune system helps the body fight off infections. However, with certain diseases, the immune system attacks healthy cells instead.

The chronic types can be caused by the same disease that can cause the acute type. Sometimes, chronic glomerulonephritis is caused by Alport syndrome, an inherited genetic disease that damages the kidneys.

In some cases, glomerulonephritis can be caused by certain drugs. For example, analgesic nephropathy is caused by heavy and prolonged use of certain pain relievers (analgesics), including nonsteroidal anti-inflammatory drugs (NSAIDS), like Ibuprofen and Naproxen."

– National Kidney Foundation; 2025

Tests to help identify glomerulonephritis

- blood tests (estimated glomerular filtration rate [eGFR] tests the kidney filtration of the blood)
- ultrasound, which can also find and identify kidney stones, blockages, and genetic defects in the kidneys.
- urinalysis (the urine albumin-to-creatinine ratio [uACR] test measures proteins in

the urine),
- genetic testing to identify gene variants linked to inherited kidney diseases.
- sometimes, a kidney biopsy to be send to a lab and examined under a microscope.

Signs of kidney infection

- Burning
- Chills
- Fever
- Blood and/or puss in the urine
- Back and/or side pain around the level of the lower ribs
- Nausea
- Vomiting
- Having to urinate often, or continually feeling the urge to urinate
- The urge to urinate can interrupt your focus and sleep
- The pain of having a kidney infection can get intense

Kidney infections can be caused by a bacteria getting into the urethra, causing cystitis in the bladder, and spreading up one or both ureter tubes into the kidney. This can be caused by kidney dysfunction, and unsanitary conditions, and possibly by oral sex.

Urinary tract, bladder, and kidney infections

These are more common in women, as they have short urethras. But men also get urinary tract infections (U.T.I.s).

There are many reasons U.T.I.s happen, including after oral sex. You can research this issue to learn more.

U.T.I.s can increase kidney problems.

I had some bladder infections (cystitis) decades ago that resulted in kidney infections (pyelonephritis). Those are painful.

Sometimes a person with a U.T.I. will experience blood in the urine (hematuria), which could be considered normal for the condition. But is a condition that needs addressed ASAP: See a doctor.

Heavy blood in the urine could be a sign of something more serious, anything from kidney stones, an infection, injury, birth defect, cyst, or cancer.

In men, blood in the urine could also mean prostatitis, a prostate infection, inflammation, injury, or an immune system disorder.

If you notice blood in your urine, see a general doctor, nephrologist, or a urologist.

Both blackberry and cranberry juice can help prevent bacteria from adhering to the bladder wall. Use organic, unsweetened cranberry juice or cranberry powder products, and drink more water. Coconut water can help to maintain electrolytes.

There are also blackberry and cranberry teas. These can be good to use regularly, especially if you have a history of U.T.I.s.

Sex and U.T.I.s

This will help protect your kidneys.

It is helpful to urinate soon after intercourse, and after oral sex. Or avoid oral sex – or use an oral dam.

Some people might not like this news. However: oral sex can increase U.T.I.s, prostatitis, and other issues – including cancer.

Also not so romantic – but safe – is to clean before intercourse, and to use a protective lube, and clean afterward.

As you were told, wear clean underwear, as even this can help to prevent U.T.I.s.

A doctor might prescribe antibiotics. Research the side effects of fluoroquinolone antibiotics. Quinolone or "fluoroquinolones" antibiotics can damage the connective tissues, including tendons, and result in tendon ruptures and damage to tissues in the feet and ankles.

The U.T.I. prevention drink

Bladder and kidney infections can happen quickly, and become serious in a short amount of time. It is important to do what will get rid of it – including what a doctor advises.

Luckily, I haven't had a U.T.I. in many years.

I found the following to help me clear a kidney or urinary tract infection. This doesn't mean this solution will work the same on you. I guzzle water and a quart of unsweetened cranberry juice mixed with a few heaping tablespoons of unsweetened, pure cranberry powder, and a hundred drops of grapefruit seed extract. It tastes quite nasty. I drink it quickly – truly guzzling it.

Depending on the symptoms you are experiencing in relation to a U.T.I. or kidney infection, you may need other solutions – including medical care.

Do not delay treatment for a kidney or bladder infection. Do what is best for your condition.

Hydrate!

Staying hydrated will help your kidneys, and all areas of health. This means: drink water, especially when you have been experiencing a U.T.I., or otherwise a bladder or kidney infection.

Stay hydrated. Especially when consuming high-oxalate foods. It will help reduce your risk of forming kidney stones. So will avoiding meat (including fish), and all dairy, reducing sodium, and avoiding processed sugars, and damaged oils.

No matter what your diet, DO drink water, throughout every day.

I most often only ingest nothing but water all morning, until afternoon. No food. I then keep my eating window open for 6 to 7 hours. I feel better doing this than I do when I eat breakfast. I had been doing it since I was young, because I was so poor – especially as a young adult with massively ruinous medical bills. Now, not eating in the morning is called "intermittent fasting." I was in the trend, before it was a trend.

Distilled water

If you are able, get a water distiller to help remove chemicals and other pollutants and substances from your water. This is particularly important if you have been diagnosed with any variety of kidney disorders, cardiovascular disease, or arthritis, or other autoimmune disorders.

Distilled water might taste flat, as it has been stripped of minerals and other substances you might be used to tasting when drinking water. To add more of a flavor to distilled water, you can add slices of fruits or vegetables, or wrinkled fresh mint leaves.

"Kidney stones are hard deposits of minerals that form in the kidney, and are painful when passing. Drinking distilled water decreases calcium and sodium levels in urine, and may prevent build-up that can lead to kidney stone formation.
– Is drinking distilled water good for bad for you?; MedicineNet; July 2024

Kitchen water distillers cost anywhere from hundreds to thousands dollars (look around to find a stainless steel one you can purchase second hand). It reduces the exposure to chemicals in tap water.

However, because distilled water lacks the minerals often found in water, including minerals that play roles in cellular and otherwise body functions, it is important to follow a well-rounded diet to get minerals in other ways.

Other people choose to drink filtered mineral water.

Each cell in the body is reliant on a balance of minerals and fluids obtained through food or water. This is including to maintain stable conditions within the cells and also around them in what is called the *extracellular fluid*. This plays into the management of both cellular nutrition and metabolic waste. The extracellular fluid contains a number of components, including hormones, water, calcium, phosphate, potassium, sodium, and other substances. These play roles in the permeability, structure, and the nutritional absorption and cellular waste disposal functions of the cells.

In addition to filtering the blood, eliminating waste, producing certain hormones, and playing a role in blood production and blood pressure, one of the many things the kidneys do is they help to maintain the balance of the minerals and other substances in the extracellular fluid. The kidneys respond to hormones produced by the adrenal glands located on the kidneys, and hormones produced by the parathyroid glands, and the brain.

"A cell's function depends on only on receiving a continuous supply of nutrients, and eliminating metabolic waste products, but also on the existence of stable physical and chemical conditions in the extracellular fluid bathing it. Among the most important substances contributing to these conditions are water, sodium, potassium, calcium, and phosphate. Loss or retention of any one of these substances can influence the body's handling of the others. In addition, hydrogen iron concentration (i.e., acid-base balance) influences cell structure and permeability as well as the rate of metabolic reactions. The amounts of these substances must be held within very narrow limits, regardless of the large variations possible in their intake or loss. The kidneys are the organs primarily responsible for regulating the amounts and concentrations of these substances in the extracellular fluid."
– Alcohol's Impact on Kidney Function; *Alcohol Health and Research World* journal; 1997

Your job is to supply the nutrients necessary for the kidneys, brain, heart, adrenal glands, spleen, pancreas, and other organs to be able to do their jobs. This means your choosing clean foods that keep the gut biome healthy – which plays into all areas of health.

As a person with kidney or heart disease, ask your doctor and/or nutritionist about water and mineral – or otherwise electrolyte – concerns. Including if you have headaches, muscle aches, stiffness, bone pain, fatigue, dizziness, fainting spells, and/or regular feelings of dehydration.

Drinking plain water helps your liver and kidneys to filter residues of chemicals and other impurities from your system. This reduces the risk of experiencing gout and kidney stones, while also improving the immune system.

As a person with kidney or cardiovascular concerns, drink clean water, and avoid getting into the habit of drinking canned or bottled drinks containing sugar, or artificial sweeteners, dyes, flavors, or scents, or otherwise junk drinks. Your body needs water, not cola, soda, alcoholic beverages, or chemically-laced "energy drinks," or any drink containing synthetic chemical ingredients.

As someone interested in health, avoid drinks containing added sulphites and/or phosphates.

Structuring and flavoring your water

No matter if you are drinking filtered, mineral, or distilled water, if you want your water to have some mild flavor, add things like thin slices of cucumber, pears, peaches, apples, other fruit, or strawberries, or other berries, or freshly crushed ginger root or pomegranate seeds.

You can also flavor water by adding wrinkled fresh leaves of mint, such as chocolate mint, or fresh fennel leaves, and let those soak for several minutes before drinking.

The goal is NOT to make the water into a gourmet feast, but simply to give it a lightly pleasant taste. Aim to hydrate for nutrition, not for luxury.

Lemon water, and other citrus, should be followed by rinsing the mouth with water to protect the teeth enamel.

Carbonated drinks

It is wise to eliminate carbonated drinks from the diet.

The fizzle in carbonated and energy drinks is caused by carbon dioxide gas infused into the liquid. Ingesting these drinks can increase blood pressure, stressing the kidneys, and also increase the risk of kidney stones.

The inorganic phosphate additives in cola can especially be problematic for those with compromised kidneys, and lead to bone damage, and other issues.

"Carbonated beverage consumption has been linked with diabetes, hypertension, and kidney stones, all risk factors for chronic kidney disease. Cola beverages, in particular, contain phosphoric acid and have been associated with urinary changes that promote kidney stones.

Drinking 2 or more colas per day was associated with a 2-fold risk of kidney disease compared with the reference category, after adjusting for age, race, sex, proximity to study hospital, BMI, income, proxy respondent statues, education, analgesic use, and diabetes. Estimates for regular colas or artificially sweetened colas were similar.

260

Cola beverages are generally acidified using phosphoric acid. Phosphorus may have an effect on the risk of kidney disease. Case reports have linked sodium phosphate bowel cleansing preparations to acute and sometimes irreversible renal failure, characterized by calcium phosphate deposits in the distal tubules and collection ducts or nephrocalcinosis. Although the level of phosphorus from colas is far lower than that from bowel preparations, long-term cola intake may lead to kidney damage, especially in the presence of underlying renal dysfunction."
– Carbonated Beverages and Chronic Kidney Disease; *Epidemiology* journal; Sept. 2012

Sugars and chemical sugar-free sweeteners

The sugar in cola drinks can increase the risk of diabetes, as it triggers the pancreas to produce more of the insulin hormone, which increases ingested sugar to move into the blood. This can increase the risk of pancreatic cancer, which is one of the most aggressive forms of cancer.

Consuming sugary drinks also increases the risk of cardiovascular disease, heart attack, and stroke.

Those who consume carbonated drinks also have an increased risk of liver damage, obesity, and Alzheimer's.

As mentioned elsewhere, colas and some other carbonated drinks contain caffeine, which, in excessive amounts, can damage the kidneys.

Energy drinks are basically liquid caffeine pills. Avoid them.

"An important new finding has been reported from the Nurses' Health Study, which is a long term study that found diets high in sodium (salt) were hard on the kidneys, and gave other information about heart disease, cancer risk factors, and the use of hormone treatments after menopause.

Kidney function declined over two decades in women who drank several diet sodas a day, according to researchers from the prestigious Nurses' Health Study. In fact, compared with women who did not drink diet soda, soda-drinking women had a 30% greater reduction in kidney function in 20 years.

The diet-soda drinkers experienced a drop in their glomerular filtration rate (an important measure of the kidney function). With age, the glomerular filtration rate tends to decline a bit. But in diet-soda drinkers, the rate of decline was 3 times as much as for women who didn't drink diet sodas. Women who didn't drink sodas experienced a decline in glomerular filtration rate of about 1mL per minute per year after age 40. But the women who consumed diet soda, glomerular filtration rate decreased by 3mL per minute per year."
– Say No to That Diet Soda?; National Kidney Foundation; Aug. 2014

To avoid kidney issues, and help heal the kidneys, avoid both regular and sugar-free colas, as well as energy drinks, and all carbonated beverages. Doing so will also help to protect your brain, heart, spleen, pancreas, liver, stomach, intestines, gut microbiome, bones, and all areas of your health.

"Excessive consumption of sugar has been associated with a variety of negative health effects, including increased risks for obesity, cardiovascular disease, type 2 diabetes, and dementia. In order to limit sugar intake, many people turn to low or no calorie sweeteners. However, there have been reports linking the consumption of some of these non-nutritive sweeteners to the risk of many of the same adverse events, such as insulin resistance, or cardiovascular disease."

– Are Artificial Sweeteners Bad for the Brain?, by Betsey Mills, PhD; *Alzheimer's Discovery* journal; Sept. 2023

"After adjustments for age, sex, education (for analysis of dementia), caloric intake, diet quality, physical activity, and smoking, higher recent and higher cumulative intake of artificially sweetened soft drinks were associated with an increased risk of ischemic stroke, all-cause dementia, and Alzheimer's disease dementia."

– Sugar and Artificially Sweetened Beverages and the Risks of Incident Stroke and Dementia: A Prospective Cohort Study; *Stroke* journal; May 2017

Want something sweet? Eat a piece of fruit.

Coffee

"Tea and coffee in moderation are not a problem. While tea and coffee do contain some oxalate, the extra fluid outweighs any possible disadvantages. In fact, some studies suggest that drinking moderate amounts of tea and coffee can actually lower the risk of kidney stones. In general, if you do drink caffeinated beverages, keep your daily amount of caffeine to no more than 400 milligrams. That's equal to four or five cups of regular coffee."

– How do you avoid kidney stone attacks?, by Howard LeWine, M.D.; *Harvard Men's Health Watch*; Feb. 2021

Who drinks four of five cups of coffee per day? I'd feel as if I were on crank. It would give me the caffeine shivers.

While I sometimes do drink some coffee, I limit it to about a cup. I often go for days, weeks – and sometimes months – without having coffee.

"An 8 ounce cup of black coffee has 116 mg of potassium. This is considered a low potassium food. However, many people drink more than one cup of coffee each day. Three to four cups of coffee a day is considered high in potassium, and could raise your potassium levels. Adding creamers or milk can further raise your coffee's potassium content. Drinking less than three cups of coffee/day is generally considered safe. Phosphorus, sodium, calories, carbohydrates, and protein are minimal in black coffee, and not of nutritional consideration.

Caffeine causes a short but sudden increase in blood pressure. Those struggling with blood pressure control may need to drink less than three cups per day."

– Coffee and Kidney Disease: Is it Safe?, by Jessianna Saville, kidney dietitian; National Kidney Foundation; Oct. 2017

It is the caffeine in coffee that is a stimulant that cranks up the central nervous system. Caffeine speeds up the information shared between the brain and heart, and the brain, stomach, and intestines, which increases alertness.

Caffeine is abundantly used as an additive in "energy drinks." These drinks contain more caffeine than coffee. There have been cases of people who have essentially overdosed on energy drinks, including those who have gone into kidney failure, have had a heart attack, or have experienced a stroke – and some have died.

In addition to coffee and energy drinks, caffeine is in certain teas, and in cocoa, and chocolate.

Caffein increases the heart rate and body temperature, and can trigger headaches, dizziness, restlessness, jitters, twitching leg muscles, insomnia, and heart palpitations.

Because caffeine increases blood flow, it can increase stress on the kidneys, which can increase blood pressure. For someone with damaged or otherwise compromised kidneys, it is best to avoid – or limit – the intake of caffeine.

Caffeine can increase urination. When the person doesn't increase their water intake when drinking coffee, it can cause kidney dehydration. For this reason, it is good to practice this step: when you drink a cup of coffee, also drink a cup of water.

It is the things people add to coffee that can be a problem, including by adding calories, sugar, and synthetic chemicals.

The popular "non-dairy" creamer sold in stores is rich in toxic chemicals and processed oils. Read the ingredients. Avoid food products containing garbage ingredients, or all of those ingredients will end up in your blood, and will have to be filtered by the liver and kidneys.

When I do have coffee, I don't use sugar, honey, or other sweetener that would add calories, or play with my blood sugar. I use either no sweetener, or I use organic stevia. A little date sugar is sometimes my choice.

If I add something to coffee, it is pure raw chocolate powder, maca root powder, nutmeg, cinnamon*, and a vegan milk I make by simply blending a banana* with hemp seeds, vanilla, and water (and sometimes a teaspoon of lucuma fruit powder, and/or maca powder).

(*Cinnamon is rich in a variety of antioxidants that help fight inflammation, and nutrients that work against cancer, diabetes, and heart disease. Cinnamon also can help balance blood sugar. But don't overuse cinnamon, as it contains coumarin, which can cause liver issues in high amounts. The most common cinnamon is Cassia cinnamon, which contains higher amounts of coumarin. Ceylon cinnamon isn't as sweet, but contains lower amounts of coumarin.)

(**A large banana can have about 490 milligrams of potassium. If you have kidney or cardiovascular disease, that amount of potassium may be more than twice as much potassium as you've been told to get in one meal. Cut the banana into a third.)

Relating to coffee and kidney disease, there is also the bit of information from the National Kidney Foundation:

"A new study published today in the *American Journal of Kidney Disease* provides evidence that coffee consumption has beneficial effects on kidney function, and could potentially be used in prevention strategies.

Coffee Consumption and Kidney Function: A Mendelian Randomization Study, authored by a team in the United Kingdom, looked at the relationship between coffee consumption and chronic kidney disease. The investigators were stimulated to pursue this by the fact that chronic kidney disease is a leading cause of morbidity and mortality worldwide, with limited strategies for prevention and treatment.

The authors examined data from hundreds of thousands of study participants and found that coffee conferred a protective effect against CKD. Drinking an extra cup of coffee per day was associated with lower incidence of CKD stages G3-G-5, higher estimated glomerular filtration (eGFR) rates, and lower albuminuria (ACR)."

– Popular Beverage Protects Against Kidney Disease; National Kidney Foundation; Dec. 2019

"Coffee is a commonly consumed beverage comprising a complex mixture of compounds, including caffeine, chlorogenic acid, and diterpenes. These have a range of in vivo properties, including anti-inflammatory, antioxidant, and antifibrotic effects. Worldwide, more than 2 billion cups of coffee are consumed daily, so small physiologic effects may have substantial public health implications. Epidemiologic studies indicate that coffee may protect against liver, neurologic, cardiovascular, and metabolic disease; all-cause mortality; and various cancers.

Several epidemiologic studies report lower risks for reduced estimated GFR (eGFR) and CKD among regular coffee drinkers.

The active ingredient in coffee that may be responsible for the results of this study is unclear. Noncaffeine chemical constituents (e.g., chlorogenic acid and diterpenes) reduce inflammation and oxidative stress, which are causative in CKD onset and progression.

Additionally, coffee may protect against CKD risk factors, including diabetes, cardiovascular disease, and obesity."

– Coffee Consumption and Kidney Function: A Mendelian Randomization Study; National Kidney Foundation; May 2020

Do you need coffee to survive, or to help you survive – or to prevent – kidney disease? No. But apparently it isn't something you need to avoid, if you have kidney problems.

As the studies seem to indicate, a cup or two of coffee per day is okay, as long as you don't load up the coffee with unhealthful ingredients. Also, stick to drinking at least a cup of water every time you drink a cup of coffee. And, drink it earlier in the day – to avoid insomnia.

Drinks, diabetes, cardiovascular, and kidney disease

You have been diagnosed with a chronic and degenerative disease that can debilitate you. Keep clear of all the problematic drinks.

Avoid energy drinks as they are loaded with what can be a problematic amount of caffeine, and health-dulling additives. It doesn't matter if these products are sold. Simply because it is a product you can buy in a food store doesn't mean the product is safe. They are especially not something to be consumed by people wanting to experience the best of health.

Avoid drinks containing added clarified sugars or artificial sweeteners.

Avoid colas, and drinks containing phosphate additives, as these are not good for the bones, kidneys, parathyroid, nerves, cardiovascular system, and other tissues – especially if you already have compromised health.

Be aware of how much sodium is in bottled and canned drinks.

Rather than drinking fruit juice, eat a piece of fruit for all of its nutrients, including the fiber.

If you do have fruit juice, water it down a little. Also, don't drink fruit juice containing added "natural" sweetener, or artificial dyes, sweeteners, flavors, scents, or preservatives.

Avoid drinks containing oils, including canola, palm, corn, and others.

Go for organic juices in glass jars, rather than in plastic bottles, or cans, or paper coated with chemicals.

Consider raw, organic veggie juices. One I like to make is a juice mix of carrot, fennel, celery, and cucumber, then blended with diced ginger root. Sometimes I blend in a spoonful of Infinity Greens powder. Or things like a half teaspoon of freshly ground fenugreek, freshly ground flax seeds, or fractured hemp seeds. (If you put lemon in your juice, always rinse with water after dinking, to protect teeth enamel.)

It is wise to avoid alcohol.

The best drink is water.

Consider getting a water distiller to help clear your water of chemicals, heavy metals, microorganisms, sediment, and other impurities. See the earlier information about distilled water and concerns of minerals.

Fresh coconut water is also good, including because it contains electrolytes.

Medications and kidneys, and interstitial nephritis

It is important to let your doctor know about any and all prescription and/or over-the-counter medicines or nutritional supplements you are taking. Some medications and supplements can interfere with kidney function, and some might interact with other medications.

Report any adverse reactions of any drug or supplement you take.

Over-the-counter pain pills (NSAIDs = non-steroidal anti-inflammatory drugs), including the overuse of Tylenol and aspirin, can damage vessels in the kidneys. These drugs can cause bleeding in the intestines, and contribute to leaky gut syndrome – playing roles in arthritis and other autoimmune disorders.

Long-term use of drugs like aspirin (above 325 mg per day), ibuprofen (Advil, Motrin), and naproxen (Aleve) can lead to a chronic kidney condition called interstitial nephritis. It causes inflammation, and decreases the ability of the kidney tubules to filter impurities and waste products from the blood.

"Interstitial nephritis is a kidney disease that lowers your kidneys' ability to clean your blood and make urine. It is a disease that causes inflammation (swelling) around parts of your kidneys' filters called tubules. Usually it is caused by a reaction to the medicine you take, and stopping that medicine solves the problem.

Acute interstitial nephritis lasts a short time. This is the most common type of interstitial nephritis.

Chronic interstitial nephritis lasts longer: weeks, months, or years.

The most common symptom of interstitial nephritis is urinating less than normal. Other symptoms can include:
• Blood in the urine
• Fever
• A rash

265

- Feeling tired or confused
- Feeling sick to your stomach and throwing up
- Swelling in your hands, feet, or other parts of your body
- Weight gain
- High blood pressure"
– American Kidney Fund; June 2024

The American Kidney Fund lists medications that can play a role in acute interstitial nephritis. They include antibiotics, the over-the-counter nonsteroidal anti-inflammatory drugs (NSAIDS), and medicines used to treat excess stomach acid called proton pump inhibitors (PPIs).

As a person with kidney or cardiovascular disease, and autoimmune diseases, including diabetes and arthritis, always research the side effects of medications, before taking them. This includes everything from meds that treat aches and pains, allergies, cold and flu, congestion, constipation, diarrhea, fever, fungal issues, hair and nail growth, heartburn, infection, motion sickness, nausea, sinus issues, skin issues, sleep issues, and viral infections. Discuss concerns with your doctor, and consider alternatives.

"Your kidneys may not be able to get rid of the extra aluminum, magnesium, and sodium in Maalox and Mylanta. Limit taking antacids to no more than 2 weeks. If you're on dialysis, you may not be able to take some of these medications, so talk with your doctor."
– Managing over-the-counter medications with kidney disease; *Fresenius Kidney Care*; 2025

"While some medicines should be avoided with CKD, many can be used safely at lower doses and/or with less frequent use. Working with your healthcare professional is important to make sure your medication regimen is safe for you and your specific health needs. Regular monitoring of your estimated glomerular filtration rate (eGFR) can help inform with medicines(s) may need to be adjusted and/or switched to something different."
– Safe Medication Use with Chronic Kidney Disease; National Kidney Foundation; 2025

According to the American Kidney Fund, causes of chronic interstitial nephritis are "usually caused by another health problem you have. Problems that can cause interstitial nephritis include: Autoimmune disease such as lupus, as well as low levels of potassium in the blood, levels of calcium in the blood being too high, sarcoidosis [a disease that causes inflammation, most commonly in the lungs and lymph nodes], and some infections."

The so-called "temporary" or acute interstitial nephritis can cause permanent kidney damage.

Some people who have experienced acute interstitial nephritis are put on temporary dialysis, until tests show the issue has resolved. Treatment will likely include medications to reduce inflammation, and control blood pressure. Permanent damage from interstitial nephritis could lead to long-term dialysis, and a kidney transplant.

Years ago I had an exchange with a pro athlete whose doctors told him he permanently damaged his kidneys by using so many common, over-the-counter painkillers for years and years. He ended up getting a kidney transplant.

Because of my genetic kidney disorder with its thin tissues and malformations, and prior history of bleeding when I was following an unhealthful diet, I've been told by my doctors that using acetaminophen (Tylenol) should be limited. Luckily, I've had relatively few times where I felt I needed a pain killer for things like sprains, or other random injuries.

With the leaky gut condition that can be caused by painkiller use, as explained elsewhere in the book, undigested proteins getting into the blood through a damaged intestinal tract can also cause kidney damage – and inflammation in the joints and other tissues throughout the body.

Erythropoietin hormone, vitamin D, and red blood cell production

The kidneys create hormones, including erythropoietin, and, by conversion of vitamin D from food or sunlight, the active form of vitamin D.

Erythropoietin (EPO) stimulates the bone marrow to create red blood cells, which then absorb and transfer oxygen throughout the body. When the kidneys detect low oxygen in the blood, the kidneys produce more of the hormone to trigger the production of more red blood cells.

People with severe kidney disease are often prescribed EPO, which helps them avoid anemia. Those with anemia could experience fatigue, shortness of breath, and weakness, and have abnormal blood counts.

"EPO treats [anemia] by imitating the action of the hormone erythropoietin, stimulating the body to produce more red blood cells. Patients who may benefit from EPO therapy include those with chronic kidney disease, those who are anemic from AIDS, or from a wide variety of hematologic disorders (including multiple myeloma and myelodysplastic syndromes), and some cancer patients who are anemic from receiving chemotherapy. In selected patients, EPO may be used to reduce the need for blood transfusions in surgery.

In the early 1960s came the development of hemodialysis, a method of removing waste products from the blood when the kidneys are unable to perform this function, to sustain the lives of patients with end-stage kidney disease. As a result of this treatment advance, these patients were able to survive the underlying disease, but their damaged kidneys could no longer make erythropoietin, leaving them severely anemic, and I desperate need of EPO therapy.

In 1983, scientists discovered a method for mass producing a synthetic version of the hormone. Experiments were conducted to test the safety and effectiveness of the new drug, EPO, for treating anemia in patients with kidney failure.

Patients who had been dependent on frequent blood transfusions were able to increase their red blood cell levels to near-normal within just a few weeks of starting therapy. Patients' appetite returned, and they resumed their active lives. It was the convergence of two technologies – long-term dialysis and molecular biology – that set the stage for anemia management in this group of patients."

– The Story of Erythropoietin; Hematology.org; Dec. 2008

When EPO levels are too high, there can be an overproduction of red blood cells. This could because someone has gone to a high elevation, needing more red blood cells to transport oxygen, or it could be related to a tumor creating high EPO levels.

Sun exposure is important for the creation of vitamin D. It plays a role in bone health, in calcium absorption, and in the immune system – and in reducing both inflammation, and the symptoms of autoimmune disorders.

Bone health

Those with kidney disease are more likely to have fragile bones (osteoporosis and osteopenia [decreased bone mineral density]). Damaged kidneys are less likely to regulate certain hormone and minerals as they should, or convert vitamin D into calcitriol, which all plays a role in bone health. Damaged kidneys don't manage blood phosphorus levels the way they should, which also weakens the bones as the parathyroid glands release more hormones into the blood, which then results in calcium from the bones being released into the blood. The imbalance of minerals can cause calcifications in the blood vessels, damage the heart, and degrade the microvessels, including in the eyes and kidneys, increasing the risks of vision problems, possible blindness, and more severe kidney problems. This condition can also cause the hormone FGF23 produced by the bones to become imbalanced, causing more damage to the bones and vascular system.

A blood test in relation to kidney disease can check the levels of vitamin D, parathyroid hormone, and levels of calcium, potassium, phosphorus, and other nutrients. Computed tomography scan (CT scan) in relation to kidney disease could help detect calcifications in the heart and bone damage.

All of the tests can also play into what a doctor recommends, including medications, dietary changes, removal of one or more of the parathyroid glands (parathyroidectomy – one is usually left in to maintain parathyroid levels), as well as dialysis, and/or a kidney transplant.

A doctor might prescribe medications for hyperparathyroidism (for PTH levels), as well as phosphate binders (not recommended for those on dialysis with CKD or terminal kidney disease, or non-calcium phosphorus binders may also be used to prevent increasing calcium), and/or synthetic calcitriol, and calcium and vitamin D supplements.

Part of weakened bones in kidney disease patients also relates to nutritional choices, as the same garbage and unhealthful foods playing into kidney issues are also not good for the bones.

Smoking and alcohol use can also be factors, as both damage the bones, cardiovascular system, liver, and kidneys, and other tissues, including collagen in the bones. The microorganisms of the gut biome are also negatively impacted by alcohol and tobacco use.

"Phosphorus is a mineral found in bones. Along with calcium, phosphorus helps build strong, healthy bones, and keeps other parts of your body healthy.

Too much phosphorus in your blood can cause changes that pull calcium out of your bones, making them weak. High phosphorus and calcium levels also lead to dangerous calcium deposits in your blood vessels, lungs, eyes, and heart."
– Kidney.org; 2025

Ways of reducing phosphorus in the diet include using nondairy milk (and getting dairy products out of your diet), reading labels to check for phosphorus levels (many labels do not include this, so you will need to learn which foods do and do not contain troublesome amounts of phosphorus), knowing which food additives contain phosphorus, including everything from breads, cookies, cakes, and other baked foods, and pastas. Also, learn about which foods are high in sodium (salt), and potassium.

Foods higher in phosphorus include certain grains, nuts, and seeds, peanuts and other legumes, and beans, beer and ale, and chocolate, and colas.

The worse condition the kidneys are in, the more likely bone health is degraded. This includes because bones continually rebuild, weaken, and strengthen in relation to things like diet, exercise, stress, sleep, and general physical activities – and parathyroid, liver, heart, and kidney function.

Bone health can degrade along with kidney health to the point the bones become misshapen, bone mass decreases, and the person can lose both height and strength. Bones become more fragile as osteoporosis sets in, and the risk of fracture increases. Bone and joint pain can become issues. The legs can also change shape, with the bones tilting inward or outward, in a condition called *renal rickets*.

"Mineral and bone disorder in chronic kidney disease is a disorder that can affect the bones, heart, and blood vessels of a person with CKD. Mineral and bone disease occurs when kidneys damaged by CKD can't filter blood and regulate hormones the way they should. The hormone levels and levels of minerals, such as calcium and phosphorus, then become imbalanced, leading to damage.

Mineral and bone disorder in CKD is also called CKD Mineral and Bone Disorder, or CKD-MBD.

The bone disease component of mineral and bone disorder is called renal osteodystrophy."
– Mineral and Bone Disorder in Chronic Kidney Disease; National Institute of Diabetes and Digestive and Kidney Diseases; 2025

These are more reasons to pay attention to kidney health, to eat a clean diet, to get adequate daily exercise, and maintain a healthy sleep pattern to help keep the bones strong.

Phosphate binder medications can help prevent bone loss in those with kidney disease, on dialysis, or who have had a transplant. But those on dialysis or with terminal kidney disease may not be given phosphate binders. (Consult with your doctor and dietician. Phosphate binders should also be free of aluminum – formerly used in older medications.)

See the parts of this book about vitamin D, osteoporosis, and dairy.

Consider consulting with a vegan nutritionist

Access: PlantBasedRDs.com.
VegNews.com also features a list of vegan dieticians.
Search: "Vegan nutritionist near me."

FODMAPs

FODMAPs stands for fermentable oligosaccharides, disaccharides, monosaccharides, and polyols. They are short-chain carbohydrates absorbed poorly by the small intestines. People sensitive to FODMAPs, or have FODMAP intolerance, are susceptible to experiencing IBS, involving bloating, constipation, diarrhea, or all. One person might be more susceptible to high FODMAP foods.

A FODAP diet limits certain foods, and is done for a certain length of time to help identify problematic foods. After the foods are eliminated for several weeks, they are re-introduced one at a time to identify which food might be a problem.

"FODMAP stands for fermentable oligosaccharides, disaccharides, monosaccharides, and polyols, which are short-chain carbohydrates (sugars) that the small intestine absorbs poorly. Some people experience digestive distress after eating them. Symptoms include: cramping, diarrhea, constipation, stomach bloating, gas and flatulence.
– FODMAP Diet: What You Need To Know; HopkinsMedicine.org

The process relating to the FODMAP diet is something you likely will be consulted about upon diagnoses with digestive issues, including those that can be experienced in combination with kidney problems.

Fermented foods

Here we are, again, mentioning fermented foods. These include kimchi, sauerkraut, kombucha, coconut yogurt, and coconut kefir. And sourdough bread made the old fashioned way, which ferments the dough. These can promote digestive system and kidney health. That is – other than sourdough bread – **IF** they are raw, not heated, not pasteurized. When you purchase these items, make sure the label says they are both raw and organic. You can also learn how to make them. (Search YouTube videos: Raw vegan fermented foods. Also search: how to make sourdough bread from scratch.)

I don't like kimchi, although many people do.

I do have a crock with a water moat to allow gasses to escape from the lid, and make sauerkraut.

If sauerkraut is canned, it has been pasteurized, and is missing many of the beneficial components. Jarred sauerkraut may be raw, but look for the words "raw" or "unpasteurized" on the label.

I do like raw sauerkraut, and fermented coconut yogurt, and coconut kefir.

People with sodium issues will need to rinse the sauerkraut to reduce the salt.

I'm not big on kombucha, but will sometimes have it. The caffeine can be a bit much, so it is best to have it about an hour or two after waking up, not late in the day. GT's kombucha is a better brand, because I know he makes it using high-quality vegan probiotics. He does the same with his coconut yogurt.

You can also purchase vegan probiotics, and use those in your smoothies, and mix them into things like raw hummus, guacamole, and as an ingredient in raw vegan cheeses. (See recipes for raw, fermented, vegan cheeses on YouTube.)

I also make raw, fermented pine nut cheese using fermented water from soaking buckwheat.

Potassium is important for kidney health

If you have severe, or end-stage kidney disease, follow doctor and nutritionist guidelines for potassium intake.

Potassium is an essential mineral, and helps to balance sodium. The balance of both are partially managed by the kidneys.

Potassium is in whole fruits and vegetables, and in electrolyte powder, and can help protect the kidneys.

The electric charge of potassium plays a role in cell, nerve, kidney, and blood vessel function, as well as blood pressure, and muscle contraction. Potassium also plays into sodium excretion.

Potassium helps to balance inner cellular fluid.

Sodium helps to balance fluids outside of the cells, including the blood and lymph.

People following high sodium and low potassium diets have increased rates of cardiovascular disease, strokes, and heart attacks.

A key to better health is to reduce salt intake, while consuming more unprocessed fruits and especially vegetables. This means, cutting out salty foods, including salty cheese, meat (including fried chicken, bacon, processed meats, and jerky), butter, processed foods, salty crackers, salty snacks, and other foods likely to be high in salt.

Because salt fortified with iodine can be a chief way in which people get iodine, people cutting out salt also need to make sure they maintain adequate iodine in their diet, or take a iodine supplement. As someone with kidney disease, the iodine issue is something to discuss with your doctor and/or dietician, or nutritionist.

Potassium-rich foods include acorn squash, almonds, apricots (especially when dehydrated), avocadoes, bananas, beans, broccoli, butternut squash, cantaloupe, cashews (use only unsalted nuts with no added oil), coconut water, leafy greens, lentils, oranges, potatoes, and raisins.

Beet and spinach leaves are high in potassium, but they also are high in oxalates. Drink additional water, and avoid oily foods, when eating spinach or beet leaves.

Dandelions are kidney friendly

I include dandelion as part of a healthy kidney diet because this nutrient-dense green is a diuretic helpful for urine production.

Dandelions are beneficial for helping relieve fluid retention in the ankles, feet, arms, wrists, hands, face, and other areas.

Dandelions contain nutrients that lower blood pressure and benefit the liver.

Both the leaves and flowers of dandelion are edible, are rich in phenolic acids, carotenoids, glycosides, and coumarins, and are a source for iron.

Dandelions contain more vitamins A, E, and K – as well as more calcium and antioxidants – than spinach.

I like to leave the dandelion flowers for the bees, as they will frolic on them – and are one of their first food sources in the spring. Bees need our help in being able to survive – and they help us to survive by pollinating such a wide variety of plants.

Soaking the dandelion leaves in ice water can reduce the bitterness.

271

Young dandelion leaves taste better and are less bitter than the larger leaves. Remember this when harvesting, and get them from an area free of toxic lawn chemicals, and away from where animals defecate.

If you don't care much for the taste of dandelion, use only one leaf diced as an ingredient in a salad or smoothie, or in your morning water as a way to get dandelion nutrients. Dandelion tea is also an option.

Salt / sodium: reducing and avoiding use

A contributing factor to both kidney and cardiovascular disease can be the consumption of too much sodium.

A high-sodium diet can damage the liver, and contribute to water retention, hypertension, renal hypertension, heart failure, and stroke.

Diets high in salt also can increase weight gain, sluggishness, and diabetes, and play a role in the formation of kidney stones.

Many Americans are consuming more than 3,300 mg of sodium per day, when a healthy intake would be less than 2,300 mg per day.

Salt is in many foods and drinks sold as "healthy." Simply because a food is marketed or labeled as "healthy" does not mean it is – including many foods labeled as "heart healthy," and/or "vegan."

The longer you go without adding salt to things, the more you don't miss it. There are ways of flavoring things with herbs and spices to make them interesting. We rarely add salt to food we make. When we do, it is iodized salt.

"Diets high in salt or sodium can increase blood pressure and harm your kidneys. Flavor foods with herbs and spices, instead of salt. It tastes just as good. Your tastebuds will adjust, and you may find it easier to use less salt on your food over time."
– 10 Common Habits That May Harm Your Kidneys; National Kidney Foundation; June 2016

Salt adds up when people use bottled salad dressings and sauces, catsup, canned foods, heat-and-serve packaged foods, instant foods, fast foods, deli foods, foods from snack shops, "protein bars," and other processed and grab-n-go foods. It all adds up – to health problems.

As someone with kidney and/or cardiovascular disease, be sure to watch your sodium intake. Get used to reading labels to understand sodium content.

Learn how to make foods from scratch using less salt than the recipe suggests – or no salt.

Flavoring foods without salt could include using – depending on what you are making – herbs, spices, garlic, onions, ginger, and/or vinegar.

Making foods from scratch is less expensive, and more nutritious than restaurant, packaged, and prepared foods.

While salt is important for health, not much of it is needed by the body, and what is needed can easily be obtained by consuming a variety of vegetables.

If you use salt, choose unprocessed salts free of aluminum, but containing iodine. Or use dulse, kelp, nori powder, or nori flakes – which are seaweeds containing a variety of minerals. It depends on what you are making, and what flavor you are aiming for.

Typical table salt is heated to 1,200 degrees Fahrenheit. This process can damage the minerals. Table salt may also include additives including fluoride, aluminum, sodium bicarbonate, anti-caking agents, and other ingredients.

There is benefit in the iodine added to salt. But you can maintain a healthful iodine level in other ways, including by taking a supplement. Speak with your doctor and/or dietician, or nutritionist about this issue.

Processed foods: Sodium, sugar, damaged oils, and chemicals

Some may say this list contains everything. It doesn't. There are also many foods on the list that could be made using healthier, less problematic ingredients, and/or prepared in ways that are more healthful.

Depending on the company, the plant-based items on this list could be low-salt, or salt-free, including nut butters, and other products.

When you shop, don't go to the processed foods aisles. Go to the produce aisle, the herb and spices aisle, and get other whole, unprocessed ingredients for making healthy foods from scratch.

The more you get used to making clean food from scratch, the easier and quicker it gets.

The less you depend on ultra-processed foods, the better. Many vegan junk foods classify as being processed, and, because of their salt, oil, and sugar contents, and AGEs, not healthful.

- **Almond butter**: As with other nut butters, they should only contain one ingredient: nuts. But some brands of almond butter contain unhealthful ingredients, like canola oil, and an abundance of salt. Learn to make your own containing one ingredient: almonds.

- **Baby foods**: Some brands contain health-damaging ingredients. Some have been found to contain microplastics, synthetic chemicals, clarified sugars, and extracted oils, and are high in sodium. Learn to make them from scratch.

- **Bacon**: Processed and smoked meats are always on the list of foods that can trigger cardiovascular disease, liver disease, kidney disease, cancers, and other health problems.

- **Baked beans**: A sugar festival. What chemicals are in the can lining? If you want something like this, learn to make it from scratch. If you must use sugar, use maple syrup. As an occasional food choice. Not a regular or common meal.

- **Biscuits**: If you want them, learn to make vegan biscuits from scratch. The store-purchased ones likely contain unhealthful ingredients, including so they can stay on store shelves longer.

- **Boxed or packaged cereals**: Gluten and sugar and unhealthy oils, preservatives, and other chemicals. Learn to make breakfast foods that nurture a healthy gut biome. Overnight oats soaked together with chia seeds, then topped with berries is a better choice. Perhaps mixed with organic, raw, fermented coconut yogurt containing quality probiotics.

- **Bratwurst**: Not what you want to be eating if you want a healthy gut biome, or a healthy cardiovascular system, or kidneys, or any high level of health.

273

- **Breadsticks**: Read the ingredient label. Learn to make sourdough bread at home, and you can make your own breadsticks with the dough. Including from gluten-free sourdough.

- **Broth**: Some are healthier than others. There is at least one vegan brand that doesn't contain oil. You could also make your own broth, by boiling down a variety of vegetables and herbs.

- **Brownies**: Sugar and oil and salt and gluten.

- **Buns**: Another food you can make at home. Use fermented sourdough.

- **Cake**: Like brownies, they are sugar and oil and salt and gluten.

- **Candy**: Junk. Sugar snacks are not what you should be having if you want the healthiest kidneys, pancreas, nerves, brain, bones, cardiovascular system, or stomach or intestinal tract. Candy isn't good for your gut biome. If you want something sweet, but not health damaging, have dates, figs, dried apricots, or a piece of fruit.

- **Canned beans**: Learn to make beans at home, including soaking the beans for hours, before rinsing, then boiling. Cans are lined with questionable chemicals to protect the can from rotting.

- **Canned fish**: Often oil and salt and chemicals leached from the can liner.

- **Canned fruit**: Usually a sugar festival. Fresh fruit is the better choice, and frozen fruit is the second choice. Organic frozen fruit can be purchased at popular club stores in the U.S. Locate your local organic farmers, and know where they sell their produce. Where possible, plant fruit trees and berry bushes.

- **Canned meats**: Including anchovies, other fish, and seafood, and ham. Salt and oil and leached chemicals from the can liner, in addition to the saturated fat, and animal proteins. The opposite of health-infusing.

- **Canned soup, chili, and other canned meals**: Often salt, damaged oils, and other questionable ingredients. What chemicals are in the can lining? Likely hormone disruptors.

- **Canned vegetables**: Often high in salt, and could have other unhealthful ingredients. As always with canned foods, question what the chemicals are lining the can.

- **Caramel**: Burned sugar. How could this be good for you, or for your gut biome, pancreas, cardiovascular system, nerves, or kidneys? It isn't.

- **Ceviche**: There is no human nutritional need to eat this.

- **Cheese and cheese products**: Salt, dairy, and coagulated fat. Often containing rennet (stomach lining of slaughtered, un-weened baby cow or bull, sheep, or goat), which is why some cheese smells like vomit.

- **Chicken products**: Still contains saturated fat, and substances that aren't good for people with kidney issues. The chemistry of the chickens often includes the farming chemicals and pharmaceutical drugs used on the farms. What does ingesting that do to your gut biome? Look up the ingredients of chicken nuggets. What is it you are eating when you eat that garbage? Do you think those things are going to nurture the health you desire?

- **Chips**: Avoid fried foods. These are often also rich in salt. Learn how to make dehydrated chips using vegetables, herbs and/or spices.

- **Chocolate bars and chocolate candy**: To get the benefits of chocolate, get pure, organic chocolate powder. Use it earlier in the day, not within several hours of sleep.

- **Chorizo**: Even the vegan chorizo is of salt and damaged oils, and questionable ingredients. It is likely that you can figure out how to make some sort of healthier version out of plants, from scratch.

- **Clam chowder**: Salt and other ingredients that promote cardiovascular and kidney disease. And whatever industrial pollutants were absorbed by the clams, which are bottom-dwelling creatures.

- **Condiments**: BBQ sauce, hot sauces, gravies, ketchup, mayonnaise, mustard, soy, tamari. Salt and damaged oils, sugars and other ingredients that dull health. Some brands are much healthier than others. Some of them can be made from scratch at home – like our ancestors did, before stores started selling dressings, gravies, marinades, and sauces.

- **Cookies**: Oils and sugars and gluten, and often synthetic chemicals, including questionable additives. If you want cookies, learn to make vegan, oil-free cookies from scratch using gluten-free flour. Experiment.

- **Corn chips, popcorn, and other corn products**: Often made from GMO corn saturated with farming chemicals. Where possible, get organic corn, or grow it. Make your own corn products.

- **Crackers**: Salt and other ingredients that again dull health. Gluten and chemical additives. Learn to make your own from scratch using healthier ingredients. Explore making dehydrated crackers. Look up: how to make gluten-free crackers.

- **Croutons**: Read ingredient labels. These often are high in salt, and contain other dulling ingredients. You can learn to make sourdough at home, and make your own croutons – without the additives and preservatives.

- **Cured foods**: Often rich in salts, damaged oils, and consisting of animal protein saturated with chemicals you don't want to have in you.

- **Dairy products**: Butter, buttermilk, cheese, cheese spreads, condensed milk, cottage cheese, cream, cream cheese, ice cream, kefir, yogurt, whey, casein. See the parts of the book detailing why dairy is not good for the kidneys, cardiovascular system, or bones, and other tissues.

- **Deli meats**: Salt and saturated fats, and often varieties of synthetic chemicals. Again, processed meats are always on the list of foods that increase the risks of cancer, cardiovascular disease, liver disease, kidney disease, and other maladies.

- **Dehydrated foods**: Learn to make healthier versions at home. All sorts of fruits and vegetables, and foods made from them can be dehydrated. Slice apples as thin as possible, and dehydrate those into a snack consisting only of apples. You can also crumble them onto overnight oats.

- **Donuts**: Oil, sugar, gluten, and who knows what combination of additives. A fried food. I don't eat fried foods. I haven't had a donut since college. They are junk. Not something you want in your body if you want the best level of health.

- **Dried meats**: See cured foods, deli meats, and bacon. Triggers for cancer, cardiovascular and kidney disease, and other degenerative diseases.

- **Drinks**: The healthiest drink is water. Drinks sold in plastic bottles can contain hormone-disrupting chemicals, micro plastics, and industrial pollutants. Get a good water filter, or water distiller. Have a stainless steel or glass water bottle. Stay hydrated without relying on expensive bottled liquids.

- **Egg substitutes**: Read ingredient labels. There are a variety of egg substitutes on the market. You can also make simple egg substitutes from scratch (see recipes on YouTube).

- **Energy drinks**: Sugar or chemical sweetener, a big dose of caffeine, mixed with chemicals, including dyes, flavorings, and scents.

- **Fast foods**: Avoid all of it. More and more fast food chains are offering vegan foods. Know they are not of the highest quality, and are in the classification of ultra-processed. But if you really want some sort of food, and can't hold out until you can get something of higher quality, those are there.

- **Flavored bagels**: Could include a variety of chemicals, bleached grains, salt, and other ingredients that dull health, including potassium bromate or potassium iodate.

- **Fried foods**: French fries, chips, donuts, meats (including chicken and fish), snacks. Most often also high in salt and/or sugar, and a variety of unhealthful ingredients – in addition to the damaged oils.

- **Frozen dinners**: These are usually on the same level of fast foods, rich in salt, damaged oils, and questionable, health-dulling ingredients.

- **Granola snack bars**: Often containing questionable ingredients, from sugars to oils to salts and low-quality grains to highly heated nuts and seeds. There are healthier choices, such as Bear Bars made from organic ingredients, and no chemicals.

- **Guacamole**: Commercial guacamole can be rich in salt, and some contain questionable ingredients, including sugars, oils, and preservatives. Learn to make your own from scratch. Those on a renal diet may need to limit their avocado consumption.

- **Ham**: Always on the list of meats that increase the risk of cardiovascular and kidney disease, cancer, and other health issues.

- **"Health food" snack bars**: So many contain questionable ingredients, from canola oil, agave syrup, rice syrup, and other health-dulling ingredients.

- **Hummus**: Many commercially sold brands of hummus contain anything from canola oil to high amounts of sodium and other problematic ingredients. Hummus is easy to make from scratch, and is a food that has been made for thousands of years with basic ingredients. Rather than oil, add more water to make the hummus easier to blend. The tahini (crushed sesame seeds) already has enough oil. Add your favorite herbs and/or spices.

- **Imitation meats**: Vegan meat products can be filled with low-grade oils, high amounts of salt, and other ingredients so processed that these should not be considered healthy. Find recipes for homemade vegan burgers made from scratch. You can make a bunch of vegan burgers, and freeze them.

- **"Instant" mixes, puddings, dressings, meal helpers, sauces, and other "instant" packaged foods**: Any "instant" foods are suspect. Read ingredient labels. Likely rich in salt, and ingredients that could be problematic for those with kidney and cardiovascular disease, and autoimmune disorders.

- **Jerky**: These are often on the list of meats with high salt content. They are processed meats that increase the risk of chronic and degenerative health conditions, including kidney, liver, and cardiovascular disease, and cancer, etc. They also are not good for the gut biome.

- **Loaf breads**: Read ingredients. There are a wide variety of breads on the market, with some much less healthful than others. Make bread from scratch using gluten-free ingredients. Avoid breads containing potassium bromate and potassium iodate. Again, organic sourdough bread is a better choice.

- **Macaroni and cheese**: The ingredient label of low-quality, health depleting ingredients speaks for itself. High in salt, oil, and a variety of things like chemical flavorings, scents, dyes, texturizers, and preservatives.

- **Margarine**: Spreadable heart disease. Not good for the gut biome, or the kidneys, heart, nerves, brain, or anything. It doesn't matter what the label says.

- **Marinades**: Learn to make your own from scratch.

- **Mayonnaise**: Made with eggs. If vegan, it likely contains a variety of ingredients that aren't what you would want to consume if you are aiming for vibrant health. Probably high in salt, unhealthful oils, etc.

- **Meal "helper" foods**: More "instant" foods containing questionable and health-dulling ingredients.

- **Microwavable products**: Heat and eat foods are always questionable. Read ingredient labels.

- **Muffins**: Sugar, oil, gluten, and who knows what else. Read ingredient labels.

- **Noodle cups / ramen**: Junk.

- **Nut bars**: What is binding the nuts? It is sugar? Corn syrup? Agave? Rice syrup? Not exactly health-infusing, even if they are sold as "healthy snacks." The only nut bar brand I know of that is of pure ingredients is Bear Bar.

- **Nut butters**: They should contain one ingredient: nuts. Not added oils, or other ingredients. You can make nuts butters at home using a food processor, and one ingredient: nuts.

- **Olives**: Canned ones are usually the lowest quality. Look for organic olives sold in glass jars. Consider the sodium content, and rinse before using to reduce the salt.

- **Packaged breakfast cereals, including the instant ones**: So many contain the ingredients you don't want in your body morning, noon, or night, or for a midnight snack.

- **Pasta products**: What are the ingredients? Are they organic? Do you have an issue with gluten? What about phosphorus?

- **Peanut butter**: As with other nut butters, they should be organic, and contain one ingredient: peanuts. (Although peanuts aren't nuts, they are legumes.) You can make peanut butter at home in a food processor with dry roasted peanuts.

- **Pepperoni**: A processed meat containing what contributes to cardiovascular, liver, and kidney disease, and cancer, and other chronic and degenerative diseases.

- **Pesto**: Read ingredient labels. You can learn to make vegan pesto at home. Or some other variety of vegetable spread with herbs and spices.

- **Pickled foods**: pickles, relish, and others. Again, read ingredient labels. If you get pickles, get organic, and sold in glass jars. If you are watching your sodium intake, rinse pickles before eating.

- **Pita chips**: Read ingredient labels. Again: gluten grains, salt, and other health-depleting ingredients. Learn to make sourdough bread at home, including gluten-free sourdough. If you occasionally want some sort of chip, experiment with sourdough in various forms, including by adding herbs and/or spices.

- **Pizza**: Typical pizza is rich in salt, oil, gluten, and processed meats like sausage and pepperoni that contribute to chronic and degenerative diseases. Develop your own homemade vegan pizza. There are oil-free, vegan pizza recipes on the ForksOverKnives site. There are a variety of gluten-free crusts, made from corn, cauliflower, or buckwheat.

- **Popcorn**: If you really want it, make it without oil. Flavor with herbs and spices, and/or nutritional yeast – rather than with salt. The commercial popcorn products contain the ingredients you don't want, including trans-fats, and loads of salt.

- **Pork rinds or pork anything**: Often on the lists of foods most likely to increase the risks of experiencing chronic and degenerative diseases, including cardiovascular and kidney disease, and cancer.

- **Potato foods and snacks**: Au gratin, casseroles (funeral potatoes), chips, fries, hash browns, mashed, puffs, scalloped, skins, soup, or stuffed.

  With kidney disease and/or diabetes, or pre-diabetes, perhaps it is better for you to stick with above-ground vegetables, rather than starchy vegetables.

If you want potatoes, cut them and soak them in water, discard the water, then steam or boil. Wet cooking will avoid creating acrylamides and other inflammatory substances.

- **Pretzels**: Read ingredient labels. These are most likely filled with salt, and made of gluten grains, and perhaps chemical flavorings, preservatives, and other health-depleting substances. Learn to make sourdough pretzel-like snacks at home.

- **Processed cheese slices**: Garbage. Slices of cardiovascular and kidney disease, and health-degrading ingredients.

- **Processed meats**: Including bacon, bratwurst, deli meats, ham, fried pork skin, hot dogs, jerky, lunch meats, pizza meats (including anchovies), salami, salt pork, sausages, and turkey. All health-depleting, and on the list of foods that contribute to various health challenges. Not good for the gut biome, autoimmune system, cardiovascular system, liver, or kidneys.

- **Protein snack bars**: Read ingredient labels.

- **Pudding**: Instant and processed foods are always questionable. Learn to make vegan, oil-free puddings. Chia seed mixed with raw coconut yogurt can created a nice base to then add natural ingredients to flavor, including peaches or berries, vanilla, cinnamon, and lucuma fruit powder.

- **Quiche**: Eggs, oil, salt. See the information in the book about eggs.

- **Ramen**: Read ingredient labels. Another item likely rich in sodium, phosphates, and other ingredients not ideal for someone with kidney or cardiovascular disease, gut issues, autoimmune dysfunction, or cancer.

- **Restaurant food**: Often rich in salt, sugar, oil, and questionable ingredients. Restaurant food is usually made for eating for luxury.

   Restaurant workers aren't your nutritionist, or dietician, or looking out for your health concerns.

   While a vegan restaurant could be a place sometimes to meet someone socially, it is not something you should be depending on for anywhere near the majority of your meals.

   Restaurant food is usually several times more expensive than foods you can make at home.

- **Roasted nuts**: Often with questionable ingredients added for flavor. There should only be one ingredient: nuts.

- **Rolls**: Read ingredients. Avoid those made of low-quality and questionable ingredients. If it isn't good for your gut microbiota, it isn't something good for your health. Store-bought rolls and restaurant rolls also may have been made using additives like potassium bromate, and other chemicals.

- **Salad dressings**: Learn to make your own from scratch, and preferably without oil. See the ForksOverKnives site for recipe ideas.

- **Salami**: A processed meat on the list of foods that can increase the risks of experiencing cancer, and other chronic and degenerative diseases. As with other meat, it isn't going to nurture a healthful but biome, cardiovascular system, or kidneys.

- **Savory snacks**: Learn to make your own with natural ingredients. The company called Bear Bar does sell organic savory snack bars that can also be crumbled to add crunch to salads. These can be helpful to have when traveling.

- **Shrimp**: Cholesterol pills that are really creatures best left to live their lives in the seas, where they help support other life forms in the network of wildlife.
    Shrimp are the roaches of the sea. Leave them alone. Their purpose is in the circle of life within the oceans.

- **Snack foods**: Processed foods are not your friend. Snack foods sold in common grab-n-go stores are usually filled with what depletes and dulls health.

- **Soups and soup mixes**: Canned soups contain the chemicals leached from the can lining. They are also likely to contain damaged oils, salts, and various other ingredients not good for your digestive tract, and that play a role in health challenges.

- **Soy sauce**: If you must have it, look for an organic brand that does not contain MSG, or other questionable ingredients. If you can find that product. Some use coconut liquid aminos, which may also not be something to rely on as a regular food ingredient, but used sparingly once in a while.

- **Sports drinks**: Sugars, or synthetic sweeteners mixed with chemical flavorings, scents, and dyes. Questionable ingredients all around. If you find yourself short on electrolytes, these can be helpful in an urgent situation. Otherwise, rely on water to hydrate.

- **Spreads**: Learn to make your own from natural ingredients. Depending on what sort of taste sensation you are going for, you could likely use a mix of herbs and spices, and a base of water soaked pine nuts blended into a creamy texture with nutritional yeast. Look up recipes for spreads on the ForksOverKnives site.

- **Tapenade**: You could make this from scratch using natural ingredients. One version consists of olives (rinsed in water to reduce sodium), capers, garlic, grated lemon zest, vinegar, herbs (basil, oregano, thyme, rosemary or sage), black pepper, all pulsed in a food processor. The commercially-sold products likely don't contain ingredients that are good for your gut biome.

- **Tofu**: I rarely eat it. If you do, go organic.

- **Tomato juice and sauces**: Learn to make your own from scratch. The store-bought products likely are high in salt, and contain sugars, oils, and other questionable ingredients.
    Because tomato products are high in potassium, as a kidney patient you may have been advised to limit your intake of tomatoes. This could be especially true with concentrated tomato foods, including tomato sauce and catsup – which might also be high in salt.

A cup of tomato sauce can contain about 725 milligrams of potassium, over 2 times the limit.

Fresh, uncooked tomatoes are not concentrated, and you can eat them with less concern about going over the daily potassium limit.

- **Tortillas, tortilla chips, and tortilla soup**: Salt, oil, GMO corn carrying farming chemical residues. If you have space, grow your own corn, and experiment with what you can make from your harvest.

  Corn has been used for thousands of years as a food made using the most simple tools. If it could be done thousands of years ago, you could do it at home.

- **TV dinners**: Junk. Salt, oil, phosphates, and questionable ingredients. Typical for processed, heat-and-eat foods.

- **Vegan junk foods**: There are tons of those in stores and for sale online. Many vegans eat an abundance of them. Those people might say they are only "vegan for the animals," not for other concerns. But maybe they don't value their health. All of the salt, sugar, gluten, and damaged oils, and other questionable ingredients in vegan junk foods can contribute to a variety of health problems, including cardiovascular and kidney disease, and cancer, and nerve degradation, a degraded gut biome, and autoimmune disorders.

- **Vegan meats**: Some of these are so rich in salt, damaged oils, and processed ingredients they can't be considered healthy. But they are there for those who wish to avoid eating animals, and do not want to support the animal farming industry. Also, they can be used to make food for people who insist on eating meat, but who don't know you are using imitation vegan meat products.

- **Veggie burgers**: The store-bought ones could contain a variety of questionable ingredients. But they are there for those who want to avoid eating animals and supporting the animal farming industry. And for those who are feeding someone who really wants the taste, flavor, texture, and smell of meat.

  Veggie burgers are easy enough to make at home using healthier ingredients. They can be frozen for future use. Explore vegan burger recipes online – including on ForksOverKnives.

Artificial sweeteners

I never use artificial sweeteners. These include Equal, Splenda, NutraSweet, Sunette, or any other brands. These typically consist of or contain things like acesulfame, aspartame, saccharin, sucralose, or xylitol. Human nutrition has NO need for any of those substances.

Depending on the type of artificial sweetener, it can increase the risk of experiencing diabetes, stress, inflammation, headaches, learning disabilities, sluggishness, weakness, lack of focus, and kidney disease, cardiovascular disease, heart attack, stroke, neurodegeneration, and cancer.

"In recent years, artificial sweeteners have gained popularity in India's food and beverage sector, largely due to rising concerns about obesity and diabetes. These sweeteners offer benefits such as reduced calorie intake and better blood sugar management. However, emerging research raises concerns about their long-term effects on brain health.

Research indicates that artificial sweeteners like aspartame, sucralose, and saccharin are linked to oxidative stress and neuroinflammation, disruptions to the blood-brain barrier, and changes in cerebral blood flow, which could accelerate cognitive decline. Additionally, they may disrupt the gut microbiome and impair the gut-brain axis, worsening neurocognitive issues. For individuals with conditions like type 2 diabetes and obesity, the effects of artificial sweeteners may be particularly severe, increasing the risk of cognitive impairment and neurodegenerative diseases."

– Artificial Sweeteners on Brain Health: Neurovascular Changes and Cognitive Decline in Indian Population; European Society of Medicine; Apr. 2025

Many processed foods contain artificial sweeteners. They include some brands of cakes, candy, cereals, coffees, colas, cookies, energy drinks, fast foods, icings, salad dressings, snack bars, sodas, yogurt, and other foods. These are often also massively advertised.

Other products that often contain artificial sweeteners include some types of prescription and over-the-counter drugs, and some brands of gum, cough syrup, mouthwash, toothpaste, and chewable vitamins.

The words *sugar-free* on a food label often means the product contains synthetic chemical sweeteners. As in chemicals humans throughout history never ingested – until some company began marketing them.

Research "synthetic sweeteners," and you will likely find a variety of reasons why you would not want them in your body. The U.S. Food and Drug Administration has determined these toxic chemicals to be "safe" below a certain limit. Why put any of that garbage into your body? Learn to enjoy foods without them being tainted with chemicals that can complicate your health, and end you.

If you want something sweet, eat a piece of fruit. Not only the juice.

Stevia as a natural sweetener

Stevia is a plant with leaves that can be dried and crushed to use as a sweetener that doesn't increase blood sugar. Nor does stevia contain the calories of sugar.

Stevia contains anti-inflammatories, antioxidants, vitamins, minerals, amino acids, and fiber.

"Stevia has the potential for a significant improvement of some biochemical parameters in chronic kidney disease patients.

Numerous studies demonstrated that stevia extract improves glucose tolerance in both diabetic and non-diabetic humans."

– Preliminary analysis of the effect of stevia in patients with chronic kidney disease (stage I to stage III); *Elsevier: Contemporary Clinical Trials Communications* journal; Aug. 2018

Some companies sell "stevia" products containing fillers, including other sweeteners, and artificial ingredients.

"Stevia's sweetness comes from something called steviol glycoside found in the leaves. And it's up to 400 times sweeter than the main ingredient of refined sugar, sucrose.

If you want to use a sweetener that's 100% stevia, it's important to check labels."

– Stevia is sweet – But is it good for you?; ClevelandClinic.org; June 2024

Research "stevia and kidneys," and see what you learn.

If you use stevia, get organic, whole leaf powdered stevia. Not an extract, and not a product with additives.

I have grown stevia in my garden. Getting the fresh leaves is as pure as can be.

Consider also getting away from depending on sweetening your foods, including with stevia. Get your taste buds away from luxury flavor. Eat for nutrition.

Sweeteners

Simply get out of the practice of using clarified sugars, including agave, corn syrup, "simple syrup," rice syrup, white sugar, and other sweeteners. The more you avoid them, the more you will be able to taste real food.

A diet rich in clarified sugars is not good for the kidneys, liver, adrenal glands, blood, weight, teeth, bones, nerves, brain, and general health.

If you have been diagnosed with diabetes, or pre-diabetes, be especially sure to maintain a healthy diet free of clarified sugars. Maintaining health also involves daily exercise – especially for anyone with diabetes, cardiovascular, or kidney problems.

If you do want to sweeten your foods, please use minimal natural sweeteners. Maybe consider coconut sugar, date sugar, maple syrup, monk fruit powder, or lucuma fruit powder. Or stevia.

Manuka honey

Manuka honey contains a compound called methylglyoxal (MGO), which is a precursor to endogenous (made in the body) advanced glycation end products (AGEs). It can increase inflammation, oxidative stress, and alter endothelial cells (lining tissues including of the cardiovascular and lymph systems), endoplasmic reticulum (membranes inside cells), and pancreatic function, and play into high blood sugar. These are some reasons I don't use Manuka honey, which is taken from bees that pollinate the tea tree bush (leptospermum scoparium) in Australia and New Zealand. It often is sold as an ideal type of honey because of its antibacterial and anti-inflammatory properties. As something containing methylglyoxal, Manuka honey might not be what someone with kidney disease, diabetes, cardiovascular, or neurodegenerative diseases should be ingesting.

Nightshades as a possible irritant

Nightshades, including tomatoes, potatoes, peppers, eggplant, paprika, and pimentos may be eaten if they are thoroughly cooked, or avoided altogether – and reintroduced into the diet months later to see how the person reacts. Many people will find no reaction, and can continue eating them.

Those with nightshade allergies might experience breathing difficulties, congestion, diarrhea, headaches, hives, nausea, tingling in the mouth.

Research: nightshade allergies.

Almonds as a possible irritant

Those with sensitivity to almonds might find that getting truly raw almonds and soaking them overnight will relieve that issue. After they have been activated, they can be dried and stored for later use.

The liver

By using cholesterol made by your body (you do not need to obtain cholesterol from food), the liver produces the bile that helps manage the bacteria of the small intestine.

A healthy diet helps maintain a healthy liver, which helps maintain a healthy intestinal balance by preventing SIBO (small intestinal bacteria overgrowth), which helps reduce leaky gut syndrome, which then helps the kidneys – and all areas of health.

Bile from the bile ducts helps the digestive system break down foods to access the fat-soluble nutrients, including vitamins A, D, E, and K1, K2, and certain other nutrients.

The liver helps to regulate cortisol, testosterone, and estrogen.

The liver secretes four hormones or hormone precursors, including angiotensinogen, hepcidin, insulin-like growth factor, and thrombopoietin.

Insulin-like growth factor-1 (IGF-1). This hormone is involved with making proteins, with fat burning, and bone growth and maintenance.

Liver malfunction often displays in the feet and ankles. Symptoms may also include dry, scaly, itchy, burning, hot, numb feet with a bad odor, and that might also have toenail fungus, gout in the big toe joints, and callouses, and corns. The ankles swell (edema), and there might be spider angiomas and red or brown dots on the ankles. The liver might be fatty, not producing adequate bile, and not breaking down proteins, or eliminating toxins, and could be inflamed with cirrhosis that results in a swollen belly.

Other symptoms of an unhealthy liver include arthritis, an abundance of belly fat, bile sludge or stones, bloating, an abundance of burping or belching, insulin resistance, joint stiffness, pre-diabetes, diabetes, fatigue or lethargy, gall stones, hormonal imbalance, and hypothyroidism.

Drugs and alcohol

Among the substances that can damage the cardiovascular system and kidneys are drugs, and alcohol.

Those who say drinking wine helps the heart because wine contains antioxidants could be relying on slanted information specifically promoted by the wine industry. Grapes also contain those antioxidants, as do many other fruits and vegetables, sprouts, nuts, and seeds. Nobody needs to be drinking wine – and its sugar and alcohol – to be getting antioxidants, or other botanical nutrients.

"Excessive alcohol intake can lead to high blood pressure, heart failure, or stroke. Excessive drinking can also contribute to cardiomyopathy, a disorder that affects the heart muscle. What's more, alcohol can contribute to obesity, and the long list of health problems that go along with it."
– Alcohol and Heart Health: Separating Fact from Fiction; Johns Hopkins Medicine; 2025

"Alcohol-induced cardiomyopathy is a condition where consuming too much alcohol damages your heart. This damage happens because parts of your heart stretch and enlarge. That weakens your heart muscle, keeping it from pumping as well as it should. Over time, this means your heart can't pump blood as effectively, which reduces your body's available oxygen supply."
– Alcohol-induced Cardiomyopathy; Cleveland Clinic; 2025

"Certain drugs, including painkillers, antibiotics, and illegal substances, can harm your kidneys. Always follow your healthcare provider's instructions and avoid unsupervised medication use.

Every drug you put in your body passes through your kidneys. If the drug is not taken following your healthcare provider's instructions, or if it is an illegal substance, it can cause injury to your kidneys.

Your kidneys could be damaged if you take large amounts of over-the-counter medications, such as aspirin, naproxen, and ibuprofen. None of these medicines should be taken daily, or regularly without first talking to your healthcare provider. Thousands of Americans have damaged their kidneys by using these medicines regularly for too long.

Heavy drinking can hurt both your kidneys, and your liver. Alcoholics have a high risk of developing both kidney and liver failure.

In general, over-the-counter laxatives are safe for most people. However, some prescription laxatives that are used for cleaning the bowel (usually before a colonoscopy) can be harmful to the kidneys.

Some medical imaging tests involve using a contrast dye. Examples of imaging tests are MRIs and CT-scans. Contrast dyes can be harmful to people who have kidney disease. Not all imaging tests involve contrast dyes. If you need to have an imaging test or colonoscopy, let your healthcare provider know if you have kidney disease, or are at risk of getting it.

Most street drugs, including heroin, cocaine, and ecstasy can cause high blood pressure, stroke, heart failure, and even death – in some cases from only one use. Cocaine, heroin, and amphetamines also can cause kidney damage."
– National Kidney Foundation

Any sort of substance abuse combined with certain other health problems can magnify the damage to the kidneys, heart, and other organs, leading to what could be permanent conditions, and/or kidney and/or heart failure.

Any drug or substance you put in your body ends up in the blood, and being filtered through the liver and kidneys.

Drugs and alcohol can damage the stomach and intestinal walls, leading to leaky gut allowing undigested substances into the blood stream, triggering, playing a role in, or worsening autoimmune disorders, including diabetes. All of it can lead to kidney, heart, and other health problems.

Substance abuse

Methamphetamine can worsen kidney problems, and is what is called nephrotoxic. Meth can interfere with the kidney's ability to process waste out of the bloodstream, and contribute to or cause chronic/long-term, or sudden kidney and heart failure.

One way meth can cause permanent kidney damage is by limiting blood flow to the kidneys. This can cause renal tubular necrosis, a situation in which part of the kidney tissue dies, leaving the person with acute kidney injury.

Meth use can also cause changes to the heart (meth-induced cardiomyopathy), leading to arrhythmias, chest pains, hypertension, palpitations, shortness of breath, and myocardial infarction (heart attack).

Meth and cocaine use can also contribute to, or cause renal medullary angiitis, which is inflammation of the blood vessels in the kidneys. In some cases, the person might be put onto dialysis, until the drugs clear their system, and renal function improves.

"It is important to recognize drug-induced vasculitis as patients with true vasculitis often require immunosuppressive therapy, and delay in treatment can result in significant mortality. Illicit drug use (specifically methamphetamine and cocaine) should be in the differential diagnosis of vasculitis as it typically resolves with cessation of the drug."
– Methamphetamine-induced renal pseudovasculitis: Suspicion is the key; *Clinical Case Reports* journal, Dec. 2018

Meth can also damage muscles and other tissues, which can then release proteins that damage the heart and kidneys, leading to long-term health problems, or death.

Drugs like cocaine and meth can increase the heart rate, leading to renal hypertension, which can cause temporary or permanent kidney problems.

In people who already have compromised kidneys, drug-induced rapid heart rate (tachycardia) and renal hypertension can contribute to death from the use of the drugs. One way is renal failure in which the kidneys don't clear waste from the blood, another is blood clots forming within the kidneys, and playing a role in kidney failure.

Diabetes and high blood pressure can be precursors to kidney disease, worsen already compromised kidney situations, and contribute to kidney failure. Anyone abusing drugs or alcohol with those conditions is inviting kidney problems.

Luckily, I was never a drug or alcohol abuser. I've seen many people ruin their lives as they became lost in addictions, including my best friend who died of an alcohol overdose. The substances are terrible for the kidneys and heart – and the adrenal glands, blood, bones, brain, brain stem, digestive tract, liver, lymph system, lungs, muscles, nerves, and all of the organs and tissues.

If you have an addiction to drugs or alcohol, please do what is needed to get away from those substances, and to live more healthfully. Nutrition, exercise, and a healthful sleep pattern are all keys.

Alcohol

If you are a drinker of alcohol, especially if you have a family history of alcoholism, consider eliminating all alcohol. This is one way of protecting your liver, kidneys, brain, nerves, heart, and other organs, tissues, and overall health.

Alcohol and refined carbohydrates (including clarified sugars and bleached grains) are not things you want to put into your body, if you are interested in experiencing the best of health.

The kidneys filter alcohol from the blood. The more alcohol a person drinks, the more the kidneys have to work to clear the alcohol from the system. Binge drinking, even once, can cause acute kidney injury, and permanent kidney damage. Too much alcohol at one time can also shut down the heart.

"Both acute and chronic alcohol consumption can compromise kidney function, particularly in conjunction with established liver disease. Investigators have observed alcohol-relates in the structure and function of the kidneys and impairment in their ability to regulate the volume and composition of fluid and electrolytes in the body. Chronic alcohol patients may experience low blood concentrations of key electrolytes as well as potentially severe alterations in the body's acid-base balance. In addition, alcohol can disrupt the hormonal control mechanisms that govern kidney function. By promoting liver disease, chronic drinking has further detrimental effects on the kidneys, including impaired sodium and fluid handling, and even acute kidney failure."
– Alcohol's Impact on Kidney Function, by Murray Epstein; *Alcohol Health and Research World* journal; 1997

Alcohol and refined carbohydrates can contribute to a fatty liver condition, and cholesterol problems, and those then can result in kidney issues, heart issues, strokes, and heart attacks. Sugar can be converted into the problematic fat and cholesterol, leading to deposits in the body tissues.

"Heavy drinking doubles the risk of developing kidney disease, a long-lasting condition that does not improve over time. It causes the kidneys to work harder, weakening their filtering ability. Alcohol also disrupts the kidneys' ability to balance fluids and electrolytes in the body, leading to dehydration. Dehydration impairs the normal function of cells and organs, including the kidneys.
Even those who only have two drinks per day may have a higher risk of high blood pressure, a leading cause of kidney disease.
Chronic drinking can also lead to liver disease, adding strain on your kidneys. Liver disease can alter the blood flow to the kidneys, lowering their filtering ability."
– Drinking Alcohol Affects Your Kidneys; National Kidney Foundation; 2014

Search: "Alcohol consumption and cancer," "alcohol kidney damage," and "alcohol heart disease."

Fatty liver tests

A liver function blood test can help determine if you have fatty liver disease. This test can be asked for when your blood gets tested in relation to your kidney function, or heart condition.

An ultrasound can also help determine if you have fatty deposits in your liver. This can be ordered when you an ultrasound is done on your kidneys.

A "fibroscan" ultrasound may also be done on your liver.

A more advanced test involves taking a needle biopsy from the liver to be sent to a lab.

If you have diabetes or metabolic syndrome, liver tests are likely done every three years.

Liver and fats

While some healthy fat is good to have in the diet, and needed, you don't want a fatty liver. Unhealthy fats tax the liver. By eating a variety of fruits, vegetables, sprouts, nuts, seeds, and seaweed, you will get enough fat in your diet. As mentioned earlier, every cell of every plant contains oil (fat), and that is all you need – not bottled oils.

Do yourself and your liver a favor by following a lower fat diet, including by eliminating fried foods, and oil-sautéed foods from your diet, as well as dairy products, meat, and eggs.

Fatty liver increases risk of kidney disease, high blood pressure, and other issues

Ongoing fatty deposits in the liver can lead to liver dysfunction, including because of scarring. It also increases the risk of kidney disease and high blood pressure. High blood pressure can also damage the kidneys.

High cholesterol could be associated with liver dysfunction, and be accompanied by fatty liver.

Metabolic syndrome, in which there is a combination of diabetes, high blood pressure, and obesity is often present with fatty liver.

Under the conditions of metabolic syndrome, the gut biome likely is not in a healthful state, which alters nutrient absorption and metabolites, and increases the risk of having permeable intestines – which is leaky gut syndrome. All of this impacts the immune system, and increases the risk of experiencing autoimmune issues.

In women, polycystic ovary syndrome can be related to the development of fatty liver. Pregnant women sometimes also develop fatty liver, which then can be reduced postpartum through a healthy diet and regular exercise.

"The body stores fat for energy and insulation in many areas, including the liver. If the fat content in the liver is too high, it can signify fatty liver disease. Diet changes are the first-line treatment for this condition.

Sugar, alcohol, refined grains, fatty food, and meat should be avoided if a person has fatty liver disease."

– Fatty liver diet: Foods to eat and avoid; *MedicalNewsToday*; Sept. 2023

Liver damage and disease

Information on this topic can fill volumes of books.

Advanced stages of fatty liver disease include inflammation, fibrosis (scarring), cirrhosis (shrunken, inflamed, scarred, and lumpy), cancer, and liver failure.

With a severely damaged liver, a partial or complete transplant likely will be recommended. A partial transplant could be from a living donor who gives part of their liver, and the liver regenerates to its normal size.

Some people undergo both a kidney transplant and liver transplant at the same time.

Increasing the risk of fatty liver disease

In addition to smoking, and lack of exercise, things that increase the chances of experiencing fatty liver disease include high alcohol consumption (alcohol-related liver disease [ARLD]), a high-fat diet, obesity, and diseases often experienced in combination with fatty liver: diabetes, and insulin resistance.

Foods that contribute to having a fatty liver include fried and sautéed oils, red meat, processed meats, dairy products, eggs, bleached grains, and also regular consumption of sodas, colas, and other drinks and foods with clarified sugars (corn syrup, rice syrup, agave, cane and beet sugar, etc.).

In other words, follow a low-fat, clean, plant-based diet, and you will lower your risk of experiencing fatty liver.

"Non-alcoholic fatty liver disease (NAFLD) is the term for a range of conditions caused by a build-up of fat in the liver. It's usually seen in people who are overweight or obese.

High levels of fat in your liver is also associated with an increased risk of serious health problems, such as diabetes, high blood pressure, and kidney disease.

If you already have diabetes, NAFLD increases your chance of developing hearth problems."
– Non-alcoholic fatty liver disease (NAFLD); National Health Institute UK; 2025

Liver and leaky gut, enteric toxins, and macromolecules

Under conditions of leaky gut, the liver is continually being taxed by having to remove oxidized enteric toxins (occurring in the intestines) and macromolecules (the larger molecules able to pass through a damaged intestinal barrier). This can worsen the conditions of those with hepatitis, other liver issues, autoimmune disorders (diabetes, arthritis, lupus, etc.), cancer, and cardiovascular and kidney diseases.

Cleaning up the liver

One herb helpful for both the kidneys and liver is milk thistle. Read up about it. Plant some, including to help your local butterfly populations exist. Make tea of it.

Because both the liver and kidneys have to deal with eliminating toxins from the body, you would do yourself a favor by following an organic diet free of ultra-processed foods. This way you are less likely to be ingesting a variety of toxic chemicals (including fungicides, insecticides, herbicides, pesticides, miticides, synthetic food additives, and other toxins). As always, following a clean diet is better for you, and also for farmers, their communities, the environment, and wildlife.

As is recommended for kidney issues, to help your liver, follow a diet rich in fruits and vegetables, stay hydrated with water, avoid sweetened drinks, drinks and foods containing synthetic chemicals, and alcoholic beverages. Eat fruit instead of drinking fruit juice. Avoid clarified sugars. Follow a low-fat and low-salt diet. Don't use tobacco. Avoid addictive substances. Avoid processed, fried, and oil-sautéed foods. Do exercise first thing every morning, with other movement done throughout the day.

Cruciferous veggies for liver health: glucoraphanin and sulforaphane

Cruciferous vegetables – also called brassica vegetables – are often noted as being beneficial for the liver. They are rich in nutrients that protect against heart disease, kidney disease, autoimmune disorders, and nerve degeneration. These vegetables include arugula, bok choy, broccoli, Brussels sprouts, cabbage, collard greens, cauliflower, kale, and turnips, and their sprouted seeds.

Cruciferous vegetables contain chemicals called thiocyanates, which can interfere with iodine absorption. This is why it is good to not overdo it with cruciferous vegetables by including them in every meal. Steaming, boiling, using them in soups and stews, and non-oil sautéing, are ways of cooking that reduce the amount of thiocyanates. Eating some cruciferous vegetables every week is a good thing, but overdoing it can load your system with thiocyanates, and play into thyroid disorders. No need to have them in every meal – especially if they are raw. Have some raw (like kale in a smoothie), and have some heated to reduce the thiocyanates.

"It is (broccoli) sprout's high concentration of a potent substance called sulforaphane that makes them a so-called superfood, a favorite of dieticians, health bloggers, and homeopaths everywhere. Paul Talalay, a researcher at Johns Hopkins, was the one to find that the sulforaphane in broccoli – the full-grown version of the sprout – significantly increases the body's ability to fend off cancer."
– Hope Sprouts Eternal, by Ashley Stimpson; *Johns Hopkins Magazine*; 2023

Broccoli sprouts are rich in vitamin C, and contain up to half as much more glucoraphanin than broccoli. As the plant grows, the glucoraphanin content decreases. When eaten by humans, the nutrient is metabolized by the gut microbiota into sulforaphane, which helps the liver in its detox processes, as it increases liver enzyme activity, decreases oxidative stress within the liver, and is a strong anti-cancer substance. The glucoraphanin nutrient is also in other cruciferous vegetables.

Learn to grow broccoli sprouts, and include those in your weekly diet. A glass jar with a stainless steel screen top held slanted nearly upside down in a stand helps prevent mold and insects. Rinse at least once per day with filtered water, and keep the jar tilted nearly upside down for the water to drain.

Sprouts can be included in raw smoothies, blended into raw juices, tossed into salads, included in wraps and sandwiches, and used as an ingredient in dinner bowls.

Soy

When some people hear you follow a vegan diet they might say, "You must eat a lot of soy." They are exposing their misunderstanding of plant-based nutrition. It might also be in alignment with the assumption that nutrition is all about "getting enough protein," and soy is how to get protein in the vegan diet. They also might think we need to mix rice and beans to get a "complete protein."

I don't eat much soy. There is no main reason. Some avoid it because of the estradiol isoflavones, daidzein and genistein in soy, but also because of the lectins, saponins, phytates (not that phytates should always be avoided – see the phytate section), and goitrogens, and the heat-generated chemicals glycotoxins, and acrylamides formed in soy when it is cooked, and the enzyme inhibitors – including protease inhibitors – in soy that can interfere with protein digestion.

Those using soy protein powders are dwelling in the misinformation of marketing claims made by the soy industry. It is an industry successful in promoting itself as an ideal food. Most soy protein powders are from GMO plants grown using synthetic farming chemicals.

Throughout human history, not many humans ate soy. For thousands of years soybeans had been eaten in China. It's only been in recent centuries that soybeans have become a food on other continents.

Most soy grown on Earth is for feeding to farmed animals. Soy also isn't good for them. It is fed to them so they gain as much weight as fast as possible so they can be sold for as much as possible – as soon as possible.

Soy grown using genetically modified beans almost always equates to the soy products containing some level of residues of the chemicals used on non-organic farms.

One benefit of soy is as a nitrogen fixer and fertilizer for garden soil and farming. This is one reason why it is planted. On farms the added benefit is the soy can then be sold.

The soy fiasco

Some view the soy industry as having done an excellent job of promoting soy as a health food. It is, or is it not? A look into what soy may – or may not – do to human health might change your mind about soy – and, at least, help you to make wiser choices if you do consume soy.

While soy is found in many "natural" foods, and is sold at "health food" stores, it is found in an increasing amount of processed foods with claims it is beneficial to health. Or, is it? Reports are conflicting. It also depends on how that soy was grown and processed, and what else is in the foods.

"The amount in which humans use soy may come with a caveat, according to emerging research. Soybeans are the most potent source of isoflavones amongst all foods on the market today. Isoflavones are a plant compound that serves as a natural fungicide to protect the soy plant as it grows, but isoflavones have the capacity to alter epigenetics in plants, animals, and fungi alike.

In humans, isoflavones mimic the estradiol compound in the body, a precursor to the estrogen hormone, and can raise over-all serum estrogen. Elevated estrogen levels can be significant on a physiological level. Elevated estrogen can do anything from alleviate hot flashes in menopausal women, to potentially interacting with thyroid hormones, to perhaps complicating fertility and health cell growth. Elevated serum estrogen can be a cause of breast cancer among women as well.

Conflicting messages have reached the cancer community regarding soy consumption. However, there is not enough fortified research yet to support a

link between soy consumption and cancer or cancer remission."
— Soy Intake and Hormonal Health Complications, by Lynne Hebert; Montana State University; 2020

"The FDA wants to pull its support of the health claim that eating soy protein may help reduce the risk of heart disease. The agency proposed the change last fall, citing evidence that questions whether there's any real benefit to heart health. If the FDA goes through with the move, then food makers will no longer be allowed to market soy products with the claim that they can help your heart. But soy won't hurt your heart, and soy does have other benefits. 'It's high in polyunsaturated fats, fiber, vitamins, and minerals, and low in saturated fat. Natural soy products — like tofu and edamame — could replace red meat and other animal sources of protein higher in saturated fat,' says dietitian Kathy McManus, director of the Department of Nutrition at Harvard-affiliated Brigham and Women's Hospital. One caveat: some soy products contain estrogen-like chemicals that could have adverse effects. So, stay away from soy isoflavone supplement and foods made with textured vegetable protein, and soy protein isolate found in many protein powders and nutrition bars. Still, McManus says it's okay to eat whole soy foods — like soy milk, edamame, and tofu — in moderation, several times per week."
— Confused about eating soy?; Harvard Health Publishing: Harvard Medical School; Sept. 2021

"Phytoestrogens have received a large amount of attention over the past few decades, particularly because of their potential estrogenic effects. For this reason, much research has examined possible benefits of phytoestrogens on menopause symptoms, although results have been mixed."
— Is There Such a Thing as "Anti-Nutrients"? A Narrative Review of Perceived Problematic Plant Compounds; *Nutrients Journal*; Sept. 2020

There are other issues with soy that may – or may not – concern you, including:

Soy contains the isoflavones daidzein and genistein, which are known as phytoestrogens. They can mimic estrogen in the body, binding with estrogen receptors on the cells. Some people claim these play a role in breast and endometrial cancers. Studies are a bit confusing, with some concluding the isoflavones in soy are antioxidants that protect tissues, are anti-inflammatory, reduce risk of cancer as they may block the receptors from binding with more potent natural estrogen, and also act to block estrogens from forming in fatty tissue, which is one of the problems with estrogen production – especially in women who are overweight when they are past menopause.

"The quantity of phytoestrogens found in just a single cup of soy milk may reduce the risk of breast cancer returning by 25 percent."
— Dr. Michael Greger, in his book *How Not to Die*; NutritionFacts.org; DrGreger.org

Search: Benefits of soy milk.

Women and soy

Epidemiological studies have concluded that women who consume more soy may be less likely to experience breast cancer. However, other dietary issues may come into play in reducing cancer risk, such as the likelihood those who include more soy in their diet may be apt to follow a more vegetarian or vegan diet, thus reducing their cancer risk by not eating meat, milk, eggs, animal fats, or bone broth.

Men and soy

While men also are at risk for breast cancer, their concern with avoiding soy products usually revolves around the risk of the phytoestrogens daidzein and genistein playing roles in enlarged breasts (gynecomastia), decreased libido, weaker erections (E.D.), lower sperm counts, loss of body hair, and mood swings. For these hormonal reasons some men avoid soy products.

Studies concluding that men who consume soy may have lower rates of prostate cancer might overlook the fact that men who consume soy are following more of a vegetarian or vegan diet, thus reducing their risk of prostate cancer because they aren't eating animal protein.

Men who think they need the protein in soy for their workout may want to consider what soy protein powder (soy protein isolates) is doing to their body tissues and hormonal balance. Soy protein isolates may be rough on the liver, or… not…

"Soybean significantly affected liver function, fatty liver, and oxidative stress indicators. The current meta-analysis combined preclinical and clinical studies and verified that soybean could protect the liver in non-alcoholic fatty liver disease by regulating lipid metabolism and oxidative stress factors via the Akt/AMPK/PPARa signaling pathway. Soybean might be a promising therapeutic agent for treating non-alcoholic fatty liver disease."
– Preclinical and clinical evidence for the treatment of non-alcoholic fatty liver disease with soybeans: A systematic review and meta-analysis; *Frontiers in Pharmacology*; Jan. 2023

"Soy isoflavones decrease fat deposits in the liver through reducing adipogenesis and lipogenesis and activating the expression of PPAR-a to potentiate fatty acid oxidation in the liver. Hence, soy isoflavones could ameliorate the progression of non-alcoholic fatty lifer disease via decreasing ALT and improving liver structure.

Soy isoflavones have antioxidant properties via scavenging free radicals, and promoting the activity of antioxidant enzymes, and thereby leading to protection against oxidative stress damage."
– Effect of soy consumption on liver enzymes, lipid profile, anthropometry indices, and oxidative stress in patients with non-alcoholic fatty liver disease: A systematic review and meta-analysis of clinical trials; *Iran Journal of Basic Medical Science*; Oct. 2020

Soy products

If you choose to have soy milk, look at the other ingredients on the label, and consider if they are health promoting, or negating substances.

Soy milk and tofu are often mixed with unhealthful ingredients, and often have been so highly heated they are rich in AGEs.

It is good to steer clear of soy isoflavone supplements, isolated soy protein products, and textured vegetable (soy) protein.

Edamame is simply steamed or boiled immature soybeans in their pods, and may be the most nutritious form of soy.

Soy milk, plant-based milks, and cow's milk

I grew up drinking cow milk. I stopped drinking it in my late teens, as it started to taste rather disgusting. I then learned of what is in it (a certain amount of blood and puss is "acceptable" under government guidelines), and how cows are treated: mechanically raped to keep them pregnant so they produce milk. When their milk production slows, they are sent to slaughter to be turned into cheap meat – fast food burgers and taco filling.

There are also the pro-inflammatory issues of dairy, the potential for increasing or worsening autoimmune disorders, and triggering or otherwise playing a role in chronic and degenerative diseases – including Alzheimer's, diabetes, cardiovascular disease, cancer, and osteoporosis – and increasing the likelihood of skin issues, asthma, and other health maladies.

The health concerns with eating dairy include it playing a role in making kidney infections worse, and increasing the risk of developing kidney stones, and kidney disease.

The casein protein in milk can also reduce capillaries in the kidneys, slowing kidney function, and worsening chronic kidney disease.

As far as plant-based milk, I normally simply blend a half banana with water, hemp seeds, and perhaps some lucuma or maca powder and vanilla. Making such a simple milk at home is easy, less expensive, and avoids the fillers in many of the commercially available plant-based milk brands. It is also easy to make hemp seed milk, which is highly nutritious. (See YouTube videos about how to make hemp milk, and other plant-based milks..)

Consider what NutritionFacts has to say about milk, including considering what medical journals say about dairy consumption:

"'After weaning [when young children stop drinking breast milk], milk of any kind is not required, and really shouldn't be relied upon as a main source of calories. Children will be fine with water and a healthy, balanced diet.

If you are going to give children [dairy] milk, there would seem to be a better choice.

Most plant-based milks on the market have the same amount [of calcium as dairy].

More importantly, the consumption of cow's milk carries risks, 'Although cow's milk is rich in calcium, it does not appear to clearly reduce fractures, but consumption carries risks including: a potential association with type I diabetes mellitus onset; anemia in toddlers; lactose intolerance; cow's milk protein allergy; and infantile colic.'

So, the adverse effects from just normal consumption of cow's milk must be compared against the risks from plant-based milks, which are problematic mainly when used inappropriately, meaning like to the exclusion of most other foods: diets that are clearly inappropriate, like the case of [a child named} Kwashiorkor in Atlanta, because his diet was basically 99% rice milk.

Plant-based milks have the benefit of being low in saturated fat, free of cholesterol, and though the protein content is generally lower than in cow's milk, plant-based milks are richer in terms of fiber. Cow's milk has zero fiber. But the fiber content in plant-based milks can be pretty pitiful [This is: commercially available plant-based milks sold in stores: homemade plant milks can be MUCH richer in fiber] compared to the whole foods from which they were derived.

Soy milk is likely the least processed out of all plant-based milks. Soy milk has the additional benefit of reducing breast cancer risk in girls, and normalizing development. Soy milk consumption is also associated with lower prostate cancer risk in men. And interventional studies suggest improved gut health by boosting the growth of good bacteria."
– Is Soy Milk the Most Nutritious Non-Dairy Milk; NutritionFacts.org; quoting from *Maternal and Child Health Journal*; 2024

The whole thing about the hormones and industrial chemicals in dairy milk, as well as the mass breeding and continual impregnation of cows to keep them producing milk, and the role the feed crop industry plays in environmental destruction and wildlife extinction continue as problems. These are more reasons to choose plant-based milks, and skip the moo.

There are a wide variety of plant-based milks sold in stores, some more nutritious then others.

Store-bought milks including almond, cashew, hazelnut, hemp, macadamia, oat, pea protein, soy, and others. Do your research about which is healthier. Read labels and compare the ingredients, including those that might not be what you want.

Depending on ingredients, homemade plant milks could always be the most healthy, fiber-rich, and least expensive choice.

Soy and protein powders

Soy protein and other isolated protein powders are not advised for people with – or wanting to prevent having – kidney disease. The protein isolates can increase the amount of nitrogen waste in the blood. This can be harsh on the kidneys, and especially problematic for people with kidney disease.

The biggest benefit of consuming cheap, GMO soy protein powder is to the bank accounts of the stores and companies selling or marketing it.

The estradiol production issues related to soy are reasons why some men avoid it. But, are they misguided? Do your research, and do what is right for you.

The phytates in soy may interfere with the absorption of minerals.

The lectins and saponins in soy may interfere with the function of the digestive tract, and help to cause leaky gut syndrome, which can increase the risk of experiencing arthritis and other autoimmune disorders.

The protease inhibitors in soy interfere with the digestion of protein.

If you are trying to improve your health, soy protein powders are not your solution. Stick to whole soy products, not protein powders, or extracts: soy oil.

Whey and casein protein powders from cow milk are also not healthful, because consuming casein increases the risk of cancer, arthritis, Type-2 diabetes, cardiovascular disease, a weak gut biome, and other maladies.

Instead of consuming protein powders containing soy, whey, or casein, eat more leafy green vegetables and raw fruit. Plants contain the amino acids (the components of protein), antioxidants, anti-inflammatories, fiber, vitamins, minerals, essential fatty acids, and other macro and micronutrients we need.

Soy and baby formula

Soy may negatively impact the thymus gland, which plays a role in the production of white blood cells – which are key to a healthy immune system. This is one reason why soy may not be a good choice for baby formula. Infants fed soy-based formula may also have an increased risk of asthma and other health issues later in life.

If a baby does not have access to breast milk – which should always be the first choice in baby food – consider other options, including hemp milk high speed blended with chia seeds, and other types of non-dairy milk rich in nutrients, including healthy fats. Do your research to make the best decision for you and the child.

"*Consumer Reports* recently tested 41 types of powdered formula for a number of toxic chemicals, including arsenic, lead, BPA, acrylamide, and PFAS. We looked at established formulas like Enfamil and Similac, newer startups like Bobbie, popular store brands, and imported brands.

Some of the results were concerning: about half of the samples we tested contained harmful levels of at least one contaminant."
– We Tested 41 Baby Formulas for Lead and Arsenic, by Lauren Kirchner; *Consumer Reports*; March 2025

From the earliest months of their lives many babies are being fed unhealthful foods that increase the risk of a variety of chronic and degenerative conditions, including kidney and cardiovascular disease, leaky gut, metabolic syndrome, cancer, neural degeneration, and diabetes and other autoimmune disorders. If a child is already genetically predisposed to certain health conditions, what they are fed can increase the risks of experiencing them.

Whatever an infant consumes ends up being filtered through their digestive tract, liver, and kidneys.

One study looked at the marketing claims various companies have used to promote infant formula:

"Our first example is partially hydrolyzed whey protein dominant formula, which has carried claims of reduced eczema or milk allergy in many regions for many years based on selected date from individual trials and two industry funded systematic reviews in 2010. However, two rigorous and independent systematic reviews subsequently found no evidence to support this claim, and in 2016 the UK Food Standards Agency's committee on toxicity concluded there is 'no evidence that hydrolyzed formula prevents eczema or milk allergy.'

Infants and their carers are not being adequately protected from adverse consequences of claims about infant formula. The current regulatory environment is permissive and associated with poorly substantiated and potentially harmful claims."

– Health and nutrition claims for infant formula are poorly substantiated and potentially harmful; British Medical Association journal; May, 2020)

The heavy metals and farming chemical residues, including pesticides, and Melamine (given to cows to increase milk production) in mass marketed baby formula are bad enough. One glance at the ingredient list of many of the commercial brands of baby formula – including the amount of corn syrup (often listed as glucose sugar, and also other added sugars), gluten, mineral oil, palm oil (and other oils), soy protein isolate (rich in phytoestrogens that mimic estrogen), preservatives, carrageenan, synthetic nutrients (including artificially produced lutein, L-methionine, lycopene, nucleotides, and taurine), and other junk substances – is reason to do some research about what is most healthful for your child.

Enzyme inhibitors, phytates, and goitrogens in soy

In addition to isoflavones, soy products often contain an abundance of enzyme inhibitors, phytates, and also substances called goitrogens that could suppress both iodine uptake and thyroid function. Even soaking raw soybeans doesn't rid the beans of the substances; cooking them also doesn't rid them of the goitrogens. These are some of the reasons why some people avoid soy.

Research goitrogens, and see what you learn.

"Plant-derived goitrogens are another set of compounds which have received attention among nutrition researchers and health professionals. The term 'goitrogen' broadly refers to agents that interfere with thyroid function, thus increasing the risk of goiter, and other thyroid diseases. Sources of these compounds include medications, environmental toxins, as well as certain foods. Glocosinolates, a diverse class of over 120 compounds, are dietary goitrogens found primarily in the Brassica family, as well as other plant foods. Upon mastication and ingestion, the enzyme myrosinase (activated in damaged plant tissue and produced by human microflora) converts glocosinolates to a variety of other compounds, including thiocyanates, nitriles, isothiocyanates, and sulforaphane. Much research surrounding glocosinolates and associated analogues have focused on their potential to prevent cancer, induce Phase II detoxification enzymes, induce apoptosis, regulate redox reactions, and inhibit Phase I detoxification enzymes.

Overall, most human studies investigating the effects of goitrogenic foods on thyroid health display neutral effects, although some conflicting results are still present. Evidence seems to suggest that suboptimal iodine status may potentiate any negative impacts of dietary goitrogens on thyroid health. Furthermore, progoitrin content amongst the Brassica genus varies significantly. Items such as broccoli, Chinese cabbages, bok choy, broccoli sprouts, and some kale varieties generally contain progoitrin and thiocyanate-generating glucosinolates at concentrations far below those likely to cause a physiological effect. In fact, consuming these foods as part of a varied, colorful, plant-based diet should not post significant risks in healthy individuals, and, conversely, may be of great benefit. In addition to beneficial glucosinolates, cruciferous vegetables provide a plethora of other health-promoting phytochemicals, fiber, and essential vitamins and minerals. For those with thyroid disease, or at higher risk of thyroid disease, long-term daily intake of progoitrin-rich items, like Russian kale, broccoli rabe, or collard greens may decrease iodine uptake, and should be cooked with iodized salt to avoid reduced iodine uptake."

– Is There Such a Thing as "Anti-Nutrients"? A Narrative Review of Perceived Problematic Plant Compounds; *Nutrients Journal*; Sept. 2020

Processed foods and soy

Some people go for the organic, non-GMO, fermented soy products, such as miso and tamari (which can be sodium-heavy). There are non-soy versions of these products, including garbanzo bean/chickpea or brown rice miso in place of soy miso, or coconut aminos instead of tamari.

Nama shoyu is also a fermented soy product. If used, seek the unpasteurized type made from organic, non-GMO soy beans. I avoid nama shoyu, as I don't like the taste, or the way it makes me feel.

Many processed and packaged foods contain soy, including in the forms of hydrolyzed vegetable protein, lecithin, soy extract, soy protein, soy flour, soy cheese, tempeh, natto, nutrition bars, soy isolate, soy oil, and other forms of soy. Soy in some form can be found in everything from processed fruit juices to potato chips and hamburgers.

Even foods many consider to be healthy, such as certain brands of bottled so-called "natural juices," contain low-grade soy ingredients. That is, not just any soy, but genetically modified soy – which likely carries residues of toxic farming chemicals. These may be damaging to gut flora and the intestinal lining.

Soy tends to give me heartburn, so I avoid it. Especially soy oil.

Soy oil is usually hydrogenated, which is rich in transfats that promote cardiovascular disease.

Cooking soy

Cooking soy at high temperatures creates a variety of heat-generated chemicals, including acrylamides and glycotoxins, which cause an immune response, can damage the intestinal flora, and the lining of the stomach and intestines, and can contribute to degenerative diseases.

See the AGEs information in this book.

Casein = dairy is in some products sold as "vegan"

"Back in the bad old days, soy cheese companies often added casein to their products without disclosing it as a milk ingredient. This tricked quite a few vegans into eating the stuff. To this day, there are still some soy- or almond-based cheeses on the market that contain casein.

As food technology has advanced, vegan cheese companies have discovered plant-based ingredients that replicate casein's meltability. There are now several great vegan cheeses on the market that have the same stretchiness as dairy-based cheese."

– Is Casein Vegan? Milk Proteins and Vegan Cheese; Vegan.com

Casein from milk is in so-called "non-dairy" creamers, and some other "vegan" products

Consider what is in a product many people use every day, coffee creamer. Following is a list of the ingredients of Coffee-Mate as posted on LabelWatch.com.

"Coffee-Mate, fat free liquid nondairy creamer. Ingredients: Water, corn syrup solids, partially hydrogenated soybean oil, and/or cottonseed oil, (adds a trivial amount of fat), less than 2 percent sugar, modified cornstarch, dipotassium phosphate, sodium caseinate (milk derivative), not a source of lactose, color added, artificial flavor, mono and diglycerides, polysorbate 60, sodium stearoyl lactylate, carrageenan, salt, beta-carotene, color."
– LabelWatch.com

If you consider that sodium caseinate is derived from milk, you may ask why a milk product is in a product labeled "dairy-free"?

Dairy extracts are also in some other products people might think are dairy-free, and products that might be labeled as dairy-free, but they might contain sodium caseinate, whey, and other components of milk. These include some brands of margarine, chocolate, cereal bars, "non-dairy" cheeses, breads, crackers, and other baked products.

"Casein proteins can be separated from milk and used independently as a supplement, or additive to thicken, texturize, and stabilize various food products.

Because sodium caseinate is derived from cow's milk, it's not appropriate for vegan or dairy-free diets. This can be somewhat confusing, as many processed foods labeled "nondairy" contain sodium caseinate. Examples include nondairy coffee creamers, and some nondairy processed cheeses."
– What Is Sodium Caseinate? Everything You Need to Know, by Ansley Hill, RD, LD; June 2020

So-called "non-dairy" creamer containing a variety of low-grade and synthetic chemical ingredients is among the first things people put into their stomachs,

The corn syrup, cornstarch, soybean oil, and cottonseed oil in non-dairy creamers are very likely from GMO crops sprayed with a variety of toxic farming chemicals.

What are those words, diglycerides and polysorbate 60 on the label of the non-dairy creamer?

Research: carrageenan, corn syrup, soybean oil, and hydrogenated oils. You likely would not want them in your food. It should be clear why they also would not be good for the gut biome.

If you want to experience vibrant health, don't ingest foods containing synthetic chemicals, corn syrup, corn sweetener, corn oil, soy oil, casein, sodium caseinate, carrageenan, hydrogenated oils, partially hydrogenated oils, diglycerides, polysorbate, or dairy.

Distance yourself from processed foods.

If it is a chemical formulated in a lab, don't eat it.

The factory farmed animal protein industry

Considering what people are eating, and while they are thinking they are doing what is right for their nutrition, when they are eating the most toxic foods humans have ever eaten is a bit surreal. It plays out in the health of those who consume the foods. Their illnesses support the medical and pharmaceutical industries. At one point, I was becoming one of those sickly people unaware of what toxic foods were doing to me.

Some of the most problematic foods people consume are what is produced by the animal farming industry.

As corporate-produced animal protein products became common foods in the U.S. and other countries, more and more money went into breeding and raising millions upon millions – and millions more – farmed animals. Into the billions per year. This meant more and more money went into planting more and more millions of acres of feed crops to feed the massively overbred farmed animals – on every continent.

Starting in the 1950s, the industrialization of the animal farming industry went into full swing. Chemicals were used to spray the fields of feed crops – and also the crops grown for human consumption. Pharmaceutical drugs also increasingly were used on farmed animals. Feed crops, meat, dairy products, and eggs began being shipped all over the planet. Billions of dollars began flowing in and out of the global industrial feed crop, meat (including fish), dairy, and egg industries every HOUR.

With some "animal farms" breeding and containing tens of thousands of animals under one roof, the farming industry continued to grow as larger and larger facilities were built to contain more and more farmed animals – in miserable, crowded, loud, stressful, and otherwise horrible conditions.

It was found the disgusting and awful way of keeping farmed animals indoors was the most financially-convenient way to raise them. Animals were then spending their entire lives indoors, on concrete floors, and/or in cages.

The crowded conditions of the incarcerated animals increased the risk of injuries and diseases among them. More pharmaceutical drugs were used, increasing the drug-resistant strains of infectious diseases – the same illnesses that also make humans sick.

It also became common to spray the incarcerated animals with chemicals to prevent mold, fungus, and the infestation of insects. The dairy and meat from the animals contain residues of these chemicals.

With factory farming came animals experiencing injured feet, and also injuries from fighting among the stressed and frustrated animals. They truly suffer. The bodies of farmed animals typically are altered. Toes and the ends of beaks of chickens and turkeys are cut off to reduce fight injuries. Pigs have teeth cut, tales removed, and other body modifications to reduce the injuries from fighting with other pigs.

The diets of factory farmed animals have been designed to enlarge the animals as fast as possible to get them to market weight.

Cows are mechanically impregnated, and kept on a schedule of impregnation and milking, impregnating, and milking. The baby bulls are sent off to slaughter, and their meat is sold as "veal."

The baby cows are kept to mechanically impregnate so they can produce milk to sell as human food in the form of milk, butter, cheese, cream, yogurt, kefir, whey, and casein. Then, after about 3 to 4 years, the cows are slaughtered for cheap meat. (Cows would otherwise normally live about 20 years.)

The animal farming industry is about money. Not about health. Not about human nutritional needs.

The animal farming industry has been good about formulating marketing and advertising campaigns to promote their products. This includes publishing materials to hand out to school kids to encourage them to eat meat, dairy, and eggs – as the industrially-produced marketing propaganda that is the "food pyramid" tells them to.

Dairy industry: refrigeration increased it

With the growth of the refrigeration industry, the dairy industry flourished. Human diseases relating to the consumption of dairy also increased.

Stockholders making money is all that matters for the largest companies so they can grow, and sell more product.

To satisfy the growing demand for dairy, the industry produced more commercials, getting people to buy more… so the industry and the stockholders could make more money. They got laws passed, and government funding funneled into the industry. Part of that included selling dairy products to public schools, jails, prisons, and the military.

The dairy industry is big into government contract work.

Corporate welfare fuels the animal farming and feed crop industries

Many politicians and those in government make money in some way from the dairy, meat, egg, and feed crop industries. They help to get the industries funded with what amounts to corporate welfare. The money and services the government provides for the industries hides how expensive meat, dairy, and eggs truly are. If it weren't for the corporate welfare, meat, dairy, and eggs would be much more expensive than what people pay for them in grocery stores and restaurants. Without the government funding all the expenses of raising millions upon millions of acres of crops, and billions of animals would be included in the prices people pay for the meat, dairy, and eggs.

"In most of the countries, the meat industry gets more subsidies from the government than the fruit and vegetable industries, though the same governments recommend their citizens to eat more vegetables and fruits.

The U.S. government spends $38 billion each year to subsidize the meat and dairy industries, but only 0.40 percent of that (i.e. $17 million) each year to subsidize fruits and vegetables. A $5 Big Mac would cost $13 if the retail price included hidden expenses that meat producers offload onto society. A pound of hamburger will cost $30 without any government subsidies."

– Saving the Planet: The Market for Sustainable Meat Alternatives; Pantas and Ting Sutardja Center for Entrepreneurship & Technology, Berkely Engineering; Nov. 2015

As years have gone on, more and more of the industrial dairy, meat, and feed grain industries have become reliant on money from the governments of various countries. This includes to build infrastructure to serve the animal farming and associated industries, including roads and bridges, water systems, and power sources.

The U.S. government also kills off millions of wild animals that could harm feed crops, or that might kill farmed animals. This is the chief reason why predator animals like bears, wolves, bobcat, cougar, jaguar, and others have largely been killed off across the U.S. It's all been about farmed animals, and food industry profits – not about what is good for human or environmental health.

In the U.S., federal, state, county, and city government systems were altered or created to purchase more and more meat, dairy, and eggs for government institutions, including everything from schools to the military, and jails and prisons.

The "food pyramid" was created to sell industrial foods

The "food pyramid" was created to help people believe they need to include meat, dairy, and eggs in their daily diet. As if plants don't contain all the amino acids we need to form proteins.

Printouts of the food pyramid, and "educational" videos about nutrition were funded by the meat, dairy, and egg industries to distribute to schools. It was all done to sell products, to make money, and not to educate people on the best nutrition. It wasn't done out of concern for the health of the children. It was done to satisfy the financial desires of the animal farming industry.

Government money in the feed crop and animal farming industries

The growing of feed crops, and raising of farmed animals, and marketing of meat, dairy, and eggs has been very specifically reliant on government money in the form of "corporate welfare."

They say spending government money to support the animal farming and feed crop industries builds "American" jobs, when, in fact, the industrialization of the food industry uses more and more robotic farming equipment to grow crops on larger fields, reducing the number of people working in the industry. The factory animal farms also hold more and more animals, and rely less on workers, and more on automated feeding and other systems.

The feed crop, animal farming, and slaughterhouse and "meat processing" industries are heavily reliant on low-paid people who are willing to do the work that is some of the most high-risk labor. Workers in the animal farming industry are more likely to be injured – or killed – than workers in many other industries.

U.S. Department of Agriculture is a trade organization

The U.S. Department of Agriculture can be viewed as a concierge service for the feed grain, meat, dairy, and egg industries. Their service is promoting the products of those industries.

Food advertising mentioning a product is approved by the U.S.D.A. is meaningless, and not a way to decide what is best for your nutritional needs. People have been gullible to the marketing of the products as they fell under the impression that the U.S.D.A. approval meant the meat, dairy, and eggs products should be part of a "healthy diet." In fact, the more meat, dairy, and eggs you eat, the more likely you are to experience a variety of health challenges, including kidney and cardiovascular disease, autoimmune disorders, nerve and brain degeneration, and cancer.

Degraded nature is largely a result of human food choices

"It is widely understood that livestock have a heavy impact on the climate, and research indicates that switching to a plant-based diet is one of the most impactful steps individuals can take to reduce their carbon emissions from food. Animal products are responsible for 57% of global food-related emissions, compared with plant-based foods, which contribute 29% of the total – even though animals provide less than one-fifth of the world's total energy from food.

Low meat diets can be beneficial across a range of environmental reasons, with vegan diets having lower greenhouse gas emissions, lower water use, and lower impacts on [wildlife] biodiversity."
– How a month of abstinence can lead to "meat disgust," by Matilda Welin; BBC; Feb. 2025

We know that most cardiovascular and kidney disease, and cancers, and autoimmune disorders are directly linked to diet. So is much of the plastic and roadside pollution, environmental damage, soil degradation, deforestation, desertification, water dead zones, climate change, and the loss of wildlife diversity. This all is not a maybe, it is an absolute.

"A U.K. study has assessed the environmental impact of high-meat, low-meat, vegetarian, and vegan diets, conclusively showing that avoiding animal products has significant benefits for the planet.

Described as the most detailed research of its kind ever to be done, the study looked at the real eating habits of 55,0000 people, as opposed to using model diets like many previous reports. It found that low-meat diets have half the emissions and land use as high-meat diets, while adopting a vegan diet can halve these figures again – totaling a 75% reduction.

Plant-based diets were also demonstrated to reduce water use by 54%, wildlife destruction by 66%, and methane production by a huge 93%. Overall, the research concluded that if everyone in the UK ate less meat, the resulting drop in emissions would be equivalent to taking eight million cars off the road."
– Vegan Diets Slash Emissions by 75%, According to Most Detailed Study Yet; VegConomist.com; July 2023

Animal farming is a breeding ground for diseases

In addition to the environmental and animal suffering issues related to the animal farming and feed crop industries, there are the disease situations created by breeding billions of animals every year, and keeping them by the thousands in factory farming situations on every continent. It presents a breeding ground for diseases, increasing the spread of viruses into wild animals, and among humans. Study what is happening with the 2025 spread of the bird flu into wildlife, and you will begin to undertint what the animal farming industry is responsible for.

Farmed animals fed to farmed animals spreads disease

One reason for the spread of diseases among farm animals is that animals in factory farms are often fed with what consists of other farmed animals and/or their waste. In this situation, parts of pigs, cows, chickens, turkeys, and other farmed animals – including organs, feathers, afterbirth, and miscarried animals – may be used in what is fed to the farmed animals.

The forced cannibalistic practices of feeding farmed animals to farmed animals have played roles in the spread of swine flu, bird flu, and mad cow disease (bovine spongiform encephalopathy). All these diseases, and antimicrobial-resistant contagions able to multiply in factory-farm conditions can then spread to humans, and to wildlife – including through insects, migrating animals, contaminated water, dirty farm and shipping equipment, and foods sold or served in stores, restaurants, cafeterias, hotels, cruise ships, prisons, the military, schools, and other settings.

Re-wild Earth

The land used to grow feed crops could be given back to the wilds of nature, where wildlife can thrive. Less than 20% of the current feed crop land would be needed to grow fruits, vegetables, beans, legumes, grains, nuts, and seeds for human consumption. Wildlife diversity would improve, as would the soil, air, water, and climate, and the world would be healthier. It would be a process of re-wilding Earth.

Eggs, fish oil, and human disease

I hear people say they are vegetarian, but they also eat eggs and take fish oil supplements.

Eggs and fish oil aren't vegetation. They don't grow on trees, bushes, or vines, nor are they leafy greens, or root vegetables. Chicken eggs come out of the reproductive organs of chickens. Fish oil is extracted from the body tissues of killed fish.

Eggs

Every year billions of male chicks are killed soon after hatching. This is because the male chicks aren't of any value to egg farms. Male chicks are killed within hours or days of hatching, and their dead bodies are treated as trash.

Some egg farms simply toss the baby male chicks into grinder machines – by the hundreds, or thousands. Some hatcheries toss the baby male chicks into grinders by the thousands, every day. Some toss them into plastic bags, suffocating them. Some gas them. Simply because they are born as male. Globally, this amounts to billions of male chicks killed every month.

Billions of female chicks are kept and raised for egg production. Billions are put through forced molting, which involves withholding water, food, and light from the egg-laying hens so they produce larger eggs. When their egg production slows, those incarcerated, egg-laying birds are sent to slaughter, cut into pieces, and their muscle is sold as "chicken" – as in chicken sandwiches, chicken salad, chicken hot dogs, roasted chicken, chicken soup, chicken breast, chicken nuggets, fried chicken, buffalo wings, chicken gumbo, kung pao chicken, etc.

Today, billions of chickens spend their entire lives in cages, unable to spread their wings. Stuffed two, three, or four chickens to a cage, and stacked two, three, or four, or more levels on top of each other. The chickens in the top level defecating onto the chickens in the lower cages. Many of the birds spend their lives covered in poo.

That is the egg industry. It is a filthy, smelly industry rife with abuse, and billions upon billions of stressed, sickly animals being raised in cramped cages, then killed, and sold as human food.

It is no surprise that chicken meat is often found to harbor bacteria that can make people sick, can cause kidney and other organ failure, and can send some people to the grave. This is why it is advisable to practice cleanliness when preparing chicken meat in your kitchen, and to be sure to cook those carcass bits at high enough temperatures to kill harmful bacteria. Unfortunately, cooking that meat also creates free radicals, rancid fats, denatured amino acids, and heat-generated chemicals that also are not good for human health, trigger immune-system responses, and increase the risk of tissue damage, cancer, and diseases – including of the liver, kidney, and heart.

Chicken eggs and human diseases

As science is proving, one thing eating chicken eggs increases the risks of experiencing heart disease, stroke, cancer, and kidney and autoimmune diseases. Cooked eggs are also rich in the free radicals that damage and age tissues, including the delicate macula area of the eyes, helping to degrade vision, and the fine blood system within the kidneys, slowing their function.

The lecithin in eggs breaks down into choline. What is found concentrated in human cancer cells? Choline. It is more present in people consuming eggs.

The choline situation is only one of the reasons eggs increase the risk of cancer.

Egg consumption raises the presence of TMAO (Trimethylamine N-oxide) in the blood. High levels of TMAO increase the risk of heart attacks, strokes, and cancers, such as cancers of the brain, breasts, uterus, ovaries, prostate, colon, kidneys, and bladder.

"Eggs are high in choline. Choline is converted in the gut into trimethylamine (TMA), which, after being oxidized by our liver into TMAO, may promote inflammation and result in cancer progression.

Since choline and carnitine are the primary sources of TMAO production, the logical intervention strategy might be to reduce meat, dairy, and egg consumption.

And if we eat plant-based food for long enough, we can actually change our gut microbial communities such that we may not be able to make TMAO, even if we try."
– Do Eggs Cause Cancer & What Explains This Connection?, by Michael Greger M.D.; NutritionFacts.org; 2021

The concentrated protein and the cholesterol in eggs also increase the risk of cancer, heart disease, strokes, erectile dysfunction, and vision degradation. They can help trigger autoimmune disorders, including arthritis.

Did you notice that, men? Eggs increase the incidence of both erectile dysfunction and prostate cancer.

"Although eggs are lumped into an overall healthier dietary pattern in some prospective studies (chicken, eggs, legumes, nuts), there are other studies suggesting concern around egg consumption and increased cancer risk. For prostate cancer in particular, there are several studies which found an increased risk. According to a prospective study published in *Cancer Prevention Research*, healthy men who consumed 2.5 or more eggs per week had an 81% increased risk of lethal prostate cancer compared with men who consumed less than 0.5 eggs per week. The authors hypothesized that this was due to a high level of cholesterol and choline in the eggs, which are both highly concentrated in prostate cancer cells. In 2012, the authors looked specifically at choline content and found that men in the highest quintile of choline intake had a 70% increased risk of lethal prostate cancer. Although choline is found in all animal foods, it is more highly concentrated in eggs at 250 mg per egg."
– Animal Protein and Cancer Risk; Osher Center for Integrative Health of the University of California San Francisco; 2025

Other cancers more common in those who consume eggs include breast cancer, colon cancer, and bladder cancer.

Eggs contain phosphorus and choline, which is a trimethylamine N-oxide precursor. Egg yolks are abundant in cholesterol. These substances can be problematic for those with advanced stages of kidney disease.

Some say you need to eat eggs to get lutein. But this nutrient is in everything from bell peppers to broccoli, Brussels sprouts, carrots, corn, kale, parsley, peas, pumpkin, romaine lettuce, and spinach, and many other edible plants.

People say we need to eat eggs to get zeaxanthin. This nutrient is in asparagus, broccoli, carrots, corn, peas, pumpkin, summer squash, and other edible plants.

Some people say we need to eat eggs to get vitamin D. There are plenty of other ways to get vitamin D that do not contain the cholesterol or other problematic components of eggs, and don't support the terrible industrial chicken farming industry.

Some people say we need to eat eggs for the protein. The amino acids we need for making protein are in edible plants, including fruits, vegetables, sprouts, nuts, legumes, seeds, and seaweeds.

You know what has more protein <u>per calorie</u> than an egg? Green leafy vegetables.

Fiber is not in eggs, meat, or dairy

Eggs do not contain fiber.

Milk and meat also do not contain fiber.

A low-fiber diet is associated with increased risk of heart disease, strokes, cancer, macular (vision) degradation, erectile dysfunction, varicose veins, leaky gut, kidney disease, and other debilitating, degenerative, and chronic health conditions.

What does contain the fiber so beneficial to health, and that prevents disease? Fruits, vegetables, sprouts, nuts, beans, legumes, seeds, and seaweeds.

Eggs and omega-3 fatty acids

People say eggs are a good source of omega-3 fatty acids. Really? Maybe they would like to reconsider that claim.

The egg industry started promoting eggs as "rich in omega-3s" after they started feeding flax seeds and/or fishmeal to the chickens. Clever.

To get omega-3s, you can skip eating the eggs. You will get omega-3s by eating a diet of salads, smoothies, hummus, dips, fresh vegetable juices, dehydrated seed and veggie crackers, and other fruits, vegetables, nuts, beans, seeds, sprouts, and seaweeds. Flax, hemp seed, chia seed, kidney beans, peanuts, seaweeds, walnuts, edamame, and sprouts are some of the sources of omega-3s.

Feeding fish to chickens to get omega-3s is ruinous

Feeding fish meal to chickens to get omega-3s is a rather obtuse, and energetically insufficient way of obtaining omega-3s.

Taking fish from the sea to form into feed for farmed chickens that would otherwise never be eating sea creatures, is also a bit strange, and energy intensive.

Overfishing the oceans to feed farm animals is obscene

The billions upon billions of fish being pulled from the oceans and turned into feed for farmed animals, and to sell into the restaurant and grocery store chains is causing overfishing, and the regional – or total – extinction of species. It is depleting the oceans of food for other creatures that rely on those fish. Sea turtles, sealions, seals, dolphin, whales, predator fish, marine birds, and other animals are all being impacted by overfishing. So are the smaller creatures living at the bottoms of the oceans damaged by trawling – dragging use fishing nets along the bottoms of the seas.

Why are we feeding an increasing number of billions of sea creatures to massively overbred pigs, cows, sheep, goats, turkeys, chickens, and other animals that would never naturally ingest sea creatures? It's an obscene disrespect of other animal life.

As it is today, tremendous amounts of fuel and other resources are used to send ships into the oceans to kill billions creatures. They are turned into "high protein" feed for farmed animals. They it is transport into the continents, where it is fed to farmed animals.

Getting omega-3s

We do not need to be feeding fish meal to chickens so we can then claim the eggs those chickens produce are "rich in omega oils."

Fish get the omega-3s from the greens they eat, as in seaweeds and algae.

You can skip eating the fish, and simply add some seaweeds (including nori, dulse, kelp, and Irish moss) and algaes (such as chlorella, spirulina, and blue-green algae) to your foods.

If you aren't into seaweeds or algaes, you can also get omega-3s from fresh raw greens (including asparagus, basil, beet greens, broccoli greens, cabbage, celery, chard, cilantro, collards, dandelion greens, fennel greens, kale, lettuces, mustard greens, oregano, parsley, spinach, and other greens.), raw fruit, raw sprouts, and raw germinated seeds (such as chia and buckwheat).

You can also obtain omega-3s from flax seeds and hemp seeds. And from raw walnuts. The common weed purslane is also a source, but purslane is high in oxalates, which you might be avoiding.

Fish oil and toxins

Consuming fish oil isn't a good way of obtaining omega-3s. The oil also contains the industrial pollutants, heavy metals, and other toxins the fish was exposed to in the water it swam in, and in the substances it ingested.

Unfortunately, even fish caught in the Arctic and Antarctica are found to contain industrial pollutants, including fire retardants, heavy metals, PCBs, and other toxins. These pollutants are harming seals, whales, dolphins, porpoises, sea turtles, bears, foxes, marine birds, coastal birds, and other animals that eat fish. An increasing number of wild animals are found to have cancer, to have difficulty carrying to term, to have babies with deformities, and to be underweight.

Lies of fish oil supplement companies

You may notice a fish oil supplement company claiming their product is obtained from fish swimming in pristine waters. Really? Where are those waters? If the fish of the Arctic and Antarctic are found to contain a variety of industrial pollutants, where on the planet do you think those companies are obtaining these fish – especially if the seas most distant from cities are found to contain fish with measurable residues of heavy metals, industrial pollutants, fire retardants, PCBs, pharmaceuticals, and other toxins?

The marketing claims of the fish oil supplement companies may sound all nice and pretty, but they are a fantasy, and nothing but a sales pitch. Even fish captured off the most remote islands of the planet are found to contain industrial toxins. It is what humans have done to the planet.

Risks of fish oil supplements

Fish oil supplements increase the risk of bleeding, such as from cuts, injuries, and cardiovascular events like strokes.

People who are taking blood thinners should avoid taking fish oil supplements as it could increase the risk of strokes and uncontrolled bleeding.

Anyone planning on undergoing surgery will need to stop taking fish oil supplements.

For some people, hemorrhage a risk factor of taking fish oil supplements.

If someone already has bleeding problems with their kidneys, taking fish oil supplements can increase the risks of bleeding.

A friend of mine in his 30s had a cerebral hemorrhage doctors attributed to his overuse of fish oil supplements. He thought more was better, including the misconception that fish oil lubricated his muscles before working out.

My friend was in the hospital for three months. After insurance, he was left with a $140,000 hospital bill, in addition to the cost of a variety of pharmaceuticals. He spent months going through physical therapy to regain his muscle coordination and strength. The experience devastated his life.

As mentioned earlier, omega-3 fatty acids are in seafood. But they are also in plants. Eat a variety of raw greens, sprouts, and fruit, and you will get the essential fatty acids you need for nutrition. We can synthesize omega-3 fatty acids from vegetables.

I can understand eating fish, if you live on an island where fruits, vegetables, and other foods aren't easy to get.

Fish isn't going to contain all of the nutrients a person can get by eating a variety of fruits, vegetables, sprouts, beans, legumes, nuts, and seeds. These include vitamins, minerals, essential fatty acids, amino acids, antioxidants, anti-inflammatories, fiber, carbohydrates, and other nutrients your body needs to thrive.

Many times the fish oil supplements are rancid and rotting, and far past being of a beneficial quality.

"The market in this prized commodity is worth billions – but are the supposed benefits worth the cost to global ecosystems?

While some fish oil is made from cod, mackerel or sardines, most comes from Peruvian anchovetas, a type of anchovy. These silvery fish are an important source of nutrition for the wildlife in the Humboldt Current, one of the most productive marine ecosystems on Earth.

As the world's largest fishery, the anchoveta catch in Peru is enormous – exceeding 4 m tons a year. Some of the haul is frozen and canned for human consumption, but it is mainly used to feed pigs, poultry, and farmed fish.

'We're extracting millions of tons from an ecosystem that depends on that fish. The ecosystem is being impoverished and losing its resilience to big changes brought about by El Niños and climate change,' says Patricia Majluf [vice-president of Oceana Peru, a group which works in international conservation to protect and restore the oceans].

Independent tests show that an alarming amount of fish oil supplements, at least 10%, are rancid. Some products reached 11 times higher than international voluntary limits for rancidity."

– 'It's mind-boggling': the hidden cost of our obsession with fish oil pills, by Richa Syal; *The Guardian*; Jan. 2022

The environmentally ruinous fish industry: overfishing and ocean life collapse

One of the problems with the fish oil industry is the amount of pelagic fish being killed. These variety of fish are known as keystone fish because they eat smaller things in the oceans, and then the larger fish eat those keystone fish, which is how the larger fish survive. These keystone fish live at a certain level of the ocean, and consume algae, and/or plankton and phytoplankton – which is where the anchovetas, anchovies, capelin, herring, and menhaden fish get their omega-3s.

The supplement industry is also removing tremendous numbers of krill (an animal in the crustacean family) from the seas, and this is reducing the food relied on by seals, whales, and penguins. All of these animals play roles in the fertilization of the oceans, and the growth of seaweeds, which then produce much of the oxygen breathed by sea mammals, marine birds, and other birds, and land animals.

Most of the air you rely on is produced by plants that exist in the oceans.

Tremendously unsustainably enormous quantities of keystone fish are removed from the oceans and turned into pellets to feed farmed pigs, cows, poultry, and farmed fish. This farmed animal feed practice is causing vast damage to the oceans and sea life. Additionally, enormous amounts of fish taken from the seas are also being used as fertilizer to grow crops to feed farmed animals. It's all ruinous to the environment and wildlife. Even more fish are being killed to sell into the multi-billion dollar fish-oil supplement industry. It's causing vast amounts of damage to wildlife, the quality of the ocean water, and the stability of the climate.

Instead of fish oil, if a person really wants an omega-3 supplement, they can take algae-derived DHA and EPA supplements, and avoid contributing to overfishing. Skip the fish oil, and choose the algae-based supplements.

It is through plants that you can get essential fatty acids. Companies selling fish oil supplements don't want you to know this.

Humans are herbivores, not carnivores, or omnivores

The teeth and mouths of humans are different from the teeth and mouths of carnivores, such as animals in the cat, dog, and bear families. Carnivores have sharp teeth and wide mouths framed by snouts, and can bite, lock, and tear at meat.

Some people say the omnivore shape of human teeth suggests humans are meant for a diet of both plant and meat content. Other people say that because human teeth are short and smooth, the human jaw swivels in a grinding motion, and the mouths are small and relatively weak, humans therefore are more structured for eating plants. (Animals that eat plants are known as herbivores.)

"You can't tear flesh by hand, you can't tear hide by hand. Our anterior teeth are not suited for tearing flesh or hide. We don't have large canine teeth, and we wouldn't have been able to deal with food sources that required those large canines."
– Dr. Richard Leakey

Carnivores and herbivores teeth and mouths

Carnivores eat meat when it is raw. Humans are not natural meat eaters. When humans do eat meat they do so only after it has been tenderized or ground, most often softened even more by cooking with high temperatures – and then, at last, sliced. It is then often saturated with flavoring, like catsup, mustard, hot sauce, fruit juice, or herbs and spices. Humans hide the flavor of meat – including by flavoring and cooking it.

Even after preparing, cooking, and cutting meat, humans often have a hard time chewing and swallowing the stuff – sometimes losing teeth and gagging to death during the process.

The human mouth structures are only part of the picture. Those who say humans are meant to eat a plant-based diet may have their beliefs verified by taking the human digestive tract into consideration.

Human intestine length, structure, and acidity

Human bowels are different from the smooth and relatively straight bowels of meat-eating animals. The human digestive tract is more than 10-times body length. Carnivores have a digestive tract that may be as long as their body. The puckered, long, and curved structures of the human digestive tract indicate humans are more attuned to eating a fiber-rich plant-based diet. The stomach acids of the human are also much weaker than those of carnivores, and are more in balance with the stomach acid levels of herbivores.

Carnivore and herbivore saliva differences

Carnivore saliva is acidic. Carnivore saliva does not contain ptyalin.

Human saliva is alkaline and human salivary glands produce ptyalin. Ptyalin breaks the hydrolysis of dextrin and starch, turning the long-chain sugars into smaller soluble sugar fragments. This is key to a creature meant to consume a diet based on starch – not meat, or eggs.

Humans need fiber

Humans need fiber to help digest food. Meat, dairy, and eggs do not contain fiber. Humans who do not eat enough fiber have higher rates of a variety of diseases, including cardiovascular disease, colorectal cancer, breast cancer, diabetes, and kidney disease, and also are more likely to have strokes and heart attacks. A vegan diet rich in raw fruits and vegetables easily contains an abundance of fiber.

Fiber in the human digestive tract is fermented and creates a number of nutrients, including the vital short-chain fatty acids that play a role in many processes throughout the body, including protecting against colon cancer.

A diet rich in animal protein increases risks of colon cancer.

Uricase oxidase produced by liver of carnivores

The carnivore liver produces uricase (uricase oxidase), which metabolizes the uric acid that is a byproduct of the breakdown of purines in meats. Organ meats are rich in purines, so are anchovies, herring, mackerel, mussels, sardines, and scallops. Carnivores love organ meats. Other meats, including beef, pork, game meats (deer, etc.), shellfish, fish, and poultry all contain purines. So does meat gravy.

311

Human don't produce uricase. When uric acid builds up in humans, they can end up with an abundance of urate crystals in their system, and results in or contributes to situations including varicose veins, cardiovascular disease, bursitis, arthritis, gout (a type of arthritis), diabetes, kidney stones, and kidney failure.

Purines

While some purines can be found in plant sources like asparagus, cauliflower, green peas, lentils, oats, and spinach, the alkaline diet that is a low-fat vegan diet rich in raw fruits and vegetables protects against the health problems associated with a diet rich in meats. Because of accompanying components in plants, fruits and vegetable purines are excreted more easily than are purines from meat sources. Vegans typically have a low level of uric acid in the bloodstream.

Claws of carnivores and human prehensile hands

Unlike carnivores, humans do not have claws that can tear into another animal to kill it and rip it open. Humans have prehensile hands, with soft fingers topped by fingernails perfect for peeling fruit.

Carnivores can survive perfectly on raw meat and water.

"Man's structure, internal and external compared with that of other animals, shows that fruit and succulent vegetables are his natural food."
– Carolus Linnaeus

Accelerating atherosclerosis and inflammation

"A recent study by Smith found that high-fat, high-protein, low-carbohydrate (HPLC) diets (which are usually high in red meat, such as the Atkins and Paleolithic diets) may accelerate atherosclerosis through mechanisms that are unrelated to the classic cardiovascular risk factors. Mice that were fed an HPLC diet had almost twice the level of arterial plaque as mice that were fed a Western diet, even though the classic risk factors were not significantly different between groups. The mice fed the HPLC diet had markedly fewer circulating endothelial progenitor cells and higher levels of nonesterified fatty acids (promoting inflammation) than mice fed the Western diet."
– Dr. Dean Ornish, Holy Cow! What's Good For You Is Good For Our Planet: Comment on "Red Meat Consumption and Mortality," *Archives of Internal Medicine*, March 2012. Ornish founded the Preventative Medicine Research Institute, PMRI.org

Eating animal protein decreases beneficial gut bacteria

As explained earlier in the book, a diet rich in animal protein decreases both the beneficial microorganisms in the gut, and the variety of microorganisms in the gut. Animal protein also nurtures bacteria that result in TMA, TMAO, indoxyl sulfate, and p-cresyl sulfate, which all negate health. Specifically, the gut organisms animal protein encourages play a role in conditions including cardiovascular disease, kidney disease, cancer, inflammation, and autoimmune and neurological disorders.

Humans are not carnivores or omnivores. Humans are herbivores and they flourish in health on a low-fat, plant-based diet rich in fruits, vegetables, nuts, seed, beans, and legumes. The human nutritional requirement for animal protein is absolute zero.

"A vegetarian diet has been advocated by everyone from philosophers such as Plato and Nietzsche, to political leaders such as Benjamin Franklin and Gandhi, to modern pop icons such as Paul McCartney and Bob Marley. Science is also on the side of vegetarianism. A multitude of studies have proven the health benefits of a vegetarian diet to be remarkable."
– VegInfo.org/Health

Healing life

As with many people who have been badly damaged by life, nutrition is only one part of healing. The longer I've been following a vegan diet, the more I notice how many people get into plant-based nutrition as a way to help heal their life.

In 2012, as he worked to correct his ways, cancer survivor Lance Armstrong spoke of the increased energy he has experienced by switching to a lower fat, organic, mostly vegan diet. Armstrong had been training with Rip Esselstyn, an athlete and the author of *The Engine 2 Diet*, which advocates a 100 percent low-fat, vegan diet.

"Even when you're training really hard, it's normal that you would have certain things for lunch or certain things for breakfast, and then have this dip, or almost like a food coma. I don't experience it anymore. My energy level has never been this consistent, and not just consistent, but high. I'm a big napper – I couldn't even take a nap these days if I wanted to.

The other thing – I expected to get rid of the dip, but I didn't expect the mental side of it, and the sharpness and the focus I've noticed. And I was the biggest nonbeliever, I was like 'whatever, man,' and I'm in. I'm not doing dinners yet, but breakfast and lunch, I'm in."
– Lance Armstrong, speaking of following a largely low-fat vegan diet while training for a marathon; March 2012

Pro athletes thriving on a plant-based diet

"Today you have processed meats and a lot of animals suffering unnecessarily for it. Now, some people just blow it off and don't have a conscience about it, or they just don't care. They wouldn't eat their dog, but they feel that way about other animals. But for me, I decided to stop eating meat. I didn't want to contribute to all of it. I'm not trying to change the world, or wear it on my sleeve, or make a political statement, because that just turns people away. I only have control over one person, and that's myself. And I feel good about it."
– Mac Danzig, vegan mixed martial arts champ

"I've found that a person does not need protein from meat to be a successful athlete. In fact, my best year of track competition was the first year I ate a vegan diet."
– Carl Lewis, nine-time Olympic gold medal winner

"I respect all life, and if I have the option to stay just as healthy and just as strong, if not stronger, by not torturing or enslaving or causing pain for other living things, I'm all for it. With so many apps and trackers now and so many companies getting on board with making tasty and healthy vegan food, there's not a good argument not to be. It just takes a tiny bit of education."

– Andy Lally, racecar driver, three-time Grand Am class champion, five-time winner of the Rolex 24 in Daytona, and Rookie of the Year at NASCAR

"I went vegan three years ago, because the more I learned about the dairy industry, the more I knew I had to go vegan. I am happy to eat and know that I did not harm any animals for my food."

– Leilani Munter, race car driver

"I recover quicker, I sleep better. My skin cleared up. I have fewer allergies. There are just so many impacts. I'm physically in better shape than I've ever been, and I'm more successful than ever right now – and my plant-based program has played such a big role in that."

– Lewis Hamilton, racecar driver, winner of seven Formula One World Drivers' Championship titles

Restaurant ignorance

If you want to experience the best of health, you won't be regularly eating at restaurants. While they could be fun for social get togethers, relying on them for your nutrition isn't the wisest choice. The food they serve likely is rich in a variety of things not beneficial for health, including being high in salt, sugar, damaged oils, and heat-generated chemicals. The menus likely are based on flavor, texture, smell, and otherwise luxury eating. Not on providing you with any type of ideal nutrition.

Restaurant workers are not nutritionists, they are hired to make and serve food. They are there to make money to support themselves. Some enjoy working in the industry, including the social aspects of it, and being part of a community. They aren't there to safeguard your health. Selling you drinks and deserts increases the bill, and increases their tips. Their kindness is to make you feel welcome, not to pick up on you, or to validate your existence.

While some restaurants serve more healthier foods than others, making plant-based food from scratch at home is less expensive, and very likely to be far healthier.

Even if a restaurant is vegan, it doesn't mean their food is healthy, or great for your health. It's often a different version of salty, sugary food, with damaged oils, but without the animal protein.

I went to a café with a friend who the restaurant has vegan items on the menu. I wasn't hungry, and was only going to get a veggie juice. The owner told me "We have vegan options, including the tuna sandwich."

Fish are not vegetables, fruits, nuts, sprouts, seeds, or seaweeds.

Have diner gatherings, know what is in the food you make, and save money while being able to spend time with people who matter to you.

Nothing born, hatched, or spawned

Vegans don't eat anything born, spawned, or hatched. Nothing with eyes, or parents. This includes fish, crustaceans, mollusks, mammals, birds, amphibians, reptiles, and gastropods (snails). Vegans don't eat eggs, or the milk from animals.

Roots of vegetarianism

It seems reasonable to assume there have always been people who have followed a diet consisting of only plant substances. People in Persia, India, Greece, Italy, Arabia, and various parts of Africa, including tribes in Abyssinia (now Ethiopia), have a history of following what we now call a plant-based diet.

Everyone from the Arabian poet al-Ma'arri, to Italy's Leonardo da Vinci, to people of the Jainism faith in India, the Greek philosophers like Plato and Theophrastus, and the stoics, including Zeno, Seneca, Ovid, and the Roman emperor Marcus Aurelius didn't eat animals. Also the Buddhist Emperor Ashoka abstained from eating animals. As did the prophet Daniel in the Old Testament.

"Perhaps the earliest known potential evidence of at least vegetarianism goes back to 7000BCE, over 9,000 years ago, to a town called Mehrgarh, belonging to the Indus river civilization. It's widely known that followers of the Hindu religion do not consume meat, and while the exact beginning of Hinduism is vague, it's philosophical foundation reaches back potentially as far as Mehrgarh, far before any written text or scripture was made. The term Hindu is etymologically linked to the Sanskrit Sindhu, which is the ancient name for the Indus river, and was a term the Persians used to identify as people living near a river."
– Vegans In Ancient Times: The History of Veganism Part One; by Emily Moran Barwick; BiteSizeVegan.org; June 2022

No one religion or group of people seems to be aligned with being the originators of veganism or vegetarianism, as there are people of all nationalities, religions, and cultures following plant-based diets.

"Non-injury to all living beings is the only religion… this is the quintessence of wisdom; not to kill anything. All breathing, existing, living sentient creatures should not be slain, nor treated with violence, nor abused, nor tormented, nor driven away. This is the pure unchangeable law. Therefore, cease to injure living things. All living things love their life, desire pleasure, and do not like pain; they dislike any injury to themselves; everybody is desirous of life and to every being, his life is very dear."
– the Yoga Shastra, a Jain scripture; As quoted in Vegans In Ancient Times: The History of Veganism Part One; by Emily Moran Barwick; BiteSizeVegan.org; June 2022

The Bible also has it's clues to people following plant-based diets, including, as mentioned earlier, the prophet Daniel who did not eat animals. There is also what it says in the book of Genesis:

"I give you all plants that bear seed everywhere on Earth, and every tree bearing fruit which yields seed: They shall be yours for food. All green plants I give for food to the wild animals, to all the birds of heaven, and to all reptiles on earth, every living creature, it shall be theirs for food."
– Genesis 1:29-31

Donald Watson and the word vegan

The modern vegan diet is often attributed to the teachings of Donald Watson, who died at age 95 in Cumbria on November 16, 2005. He became a vegetarian after seeing his Uncle George involved in the slaughter of a pig. Hearing the pig's screams haunted him. "I decided farms – and uncles – had to be reassessed: The idyllic scene was nothing more than death row, where every creature's days were numbered."

Eventually, Watson eliminated dairy from his diet. When his elder brother and a sister also became vegetarians, his mother, who was not a vegetarian, made the comment that she felt like a hen who had hatched a clutch of duck eggs.

"We may be sure that should anything so much as a pimple ever appear to mar the beauty of our physical form, it will be entirely due in the eyes of the world to our own silly fault for not eating 'proper food.' Against such a pimple the great plagues of diseases now ravaging nearly all members of civilized society (who eat 'proper food') will pass unnoticed."
– Donald Watson, founder of veganism

As an adult, Watson formed a group of "nondairy vegetarians." They advocated the health benefits of such a diet, and taught that animal agriculture was likely to spread diseases – including the tuberculosis identified in Britain's dairy cows.

Watson concocted the term "vegan" by taking the beginning and end of the word "vegetarian." In 1944, they published the first edition of the *Vegan News*.

Sunfoodists in 1800s Scotland

People who joined Watson's Vegan Society were among those who lived in Scotland, where a group of people in the late 1800s called themselves "sunfoodists." They didn't eat animal protein, but did use honey.

Natural hygiene movement

While a plant-based diet has been practiced among people here and there throughout history, the "Natural Hygiene" movement of the 1830s is often cited as the beginning of modern-day vegetarianism.

The current popularity of a strictly or a largely raw vegan diet can be attributed to a variety of people throughout history.

Teachings of the plant-based diet

Starting in the 1980s, there have been an increasing number of books about some variety of the plant-based diet. The information and advice in many of them is not reliable, but standards are improving as scientific studies confirm the benefits of the diet. More people are also seeking information about the diet and its association with sustainable living, environmentalism, and the protection of wildlife.

There are now sites like NutritionFacts, and ForksOverKnives, and groups like the Physicians Committee for Responsible Medicine, and EarthSave providing science-based vegan nutrition information.

The food system can collapse in a matter of hours

Most people are reliant on restaurants and stores for every calorie of their food. This situation consists of relying on a food system that can collapse not only within months, or weeks, or days, but within hours.

See: ClimateHealers.org, GoVeganic.net, LearnVeganic.com, NoblePeaceTribe.org, OurPermacultureLife.com, Permaculture.co.uk, PermacultureDevelopment.org, Permaculture.org.uk, PermaclutreJournies.com, Permies.com, Spiralseed.co.uk, VeganAustralia.org.au, VeganicPermaculture.com, VeganicPermacultureSpain.com, VeganPermaculture.org, VeganOrganic.net, VeganSustainability.com, WildEarthFarmAndSanctuary.com. Search: Food forests, organic home gardening, wild food foraging,

Human food choices vs wildlife and the environment

The farming practices of the animal farming and feed crop industries play lead roles in what is now the insect apocalypse, the bird apocalypse, the plunge in land animal populations, the degradation of soil, and in desertification (which is the loss of soil organisms that support life). Animal ag and feed crops also play lead roles in the degradation of wetlands, marshes, ponds, streams, rivers, lakes, oceans, and aquifers, and in climate change.

Supporting the animal farming industry is supporting the industrial feed crop industry that badly damages every continent, and decreases populations of pollinator and migrating wildlife.

Someone might say mentioning all of this about the environment is going far off the course of heart and kidney health. But if the environmental situation doesn't radically improve, there will not be any human hearts, or kidneys – but only human bones.

The health of the environment is directly related to the health of every cell in your body, including the trillions of single-celled occupants of your gut.

From the health of the microscopic life, to the health of the largest animals and plants on the planet, it is all an interconnected web of life. If one section of the web becomes ill, it weakens, and its illness impacts the other sections of the web. The situation can lead to what can be catastrophic for the entire web.

Scientists from all over the planet agree: the web of life on earth is in danger. This is specifically because of human behaviors. Topping the list of those behaviors damaging to Earth life are human choices and practices relating to food.

"The planet cannot support billions of large meat eaters. There just isn't enough space. If we all had a largely plant-based diet, we would need only half the land we use at the moment. We must radically reduce the area we use to farm so we can make space for returning wilderness. And the quickest and most effective way to do that is for us to change our diet."
– David Attenborough, author *Life On Earth*

Learn about permaculture and growing food

- Edible weeds
- Food forests
- FoodNotLawns.com
- How to grow an organic garden
- KitchenGardeners.org
- UrbanHomestead.org
- Veganic gardening

317

- Vegan permaculture
- VegetableGardener.com
- Wild food harvesting

Explore books about growing food. Consider:
The Edible Front Yard: The Mow-Less, Grow-More Plan for a Beautiful, Bountiful Garden, by Ivette Soler.

Fruiting trees provide

While acknowledging that people may not care to limit themselves to just a few types of fruits for their nourishment, it is still interesting to consider that several fruit trees can supply a person with more food than they could possibly eat throughout their lifetime.

I have friends whose homes are surrounded by fruit trees producing so much fruit they can't give away the fruit fast enough. They get as much as they need, and abundantly more.

Bees, honey, propolis, royal jelly, pollen

Many consider honey to be not vegan. Even saying this might frustrate those who are against consuming honey. Are they sure to only eat foods that were not grown on farms where rented or farmer-managed bee hives were used to pollinate crops? Do they understand that removing honey from the hives results in the bees pollinating more crops?

However, is the richly sweet substance that is honey something you should be eating, if you have cardiovascular disease, kidney disease, diabetes, or certain other issues? Perhaps not.

Unlike some people who call themselves "vegan," I sometimes might have foods containing honey or other bee products, such as pollen, propolis, and royal jelly. I don't seek these products, but they are sometimes in something I eat.

Some people are opposed to consuming bee products because the bees clearly are gathering food for their communities. Some people view taking honey from bees as stealing. Also, there are people opposed to consuming bee products because some beekeepers kill wildlife, including bears, to protect their hives. And bees can be killed in the beekeeping and honey-gathering procedures.

When humans remove honey and pollen from a hive, the bees have to work harder to gather more food. Some people consider the process to be "enslaving bees." However, with bees collecting more pollen and nectar, the result is more flowers being pollinated, and this results in more fruits, nuts, and vegetables for both humans and wildlife, and more seeds, which means more plants.

Earth needs more plants, which filter water, help to produce oxygen, sequester greenhouse gasses, and protect, build, improve, and stabilize soil, and help to balance the climate, provide homes for wildlife, and make earth a prettier place.

Managed bee hives are used on farms to pollinate crops, including foods sold into the system from which vegans get food.

Vegans can get rid of the belief of their life being non-reliant on bees. Humans, plants, and wildlife rely on insects to survive.

If you choose to consume bee products, please use only "organic" products, and seek out the products from beekeepers who don't kill other wildlife.

Honey test

If you do choose to purchase honey, make sure that what you purchase is honey. And not corn syrup, rice syrup, or some other concoction.

Drop some into a glass of water. If it dissolves quickly, it isn't honey, but is likely corn syrup, or some other sweetener. Honey will not instantly dissolve in water.

Plant-based athletes

Follow a plant-based diet and you will be doing what many world-class athletes do. For instance, Dave Scott, who had won the Hawaiian Ironman contest six times, and who has been considered among the best athletes who ever lived, did so while following a vegan diet.

Ultramarathon champion Scott Jurek won the Western States race seven straight times. In 2005 Jurek also won the grueling 135-mile Badwater race, which begins at the lowest elevation in the Western Hemisphere, in Death Valley, California, and ends 8,300 feet up a mountain. He did it faster than anyone in the history of the race. Then he won it again in 2006. He did this while following a vegan diet.

On October 16, 2011, Fauja Singh finished the Scotiabank Toronto Waterfront Marathon in about eight hours. You may think eight hours is a slow time for completing a marathon. At the time of the race, Singh was 100 years old. He credited a vegetarian diet as being key to his longevity, stamina, and ability.

Vegan athletes include:
- Snowboarder Hannah Teter
- Basketball player Chris Paul
- Basketball player Kyrie Irving
- Football player Deatrich Wise, Jr.
- Football player Colin Kaepernick
- Football light end Tony Gonzolez
- Heisman trophy winner Desmond Howard
- Running back, Montell Owens
- Soccer player Alex Morgan
- Soccer player Chris Smalling
- Soccer player Hector Bellerin
- Soccer player Alex Morgan
- Formula One racer Lewis Hamilton
- Cricket player Kane Richardson
- Cricket player Adam Zampa
- Cricket player Peter Siddle
- Triathlete Lisa Gawthorne
- Triathlete Brendan Brazier
- Ironwoman Ruth Heidrich
- Olympic sprinter Morgan Mitchell
- Runner Fiona Oakes
- Speed cyclist Dotsie Bausch

Kidney Heart Health Nutrition

- Tennis player Martina Navratilova
- Tennis champs Venus and Serena Williams
- Tennis player Novak Djokovic
- Tennis player Nick Kyrgios
- Olympic wrestler Chris Campbell
- Mr. Universe Bill Pearl
- Gymnast Dan Millman
- Bodybuilder Evan Connelly Novacek
- Bodybuilder Kristopher Flannery
- Marathon champ Jane Wetzel
- Olympic skater Surya Bonaly
- Boxer Keith Holmes
- Boxer David Haye
- Boxer Peter Hussig
- Mixed martial arts champ Mac Danzig
- Karate champ Ridgely Abele
- Surfer Tia Blanco
- Surfer Nikki Van Dijk
- Ballet dancer Juliet Burnett
- Powerlifter Kendrick Farris
- Powerlifter Patrik Bouboumian
- … and many more.

Follow a clean, plant-based diet. Thrive in health, and in your life.

Thank you for reading my book.

Daniel John Carey

Glossary of Names

A: Glossary of names
Addis, Thomas, 49, 50; Armstrong, Lance, 313; Attenborough, David, 317; Austin, Alfred, 166

B: Glossary of names
Baker, Roxanne, 188; Barber, Janette, 43; Barnard, Neil, 135; Barry, Steve, 25; Barwick, Emily Moran, 315; Berendt, Joachim-Ernst, 135; Berkoff, Nancy D., 70; Berkoff, Nancy, 4; Bharara, Preet, 12; Blackburn, Elizabeth, 131; Boik, John, 53; Boynton, Brian M., 11; Brescia, Michael, 8; Brown, Mary Jane, 111; Bumberg, Bruce, 119, 124, 126, 254

C: Glossary of names
Camino, James, 8; Clement, Brian, 89; Cosmer, Michele, 4

D: Glossary of names
Danzig, Mac, 313; Davison, Courtney, 141; Descartes, Rene, 167; Drews, George Julius, 90

E: Glossary of names
Epstein, Murray; 287; Eququiza, Riann Jenay, 119, 124, 126, 254; Esselstyn, Caldwell, 141, 153, 154, 159, 207; Esselstyn, Rip, 160, 313

F: Glossary of names
Favo, Francesca, 21, 142, 159; Francisco, Jugo, 145

G: Glossary of names
Graber, Eric, 82; Graham, Thomas, 7; Greenhalgh, Tom, 188; Greger, Michael, 35, 52, 58, 79, 146, 158, 182, 184, 192, 292, 306; Greider, Carol, 131; Gu, Wei, 181

H: Glossary of names
Haas, Georg, 8; Halweil, Brian, 166; Hamilton, Lewis, 314; Han, Seung Hyeok, 22; Hanh, Thich Nhat, 69; Hanley, Linda, 11; Herbert, Lynne; 292; Hill, Ansley, 299; Howell, Edward, 87

K: Glossary of names
Kall, Rob, 167; Keys, Ancel, 61, 64; Kirchner, Lauren, 296; Kirsch, Matthew, 11; Klaper, Michael, 188; Kolff, Willem Johan, 8

L: Glossary of names
Lally, Andy, 314; Lang, Katharine, 75; Leakey, Richard, 310; LeWine, Howard, 262; Lewis, Carl, 313; Linnaeus, Carolus, 312;

Lum, Jon, 100; Lynch, Parker, 17; Lyons, Owen D., 216

M: Glossary of names
Mangione, Luigi, 45, 46; Mann, George V., 182; McDougall, John, 71, 78, 153; McMullan, Ciaran, 216; Mills, Betsey, 26; Moore, Mary Tyler, 251; Munter, Leilani, 314; Murthy, Vivek, 117

N: Glossary of names
Nin, Anais, 168; Norris, Jack, 198; Nunley, Kara S., 48

O: Glossary of names
Ornish, Dean, 132, 312

P: Glossary of names
Patural, Amy, 193; Pelck, Corrie, 21; Perside, Edward C., 49; Prudden, Bonnie, 24; Ptamanik, Priyanjana, 228

Q: Glossary of names
Quinton, Wayne, 8

R: Glossary of names
Ramsing, Becky, 73; Ranniger, Gwen, 120; Rochefourcauld, Francois de la, 16; Rolyson, William D., 84; Russel, Heather, 199

S: Glossary of names
Saville, Jessianna, 262; Scribner, Belding Hibbard, 8; Semple, Dugald, 90; Sher, Barbara, 168; Shields, Clyde, 8; Sinclair, David, 130, 131; Solar, Ivette, 318; Sooparth, Dira, 4, 161; Spector, Tim, 132; Spock, Benjamin, 197; Stallone, Sylvester, 34; Stimpson, Ashley, 290; Syal, Richa, 309; Szostak, Jack, 131

T: Glossary of names
Thompson, Brian, 45; Toyoda, Kazunori, 252; Truman, President, 50, 54; Tuohy, Karen M., 142; Tuohy, Karen M., 21, 159; Tuttle, Will, 166

V: Glossary of names
Viola, Roberto, 21, 142, 159

W: Glossary of names
Walker, Matthew, 217; Watson, Donald, 315, 316; Welin, Matilda, 303; Wigmore, Anne 87, 91, 134; Wilder, Russel, 177, 178

Z: Glossary of names
Zimmerman, Robert S., 252

A

INDEX AND TOPICAL GUIDE

B: Index and Topical Guide

stomach issues, 209; **burns**, 179; **burping**, 284; **burweed marsh elder**, 215; **Business and Professional Men's Study**, 61; **butter beans**, 100; **butter**, 25, 50, 71, 134, 176, 190, 197, 275, 301; **butyrate**, 20, 21, 74, 80, 149-152, 221; **Butyricicoccupos sp.**, 150

C: Index and Topical Guide

C vitamin, 95, 111, 119, 202, 222, 290; **C-monochloropropane-1-diol esters**, 109, 110, 111, 112, 113, 114, 115; **C-reactive protein**, 70, 96, 141, 221; **C. hathewayi**, 74; **C. sporogenes**, 74; **C.diff**, 72; **cabbage**, 81, 82, 85, 91, 94-96, 143, 157, 178, 236, 270, 290, 297, 308; **cadmium**, 121, 160, 172, 173, 182, 186; **cafeterias**, 36, 55, 58, 64, 304; **caffeine**, 214, 215, 229,, 261- 264, 270, 276; **cake**, 76, 139, 171, 247, 269, 274, 282; **calcitriol**, 242, 244, 268; **calcium carbide**, ripening agent, 137, 138; **calcium renal calculi**, 104; **calcium**, 2, 4, 17, 47, 60, 77-79, 93, 95, 100, 103, 104, 130, 137-139, 187-189, 193-197, 201, 203, 229-240, 242-244, 248-250, 253, 259, 261, 266, 268, 269, 271, 294; **California law against toxic foods**, 127; **calisthenics**, 209, 213, 215; **callouses**, 284; **caloric intake**, 126, 131, 133, 165, 262; **calories and protein**, 170; **calves**, stomach lining of, 172; **camu camu**, 136; **Canada removes dairy from food group**, 189, 190; **Canadian Diabetes Association**, 6; *Cancer & Natural Medicine*, book, 53; **cancer**, 1, 3, 5, 9, 16, 17, 18, 20, 22, 30, 32, 34, 35, 40, 42, 47, 48, 53-55, 59, 60, 63, 66, 67, 71, 72, 74, 75, 77, 81-86, 90-93, 107, 108, 111-119, 123-129, 132-133, 137, 139, 141, 142, 145, 148-153, 155-163, 165, 170, 172, 174-176, 179-182, 186-193, 196, 199, 201-206, 208-210, 212, 216, 218, 220, 221, 223, 224, 227, 230, 240, 245, 247, 252, 257, 258, 261, 263, 264, 267, 273, 275-281, 287-297, 303, 305-308, 311-313; *Cancer Prevention Research* **journal**, 206; **candida**, 72, 146; **candy**, 76, 128, 129, 140, 171, 274, 275, 282; **cane sugar**, 76, 225, 246; **canned foods**, 9, 106, 115, 121, 126, 128, 139, 140, 247, 260, 264, 270, 272, 274, 278, 280, 309; **cannellini beans**, 100; **cannibalistic practices in animal farming**, 304; **canola oil**, 40, 44, 51, 164, 207, 273, 277; **Capelin**, 310; **capillaries**, 65, 77, 117, 171, 184, 190, 200, 207, 208, 251, 294; **capsaicin**, 83, 84, 249; **capsicum annuum**, 84; **capsicum frutescens**, 84; **caramel**, 274; **carbendazim fungicide**, 121; **carbohydrate-binding proteins**, 92; **carbohydrate**, acrylamide, 121; AGEs and 110, 121; alcohol and, 286, 287; amylase enzymes, 91;Atkins diet and, 312; blood glucose and, 180; bread and, 245; breastmilk and, 169; caloric intake, 126; chains, 174; coffee and, 262; enzymes and, 90, 91; fatty acids and, 64; fatty liver and, 287; fermentation in gut, 20, 221; fish meat doesn't

have, 309; FODMAPs and, 236, 270; furan and, 119; kidney-safe diet, 245; metabolism, 104, 203; intolerance, 182, 183; keto diet and, 177, 180-183, 229, 312; lectins and, 92; lupus and, 145; gut biome and, 20, 73, 150, 152; organic anions and, 221; Paleolithic diet and, 312; phytate and, 104; potatoes and, 114; Prevotella enterotype, 73; refined, 140; vegan keto, 177; **carbon monoxide poisoning**, 221; **carbonated drinks**, 76, 260, 261; **carboxylase enzymes**, 66; **carcinogenic**, AGEs, 52, 112; arsenic, 182; chemicals, 52; C-monochloropropaine-1-diol-esters, 113, 114; food additives, 118; glycidyl, 114; glyphosate, 161; heterocyclic aromatic hydrocarbons, 113; meat, 52; PAHs, 118; red meat, 175; **carcinogens**, AGEs, 112-115, 118; alcohol, 116; arsenic, 182; carbendazim, 121; chemicals, 52; fiber and, 71; fried food, 17; furan, 119; glyphosate, 161; heterocyclic aromatic amines, 113; meat, 175; oxidative stress, 203; plant-based diet protects against, 53; polycyclic aromatic hydrocarbons, 118, 159, 160; potassium bromate, 107, 108; processed meat, 17, 175; triphenyltin, 125; **carcinoma**, basal cell, 48; benefits, 73; biomarker, 175; renal cell, 223; risk profiles, 142; squamous cell, 48; **cardiometabolic**, disease, 82; health, 19, 83; 156; markers, 19; **cardiomyopathy**, 203, 284-286; **cardiorenal disorders**, 153; **carnitine**, 73, 153, 158, 172, 305; **carnivore microbiome**, see TMAO, 19; **carnivores**, humans are not, 30, 31, 310, 312; intestinal length of, 311; liver of, 311; prehensile hands and, 312; ptyalin, 311; saliva and, 311; structures of, 29, 31, 310-312; **carotenoids**, 119, 218, 271; **carotid intima-media thickness**, 60; **carrageenan**, 297, 299; **carrots**, 81-83, 199, 218, 236, 237, 239, 248, 265, 306; **cartilage**, broth, 122; electrolytes and, 250; inflammation, 143; phosphorus and, 249; **casein**, allergies, 187, 191, 192; anaphylaxis and, 192; antioxidants, lack of, 219; arthritis and, 295; avoiding, 25, 50, 134; baby cows and, 301; cancer and, 182, 186, 193, 295; capillaries of kidneys, reduces, 294; cardiovascular disease and, 295; diabetes and, 295; fiber and, 71, 150; glomerular filtration and, 172, 190; gut biome and, 295; kidney filtration and, 294; leaky gut and, 192; non-dairy creamers and, 299; nutrition and, 189, 275; prostate cancer and, 193; protein, 169, 172, 186, 190, 192, 299; protein powder, 172, 295; smoothies, 182; vegan products and, 298, 299; **cashew**, calcium and, 189; cheese, 177, 197; fermented, 177; leucine, 200; living foods and, 102; methionine, 185; milk, 189, 197, 295; oxalates and, 189; phosphorus and, 248; potassium and, 271; zinc, 94; **casomorphin**, 174; **cassia cinnamon**, 215, 263; **castor bean**, 100; **catabolism**, 78; **cataracts**, 183, 191; **catechin**, 82, 96; **catsup**, 34, 137,

D: INDEX AND TOPICAL GUIDE

Experimental and Clinical Sciences Journal, 153, 212; **extinction**, 295, 307; **extracellular fluid**, 259; **extraskeletal calcification**, 196; **eye lids puffy**, 136, 225, 255; **eyes**, 3, 22, 38, 44, 51, 59, 69, 74, 80, 94, 103, 108, 118, 136, 143, 167, 168, 187, 208, 210, 214, 218, 223, 229, 248, 250, 251, 252, 255, 268, 305, 314, 316

F: INDEX AND TOPICAL GUIDE

facial swelling, 187; **factory farming**, 30, 36, 55, 56, 57, 59, 62, 64, 67, 86, 122, 126, 161, 163, 165, 166, 168, 174, 281, 291, 300-304, 317, 310; **Faecal lipocalin-2**, 79; **Faecalibacterium prausnitzii**, 74, 152; **fainting**, 38, 260; **falafel**, instant, 105; **False Claims Act**, 11; **farm workers**, 125, 160, 161, 166, 302; **farmed animals**, 30, 36, 55, 56, 57, 59, 62, 64, 67, 86, 122, 126, 161, 163, 165, 166, 168, 174, 281, 291, 300-304, 317, 310; bioaccumulate toxins, 122; bird flu among, 304; bovine spongiform encephalopathy, 304; cannibalism in feed, 304; contagious disease and, 304; chemicals used on feed crops, 161, 165, 166; corporate welfare supports, 302; diseases spread among, 304; factory farms, 56, 59, 64, 67, 300, 304; **farmed fish**, 162, 165, 309, 310; **farmers' markets**, 44, 52; **farming industry**, see factory farming, pesticides, and feed crops, 30, 33, 36, 55, 168, 281, 300-302, 304, 306, 317; **fascia**, 218; **fast foods**, advertising, 37; artificial sweeteners in, 282; avoid it, 276; chemically saturated, 23, 56, 62; city food deserts and, 54; dairy industry and, 294; dawning of industrial, 61, 62, 64, 67; factory farmed animals and, 64, 294; feeds the disease industries, 55, 56; frozen dinners and, 276; gut bacteria and, see autoimmune disorders, cancer, cardiovascular disease, fiber, kidney disease, leaky gut, and microbiome, 79; hospital food and, 59; human illnesses from, 23; **fat**, absorption, 239; AGEs and, 110, 112; avocado oil, 153, 207, 240; belly, 284; breast milk and, 169; burning, 181, 284; canola oil, 40, 44, 164, 207, 273, 277; cardiovascular disease and, 64; cells, 119-125; chicken, 159; children and, 197; cholesterol and, 59, 287; coagulated, 274; coconut oil, 87, 113, 157, 207, 240; collects toxins, 125; corn oil, 153, 207, 299; cottonseed oil, 299; dairy and, 192; dietary, 64, 65, 181; eliminating, 71; enzymes and, 90, 91, 132; excess, 10; factory farmed animal fat, 64, 161; fiber and, 71; fried, 16, 17, 23-25, 34, 40, 44, 50, 53, 65, 72, 75-77, 79, 88, 109-116, 121, 132, 134-136, 140, 143, 155, 171, 174, 186, 193,197, 207, 210, 212, 225, 228, 230, 236, 237, 239, 252, 271, 275, 276, 279, 288, 289, 305; GMOs and, 162; gut bacteria and, 79, 148, 149, 150, 155; healthful fats, 59, 296; heated, see AGEs, 132; hemp oil, 178, 240, 307, 308; herbicides and, 124; intake and cardiovascular

disease, 64, 65; kidney stones and, 240; keto diet and, 177, 179-183; liver, see fatty liver, 200, 288, 289, 293; manganese and, 203; meat and PAHs and, 112; metabolism, 119; myelin sheath of nerve cells and, 204; nitric oxide and, 208; nondairy creamers and, 299; obesogens, 119; oil extracts, 23, 113, 118, 135, 140, 152, 157, 197, 207, 210, 239, 273; olive oil, 113, 141, 142, 153, 207, 223, 240; polyunsaturated, 65, 67, 119, 292; quality of, 185; rancid, 17, 75, 93, 140, 143, 153, 154, 305, 309; safflower oil, 207, 240; saponification and, 235, 240; saturated, 22, 52, 59, 65, 73, 141, 142, 159, 170, 174, 176, 180-183, 188, 192, 197, 208, 223, 240, 274, 275, 292, 295; sauteed, 40, 65, 76, 77, 109-115, 134, 135, 174, 237; seed oils, 153, 207, 240, 299; sleep and, 213; sticky, 65; storage, 119-125, 288; sunflower oil, 207; toxins collecting in, 125, 161, 210; trans, 140, 278; ultra-processed foods, 61; unhealthy, 6, 43, 77, 273; unsaturated, 65, 159; **father of dialysis**, 7, 8; **fatigue**, 42, 136, 138, 145, 177-180, 201, 216, 220, 226, 232, 255, 260, 267, 284; **fatty liver**, 21, 70, 177, 179, 200, 287-289, 293; **feathers**, animal farming, 304; **fecal**, clostridia, 158; microbiota transplant, FMT, 253; samples, 79; **feed**, high protein, 307; feed crops, 67, 122, 126, 161, 291, 295, 300-302, 304, 317; fish, 162, 163; fungicides and miticides and, 126; GMO crops, 161, 163, 165, 166; human diseases spread from, 304; industrial fast food, 64; mad cow disease and, 304; mass breeding of, 168, 300; miscarried, 304; oats, fed, 86; overfishing and feed for, 307, 310; pharmaceuticals and, 122, 300; physically altered, 62, 300; soy, fed, 291; swine flu among, 304; viruses spread from, 304; wildlife killed to protect, 302; **feet of farmed animals**, injured, 300; **feet**, numb, 284; swollen, 136, 225; **female sexual dysfunction**, 184; **fennel**, 53, 178, 260, 265, 308; **fenugreek**, 102, 136, 265; **fermentation**, foods, 93, 101, 103; gut, 18, 19, 20, 70, 149-152, 156, 158, 221; **fermented foods**, 19, 60, 69, 72, 90, 91, 94, 95, 96, 98, 101, 103, 105, 143, 157, 178, 185, 236, 270; **fertility**, 112, 165, 291; **fever**, 76, 88, 224, 236, 255, 265, 266, 257; **fiber**, 6, 18, 19, 21, 52, 53, 59, 60, 65, 66, 68-71, 73, 85, 86, 92, 102, 133, 141, 143, 149-152, 156, 158-160, 170, 176, 178, 181, 189, 197, 208, 212, 215, 218, 221, 222, 235, 236, 245, 253, 264, 285, 292, 295, 296, 298, 307, 309, 311; **fibroblast growth factor, FGF**, 3, 241, 244, 423; **fibromyalgia**, 42, 144; **fibroscan** 287; **fibrosis**, kidney, 149, 151, 177, 200, 219, 220; liver, 83, 123, 288; **figs**, 138, 201, 238, 274; **filters**, kidneys, 26, 172, 186, 190, 200, 217, 225, 226, 250, 256, 257, 261, 266, 287; **financial profits in medicine**, 7, 9, 14, 45, 46, 50, 55; **finding a cure fundraisers**, 55; **fingernails**, 31, 312; **Fire retardants in**

G: INDEX AND TOPICAL GUIDE

XI

H: INDEX AND TOPICAL GUIDE

I: INDEX AND TOPICAL GUIDE

M: INDEX AND TOPICAL GUIDE

mitochondria and, 130; MSG, 123; myoglobin protein and, 231; nitric oxide, 207, 208; nutrition, 51; pain, 145; phosphorus and, 249; potassium 271; sleep and, 213; statins, 206; stomach, 209; strength, 19, 167; stroke and, 309; substance abuse and, 286; twitching leg, 263; weakness, 75, 243; **musculoskeletal complications**, 154; **mushrooms and vitamin D**, 195, 196; **music and rhythm**, 135; **mussels**, 118, 311; **mustard greens**, 166, 308, 311; **mustard**, 311, 275; **mutagenic effects of methyl bromate**, 107; **myasthenia gravis**, 144; **mycobacterium vaccae**, 166; **mycotoxins**, 203; **myelin sheath**, 204; **myeloproliferative neoplasms**, 201; **myfortic**, 12; **Mylanta**, 266; **myo-inositol hexakisphosphate**, 103; **myocardial infarction**, 59, 153, 212, 286; **myoglobin protein**, 231; **myositis**, 144; **myrosinase enzyme**, 297

N: INDEX AND TOPICAL GUIDE

nail polish remover, 183; **nails, discolored**, 250; **nama shoyu**, 298; **Naproxen**, 256, 266, 285; **nasal mucosa**, 138; **nasogastrically**, 253; **National Advisory Heart Council**, 54; **National Confectioners Association**, 128, 129; **National Diet and Nutrition Survey**, 248; **National Health and Nutrition Examination Survey**, 126; **national health insurance**, 46, 50; **National Heart Act**, 54, 55; **National Heart Institute**, 59, 60, 54; **National Institute of Diabetes and Digestive and Kidney Diseases**, 269; **National Institute of Environmental Health Sciences**, 129; **National Institutes of Health**, 54, 54; **National Kidney Foundation**, opening pages, 6, 48, 60, 117, 174, 247, 248, 256, 262, 263, 264, 272, 285, 287; **National Library of Medicine**, 114; **National Medical Enterprise**, 10; **National School Lunch Program**, 190; **National Toxicology Program's Report on Carcinogens**, 115; **native edibles**, 64; **native plant decline**, 162; **Natural Hygiene movement**, 316; **natural sweetener**, 282; *Nature Communications* journal, 59; *Nature Microbiology* journal, 20, 63, 150, 156; **nature provides food variety**, 63; *Nature Reviews Nephrology*, 216; **nausea**, 76, 88, 106, 136, 139, 192, 215, 231, 233, 255, 257, 266, 283; **navy beans**, 99, 100, 200, 248; **NCD Alliance**, 61; **nectarines**, 83; **neglected health**, 213; **neoflavonoids**, 85; **neoplasms**, tumors, 201, 202; **nephrolithiasis**, 177, 235, 237; **nephrologist**, 4, 11, 15, 161, 225, 226, 252, 257; *Nephrology Dialysis Transplantation* journal, 152; *Nephrology* journal, 70; **nephrology**, origins of, 49; **nephropathy**, kidney disease, 4, 149, 223, 227, 241, 252, 255, 256; **nephroprotective medications**, 2; **nephrotic syndrome**, 256; **nephrotoxin**, 107, 115, 285, 287; **nerves**, AGEs and, 111, 112; alcohol and, 84, 117, 286; animal protein and,

32, 212; anthocyanins and, 80; appetite and, 230; artificial sweeteners and, 247; B12 vitamin and, 204; clean diet and, 21, 23, 25, 30, 133, 135; cruciferous vegetables and, 290; degeneration of, 35, 290, 303; diabetes and, 225; diabetic retinal disease and, 251; DNA and, 163; D vitamin and, 194; dysfunction, 35, 128; electrolytes, 250; eggs and, 35; exercise and, 208, 210; eyes and, 251; fiber and, 69, 149, 245; food additives and, 128, 212; gastroparesis and, 209, 230; glycotoxin, 183; GMOs and, 163; gut biome, 79, 146-149; Hippel-Lindau disease and, 223; inflammation and, 183, 229; junk food and, 9, 23, 49, 281; kidney disease and, 3, 16, 51, 242, 249; linked to all of health, 244; manganese and, 203; margarine and, 277 medications and, 249; metabolites and, 208; methylglyoxal and, 183; molecules of emotion and, 252; myelin sheath and, 204; neuropathy and, 252; neurotransmitters and, 208; nutrition, 53; opioid receptors and, 229; peppers and, 83; phosphorus and, 249 phytates and, 103; polyphenols and, 82; porphyria and, 225; potassium and, 271; serotonin and, 211; short-chain fatty acids and, 149, 212; sleep and, 213; stomach lining and, 209; sugar and, 212, 264, 274, 283; tobacco and, 117; toxic drinks and, 210, 264; unhealthy foods and, 54; waking and, 215; wiring, 168; **nettle leaf**, 53, 178; **neurodegeneration**, 3, 19, 82, 84, 96, 104, 109-111, 159, 193, 204, 206, 220-222, 228, 230, 251, 281, 282, 283; **neuroepidemiology**, 222; **neuroinflammation**, 221; **neurological**, decline, 153; disorders, 5, 20, 153, 204, 212, 254, 312; health and vegan diet, 222, 228; kidney disease and, 252; system, 138; well-being, 221; **neuronal activity regulation**, 203; **neuropathy**, 144, 225, 252; **neuroprotective**, 80, 82, 91, 92, 103; *Neuroscience* journal, 166; **neurotransmitters**, 208, 222; *New England Journal of Medicine, The*, 182; **New Jersey Department of Health and Senior Services**, 108; **New Medical Life Sciences**, 228; **New York friend has heart attack**, 30; **New York Stock Exchange**, 13; **New Zealand**, 283; **Nicotinamide adenine dinucleotide molecule**, 131; **Nicotinamide phophori-bosylransferase enzyme**, 130; **nightshades**, 283; **nitric oxide**, 86, 205-208; **nitriles**, 297; **nitrogen fixer**, 291; **Nobel Prize in Physiology or Medicine**, 131; **nocturnal animals**, 214; **non-communicable degenerative diseases**, 9, 59, 151, 252; **non-dairy creamer**, 140, 263, 299; **non-flavonoid polyphenolic compounds**, 85; **non-food**, 49, 127; non-foods, are, 127; phosphates and, 241, 247; poison, is, 62; salt and, 272; sickness loop and, 23; stomach surgery and, 210; **Non-GMO Project**, 161, 163, 164; **non-Hodgkin's lymphoma**, 159, 162; **non-phenols**, 66; **nondihydrocapsaicin**, 84; **nongluten grains**,

O: INDEX AND TOPICAL GUIDE

P: INDEX AND TOPICAL GUIDE

S: INDEX AND TOPICAL GUIDE

X: Index and Topical Guide

Y: Index and Topical Guide

Z: Index and Topical Guide

The Author

Carey is a survivor of kidney failure caused by a combination of genetic defects and dietary issues.

Finding out when he was in his 20s that he has kidney disease brought him to understand why he had been experiencing pain, bleeding, and other health issues since early childhood.

Diving into learning about chronic kidney disease as he was involved in other areas of publishing lead to him helping a variety of doctors and nutritionists to research and write their books.

Now only writing his own material, Carey is the author of several books. One is a popular book about screenwriting, which has been used as a text in film schools. He runs a screenwriting workshop in Los Angeles, and overhauls screenplays for production companies.

Protect your health.
Get your medical tests.
Reduce your risks.
Follow a clean diet.
Exercise daily.
Follow a healthful sleep pattern.

"Plant-based diets can help improve blood pressure, control high blood sugar, and maintain a healthy weight. Plant-based diets can help prevent other medical problems such as heart disease, and help to manage or slow the progression of kidney disease."
– Plant-based Diet and Chronic Kidney Disease; UC Davis Health

If you found this book helpful,
please write a reader review on the Amazon page for the book.

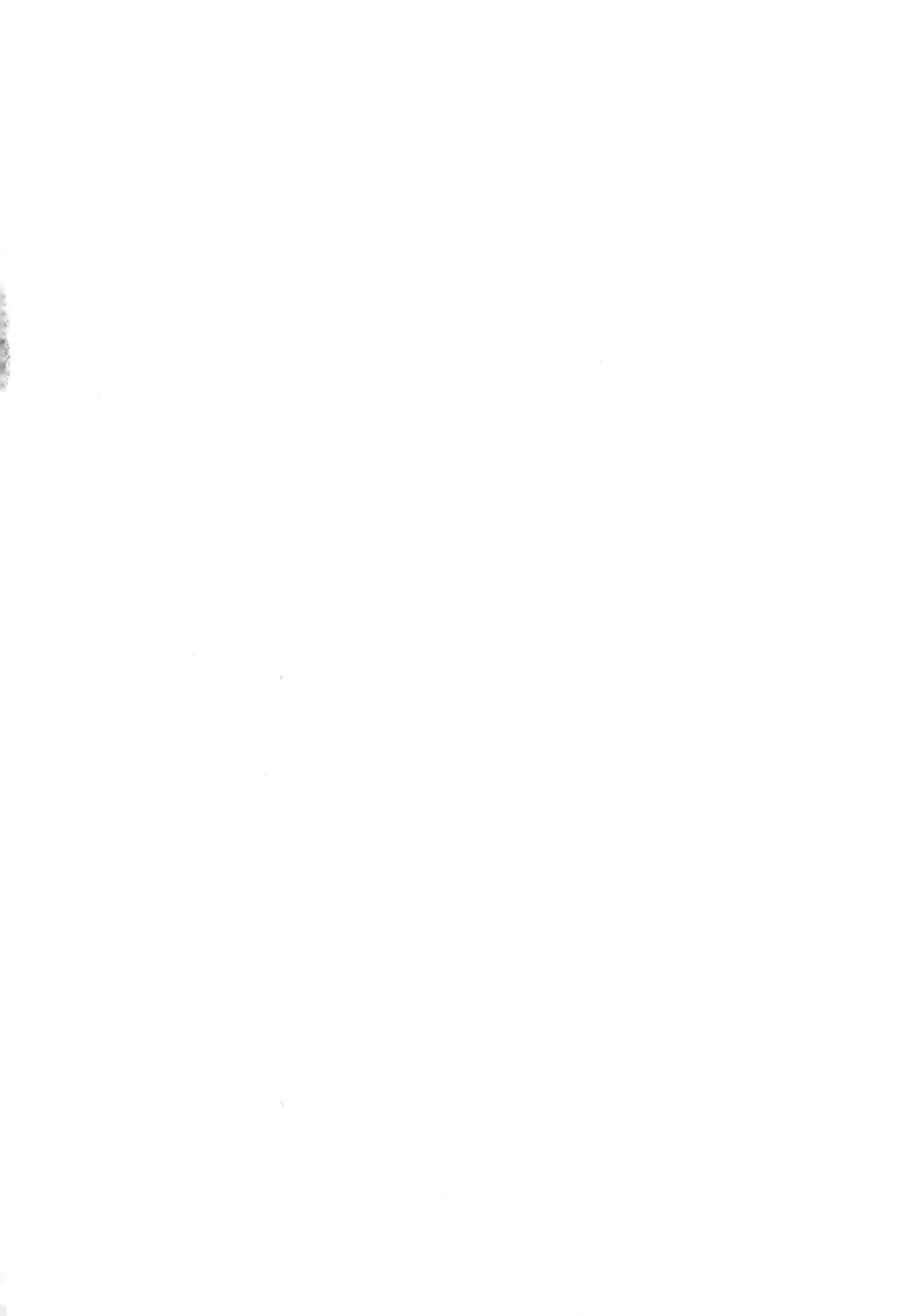